EXAMINATION OF KIDNEY FUNCTION

DEVELOPMENTS IN NEPHROLOGY

Also in this series:
Cheigh JS, Stenzel KH and Rubin AL: Manual of Clinical Nephrology of the Rogosin Kidney Center.
1981 ISBN 90-247-2397-3
Nolph KD, ed.: Peritoneal Dialysis
1981 ISBN 90-247-2477-5
Gruskin AB and Norman ME, eds: Pediatric Nephrology
1981 ISBN 90-247-2514-3
Strauss J, ed.: Hypertension, Fluid-Electrolytes, and Tubulopathies in Pediatric Nephrology
1982 ISBN 90-247-2633-6
Strauss J, ed.: Neonatal Kidney and Fluid-Electrolytes
1983 ISBN 0-89838-575-X

Examination of Kidney Function

O. SCHÜCK
Institute for Clinical and Experimental Medicine, Prague

1984 **MARTINUS NIJHOFF PUBLISHERS**
a member of the KLUWER ACADEMIC PUBLISHERS GROUP
BOSTON / THE HAGUE / DORDRECHT / LANCASTER

Distributors

for the United States and Canada: Kluwer Boston, Inc., 190 Old Derby Street, Hingham , MA 02043, U.S.A.

for Hungary, Albania, Bulgaria, China, Cuba, Czechoslovakia, German Democratic Republic, Democratic People's Republic of Korea, Mongolia, Poland, Rumania, Soviet Union, Democratic Republic of Vietnam and Yugoslavia: Avicenum, Czechoslovak Medical Press, Prague

for all other countries: Kluwer Academic Publishers Group, Distribution Center, P.O.Box 322, 3300 AH Dordrecht, The Netherlands

Library of Congress Cataloging in Publication Data

Schück, Ota.
  Examination of kidney function.
  (Developments in nephrology; v. 4)
  Includes index.
  1. Kidney function tests. I. Title. II. Series.
[DNLM: 1. Kidney function tests. 2. Kidney diseases — Physiopathology.
W1 DE998EB v. 4/QY 175 S385e]
RC904.S338   616.6'1075   82-6402
ISBN-13: 978-94-010-8997-5   e-ISBN-13: 978-94-009-5660-5
DOI: 10.1007/978-94-009-5660-5

Book information

Joint edition published by: Martinus Nijhoff Publishers Boston, USA and Avicenum, Czechoslovak Medical Press, Prague

Copyright

CONTENTS

8

GLOMERULAR FILTRATION

Historical remarks

Measurement of glomerular filtration rate (GFR) is one of the most important methods of clinical investigation of kidney function.

From a historical point of view an important conceptual bridge between physiological studies and clinical practice — which culminated in the use of clearance methods to investigate human renal function — was Rehberg's view in 1926 that GFR could be measured in man. Rehberg was the first to make the correct assumption that GFR could be measured in man when using a marker substance which would be readily filtrable at the glomerulus but not processed in any direction (other than in the direction of bulk flow) by the tubules. Using such a substance, the amount excreted (UV) would be the same as the amount filtered. If such a substance is easily filtrable at the glomerulus, its concentration in the filtrate and in plasma (P) from venous blood should be almost identical.

This condition can be expressed by the following equation:

$$UV = GFR \times P \text{ or}$$

$$GFR = \frac{UV}{P} \tag{1}$$

Rehberg felt that creatinine fulfilled the above conditions because its concentration index (U/P) was the highest of any endogenous substances then known (Fig. 1).

Present knowledge teaches us that creatinine, in man, is not excreted only by glomerular filtration, but also by tubular secretion. The latter is more significant with administration of an exogenous creatinine load. Nevertheless, Rehberg's work on the theoretical basis of GFR measurement in man, and even his choice of creatinine as the marker substance, were historical milestones for functional investigation of the kidneys in clinical medicine.

Richards, Westphall and Bott (1934) and Shannon and Smith (1935) devoted great energy to finding a better marker substance to fulfill Rehberg's conditions. Both groups arrived at the polysaccharide inulin as the ideal marker.

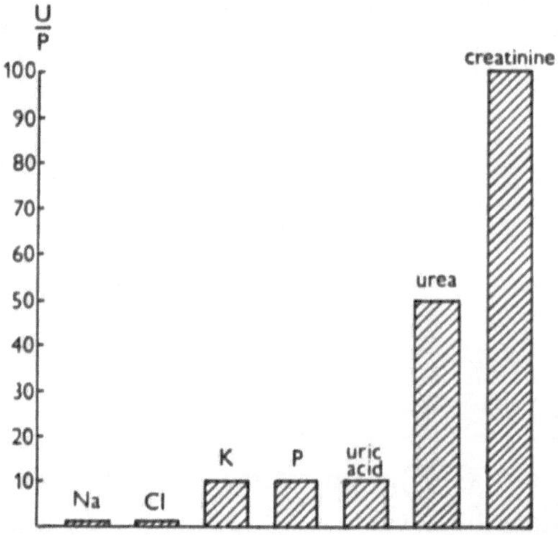

Fig. 1: Concentration index of various substances excreted by the human kidney.

Measurement of inulin clearance became the most precise estimate of GFR in man and experimental animals. Unfortunately, this measurement is neither simple nor satisfactory for routine clinical practice, and further marker substances were still sought after. Each new marker was compared to inulin which had become the reference Standard.

Out of the complex series of studies, the clearance of endogenous creatinine was finally settled on as the most appropriate for routine clinical investigation.

The relation between inulin and endogenous creatinine clearances in healthy subjects and in patients with renal disease has occupied the attention of many laboratories.

Many complications arose from the biochemical problems of determining "true" levels of endogenous creatinine versus the so-called "Jaffé positive chromogen". At present, these analytical procedures have been so unified and solved that endogenous creatinine clearance (C_{cr}) has become the clinical reference method of choice, even if it is not "exactly" the same as "true" GFR.

Since the quantitative urine collection is usually difficult, the glomerular function in routine clinical practice is usually assessed semiquantitatively by measurement of the plasma creatinine concentration alone.

In recent years there have been attempts to simplify the measurement of GFR using radionuclides. A number of substances have been suggested. Good agreement has been observed between GFR and the clearance (evaluated on the basis of the slope clearance technique) of the following substances: ^{51}Cr-EDTA, ^{131}I-Iothalamate and ^{99m}Tc-DTPA.

PHYSIOLOGY AND PATHOPHYSIOLOGY

The fluid formed in the glomerular capillaries represents a plasma ultrafiltrate, the glomerular capillaries functioning as the filter. One might assume that pores exist in the wall of the glomerular capillaries, through which filtration takes place. This has led to mathematical concepts of the properties of the glomerular filter presented by Pappenheimer et al. (1951, 1953). Flow of fluid through these pores occurs according to Poiseuille's law. These "pores" have not, however, been demonstrated by electron microscopy and the question can be raised whether such "pores" exist as stable entities, or whether the mathematical description is quantitatively valid but does not represent the morphological substratum. It is possible that gel hydration of the membrane macromolecules (Chinard 1952) allows penetration of small molecules through the aqueous phase, but stops larger molecules (for details see p. 86).

More detailed data on the mechanism of glomerular filtration based upon micro-puncture experiments has been presented by Brenner et al. (1971, 1972). In agreement with the ultrafiltration view, this process can be characterized in a single nephron (SNGFR) by the following formula:

$$SNGFR = K_f(\overline{\Delta P} - \overline{\Delta \pi}) \tag{2}$$

where K_f = the filtration coefficient, ΔP = the mean transcapillary hydraulic pressure difference and $\overline{\Delta \pi}$ = the mean transcapillary oncotic pressure difference.

The value of $\overline{\Delta P}$ is given by the difference in mean hydraulic pressure inside the glomerular capillaries (P_{GC}) and mean hydraulic pressure on the outer side of the glomerular membrane, i.e. inside Bowman's capsule (P_T).

The mean transcapillary difference in oncotic pressure ($\overline{\Delta \pi}$) is given by the difference between the mean oncotic pressure of the plasma in the glomerular capillaries (π_{GC}) and the level in the filtrate inside Bowman's capsule (π_T).

The value of K_f is given by the product of effective hydraulic permeability (k) and the filtration area (S). Therefore:

$$K_f = S \times k \tag{3}$$

Direct measurements in rats and squirrel monkeys suggest that P_{GC} ranges about 45 torr, i.e. about 40% of mean aortic pressure. Since values of P_T are about 10 torr, it would appear that under normal conditions $\overline{\Delta P}$ ranges about 35 torr. Direct measurements of afferent and efferent arteriolar pressures also show that the transcapillary hydraulic pressure difference decreases only by 1–2 torr along the length of the glomerular capillary (Brenner 1971).

The level of oncotic pressure at the afferent end of the capillary (π_A) is about 20 torr and this increases because of the ultrafiltration of protein free fluid, at the efferent end (π_E) to about 35 torr.

Local differences $\overline{\Delta P} - \overline{\Delta \pi}$ therefore decrease along the glomerular capillaries from values about 15 torr at the afferent end to values about 0 at the efferent end. From the above figures it is clear that the most rapid formation of glomerular filtrate occurs at the afferent end of the capillary — the slowest (or nil value) at the efferent end of the capillary.

The state in which $\overline{\Delta P} = \overline{\Delta \pi}$ is termed "filtration equilibrium". In animal experiments it has been shown that filtration equilibrium can occur in vivo. The rate of blood transfer into the glomerular capillaries in such cases is an important determinant of the level of GFR. Whether filtration equilibrium can occur in man is not yet known.

From data in micropuncture studies on single nephrons it can be indirectly estimated that the total value of GFR is given by the sum of values of single nephron GFR (SNGFR), i.e.

$$\text{GFR} = \sum \text{SNGFR} = \sum S \times k \times (\overline{\Delta P} - \overline{\Delta \pi}) \tag{4}$$

Pathological processes in the kidney can have various effects on these parameters which determine the rate of glomerular filtration.

Glomerular filtration can drop when $\overline{\Delta P}$ decreases. This happens in various haemodynamic disturbances. If the afferent arteriolar tone increases, and this is followed by a decreased blood flow, $\overline{\Delta P}$ can be kept unchanged only if the efferent arteriolar tone increases adequately.

In cases of peripheral circulatory insufficiency GFR decreases in relation to the $\overline{\Delta P}$ decrease. A $\overline{\Delta P}$ decrease due to increased hydraulic pressure in Bowman's capsule can result from decreased tubular solute and water reabsorption, or by a consequence of a disturbance in tubular fluid flow.

$\overline{\Delta \pi}$ decreases in patients with hypoalbuminaemia due to nephrotic syndrome. Under these conditions if the number of functioning nephrons is not reduced, GFR can reach supernormal values.

A decrease in the number of functioning nephrons produced by excision of various amounts of renal parenchyma is associated with an increase in GFR in the contralateral kidney (Hayslett et al. 1968). Micropuncture studies have suggested that an increase in SNGFR in residual nephrons in the rat after reduction of the renal parenchyma by 50–75 % can be explained by an increase in blood supply to the glomeruli. In this case the value of K_f did not show a significant change against a control group (Deen et al. 1973, Bayliss et al. 1976).

For clinical investigation of renal function it is important to know whether various pathologies change the value of k. This problem is not yet solved.

In chronic renal diseases associated with a gradual reduction in the number of functioning nephrons the decrease of the filtration area of glomerular capillaries ($\sum S$) is probably one of the most important factors responsible for a decrease in GFR.

Attention should be called to the fact that equation (4) simplifies computations in states of kidney pathology because k, just as $(\overline{\Delta P} - \overline{\Delta \pi})$; can vary from glomerulus to glomerulus.

METHODS OF INVESTIGATION

Most of the clinical methods used for estimation of GFR are derived from the clearance concept introduced into physiology by Moeller, McIntosh and Van Slyke in 1929.

In keeping with the Rehberg's formula proposed for the calculation of GFR, this renal function can be estimated as the clearance of a substance which is freely filtered by the glomerulus and is neither reabsorbed nor secreted by the tubules.

The renal clearance (C) of any substance excreted by the kidney is calculated according to the formula:

$$C = \frac{UV}{P} \tag{5}$$

(U = urine concentration, P = plasma concentration of the substance under study, V = urine flow rate). This renal clearance value indicates the virtual volume of plasma from which the substance in question has been "completely removed" during a given time interval.

CLEARANCE OF INULIN

Inulin is a polymer of fructose, the molecular weight of which is about 5500 daltons. Indirect evidence based on clearance studies is compatible with the conclusion that inulin is freely filtered and is neither secreted nor reabsorbed. This conclusion has in the past years been verified by micropuncture studies (Gutman et al. 1965, Maude et al. 1965, Harris et al. 1974).

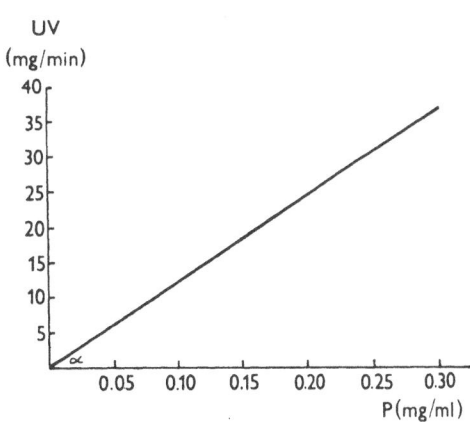

Fig. 2: Relationship between plasma concentration and urinary excretion of inulin.

The rate of urinary excretion of inulin ($U_{in}V$) is directly proportional to its plasma concentration (P_{in}) over a wide range. Equation (1) suggests that in such a linear relation if $P_{in} = 0$, the value of $U_{in}V$ is also nil. The line therefore intersects the 0-point of the graph (Fig. 2).

The measurement of inulin clearance (C_{in}) is not a routine clinical method. This method is indicated if knowledge of an accurate value of GFR is necessary.

A precise measurement of C_{in} requires the establishment of a balanced state of plasma inulin concentration for the urine collection period. The precision of the measurement is very dependent upon the precision of the urine collection and holding to all details of the infusion procedure and blood sampling. For this reason, the procedure is presented in detail.

Urine collection

In earlier years C_{in} was measured using a bladder catheter. This latter procedure is now an exceptional one, since it has been clearly shown that bladder catheterization can infect the urinary passages with possible late sequelae.

a) Urine collection by spontaneous voiding

is sufficient in most investigated subjects. Problems can arise in patients with a large volume of residual urine. Complications can also arise in patients who cannot spontaneously void at the required time (psychological factor). This latter is not necessarily a serious error, since the urine collection can be prolonged.

Collection of urine by spontaneous voiding is not associated with any degree of serious error if the rate of urine flow is adequate, so that the volume of residual urine will be negligible in relation to total urine flow. This condition can be achieved by having sufficiently long collection periods, and in addition we increase the rate of urine flow with an oral water load.

On the basis of Stříbrná's work (1973) it is clear that the so-called physiological residual urine volume in the bladder does not exceed 3 ml. If the total urine volume is, e.g. 100 ml, we are dealing with a 3 % error. Usually we use 60-min collection periods, or even longer. The collection period starts with spontaneous bladder emptying and recording the time of completion of urination. Time is also carefully recorded at the end of the collection period.

The investigation should be carried out in a separate quiet room, since psychological factors can influence the ability to void spontaneously. In order to secure a sufficiently large urine volume, the patient drinks 0.5–1.0 l water one hr before the investigation is started. The urine flow rate increases to more than 3 ml/min, so that in 60 min there will be a sample of 180 ml or more. The physiological residual volume error will than be negligible.

It should, however, be stressed that in patients with very low GFR values the standard oral water load does not result in the same degree of increase in urine flow as in normal controls or in patients with only a moderate decrease in GFR. In such cases, we have to prolong the collection period to e.g. 120 min.

b) Collection of urine by catheter

This is an exceptional procedure. In patients with voiding difficulties we usually prefer a different measurement principle which does not require quantitative urine collection (e.g. the slope clearance method, cf. p. 18).

Bladder catheterization is only too frequently associated with a spontaneous increase in urine flow rate (Miles et al. 1953, Schück et al. 1958). This is usually a Na-containing osmotic diuresis resulting from psychological stress rather than the result of direct irritation of urinary passages.

With the catheter in place, the urine collection period starts and ends with a washout using 20 ml sterile distilled water or saline heated to body temperature, and insufflation of 60 ml air. Complete emptying of the bladder is assisted by a slight pressure in the suprapubic region.

On subsequent days, the subject should be followed with urine bacteriology. If the procedure is a multiple one, such a bacteriological follow-up should be made several months later.

c) Attainment of a constant plasma concentration, and sample collection

The renal clearance of inulin is measured with plasma levels of 20 to 30 mg%. This is achieved by an initial load i.v. and a subsequent maintenance infusion. The initial load should deliver sufficient inulin into the inulin-distribution space to achieve the required concentration. This distribution space of inulin equals the volume of mobile water in the extracellular fluid (ECF), i.e. about 20% of body weight.

According to Smith (1956), 50 mg inulin/kg should be given as the load. In general, the size of this load is determined by $DV \times P$ where DV = the distribution volume and P = plasma concentration desired.

Infusion of inulin for the maintenance dose should give, per unit time, that amount of inulin excreted in the same interval.

Since inulin is excreted only by glomerular filtration, the maintenance dose is given by $GFR \times P$

P is selected as 25 mg% (i.e. 0.25 mg/ml) and GFR is estimated from C_{cr} measured on preceding days.

If, for example, C_{cr} = 40 ml/min, then the maintenance dose will be $40 \times 0.25 =$ = 10 mg/min.

The usual infusion set can be used, but an infusion pump is preferred. The infusion rate with the usual infusion set should range about 2 ml/min. When an infusion pump is used, a slower rate is usually selected (e.g. 0.3 ml/min). The infusion rate must be regulated according to the concentration of inulin used to deliver the maintenance load.

If, for example, the infusion rate must deliver 10 mg/min with an infusion rate of 1 ml/min, we have to use a 1000 mg% inulin solution. The calculated amount of inulin is dissolved in saline under sterile conditions.

Inulin is marketed as a powder which should be first dissolved in redistilled water with heating.

The times of the priming injection and the start of the maintenance infusion are precisely recorded.

The actual clearance measurement starts one hour later. This period is necessary to achieve a balanced state of P_{in} (actually, a balanced state of concentration in the entire distribution space). Blood samples are collected from the contralateral antecubital vein. Since several such samples are required, an indwelling needle should be introduced, filled with heparinized saline between uses.

With a longer (60 min) urine collection period a blood sample is collected at the start (5–10 min after starting the period), in the middle (30th min) and at the end (55th min of the 60-min period). Collection times are precisely recorded.

Investigation of C_{in} in a catheterized patient usually requires shorter urine collection periods (10–20 min). Blood samples are taken in the middle of this period. Three collection periods are usually measured.

Samples of blood and urine taken before inulin administration are required as blank values in the spectrophotometer.

d) *The time course of the investigation*

Before we measure C_{in} it is of advantage to know C_{cr} in order to estimate the maintenance dose more precisely. The test is carried out in the AM on an empty stomach, or a small tea and toast breakfast is allowed, which improves the patient's cooperation. The subject should recline, standing only to void urine. The patient should be fully informed for better cooperation.

About one hour before the test starts, 0.5–1 liter water is drunk and the following protocol gives the remainder of the procedure:

8:00 AM Bladder emptying, urine sample (U_0) taken as the blank sample.
8:05   Blood sample (B_0) to serve as the blank. Immediately thereafter the priming load is given i.v., and the maintenance infusion started.
9:05   Spontaneous voiding, start of urine collection period.
9:10   Blood sample from contralateral antecubital vein (B_1).
9:30 B_2 is taken from the same contralateral vein.

10:00 B$_3$ is taken from the same vein.
10:05 Urine is collected, the test is terminated.

e) Calculations

On the basis of P$_{in}$ concentrations, we can estimate whether a balanced concentration state had been attained during the collection period. On the basis of three values of P$_{in}$ we proceed as follows:

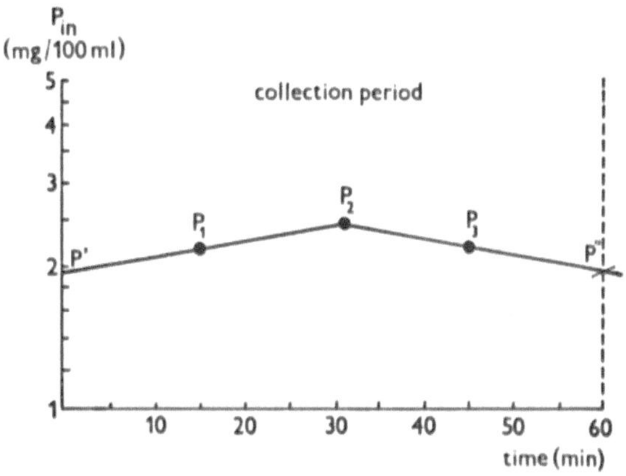

Fig. 3: Time-course of plasma inulin concentration during inulin infusion. P' and P" indicate extrapolated values of plasma inulin concentrations to the beginning and to the end of the urine collection period.

i) If all three values are approximately the same (with reference to the error of the analytical method), the situation is simple and the calculation is based on the constant value or the mean of the three close values. The clearance value is calculated according to the formula:

$$C_{in}(ml/min) = \frac{U_{in}V\,(mg/min)}{P_{in}(mg/ml)} \qquad (6)$$

There may be an irregular variation in P$_{in}$ values or a rising or falling tendency. We then calculate the area under the curve of concentration vs. time (AUC), join the points, and determine the concentration at the start and at the end of the urine collection period by extrapolating graph lines (cf. Fig. 3).
The clearance value is calculated according to the formula:

$$C_{in}(ml/min) = \frac{U_{in}V\,(total\ collected\ mg)}{AUC\,(mg\ min/ml)} \qquad (7)$$

If the collection period is short and the bladder is catheterized and a stable P$_{in}$ was not attained, we proceed as follows:
On semilog paper we determine the values which precede the mid-point of the

17

period by 2 min (cf. Fig. 4); this delay corresponds to the so-called urine transit time from the kidneys to the bladder. C_{in} is calculated according to formula (6).

The C_{in} value should then be reduced to a level per 1.73 m² of body surface area. The surface area of the subject can be read off from tables of weight vs. height (Table 1) or from a nomogram (Fig. 5a or 5b).

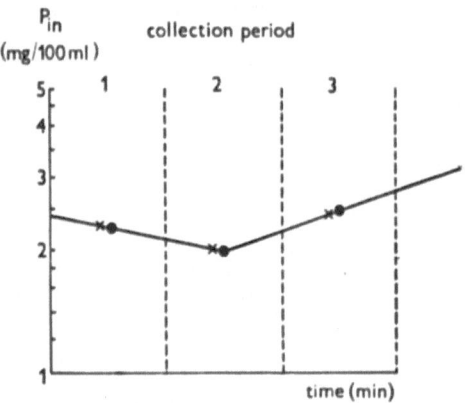

Fig. 4: Time-course of plasma inulin concentration during inulin infusion and catheterization of urinary bladder. x indicate the plasma levels of inulin 2 minutes before the middle of the urine collection period.

The corrected value of C_{in} is calculated as follows:

$$C_{in} \text{ (ml/min per 1.73 m}^2\text{)} = \frac{C_{in} \text{ (ml/min) } 1.73}{\text{body surface area (m}^2\text{)}} \qquad (8)$$

This correction is important with subjects of abnormal proportions and in children.

Slope clearance of inulin

After a single bolus injection inulin disappears exponentially so that a semilog plot of concentration vs. time gives us a straight line (Fig. 6).

After the injection of the priming dose (50 mg/kg) blood samples are usually taken after 20, 40, 60, 90 and 120 min. Extrapolation of this line to the ordinate gives the theoretical plasma concentration of inulin at $t = 0$ (P_0).

Such a graph (Fig. 6) gives the biological half-life (t 1/2). On the basis of t 1/2 we calculate the plasma clearance of inulin according to the formula:

$$C_{in}\text{(ml/min)} = \frac{D\text{(mg) } 0.693}{P_0\text{(mg/ml) t 1/2 (min)}} \qquad (9)$$

where D is the total injected amount of inulin (for details see p. 74). The accuracy of this method does not reach the level of the method based on constant plasma concentration, but the clearance value is evaluated without urinary collection.

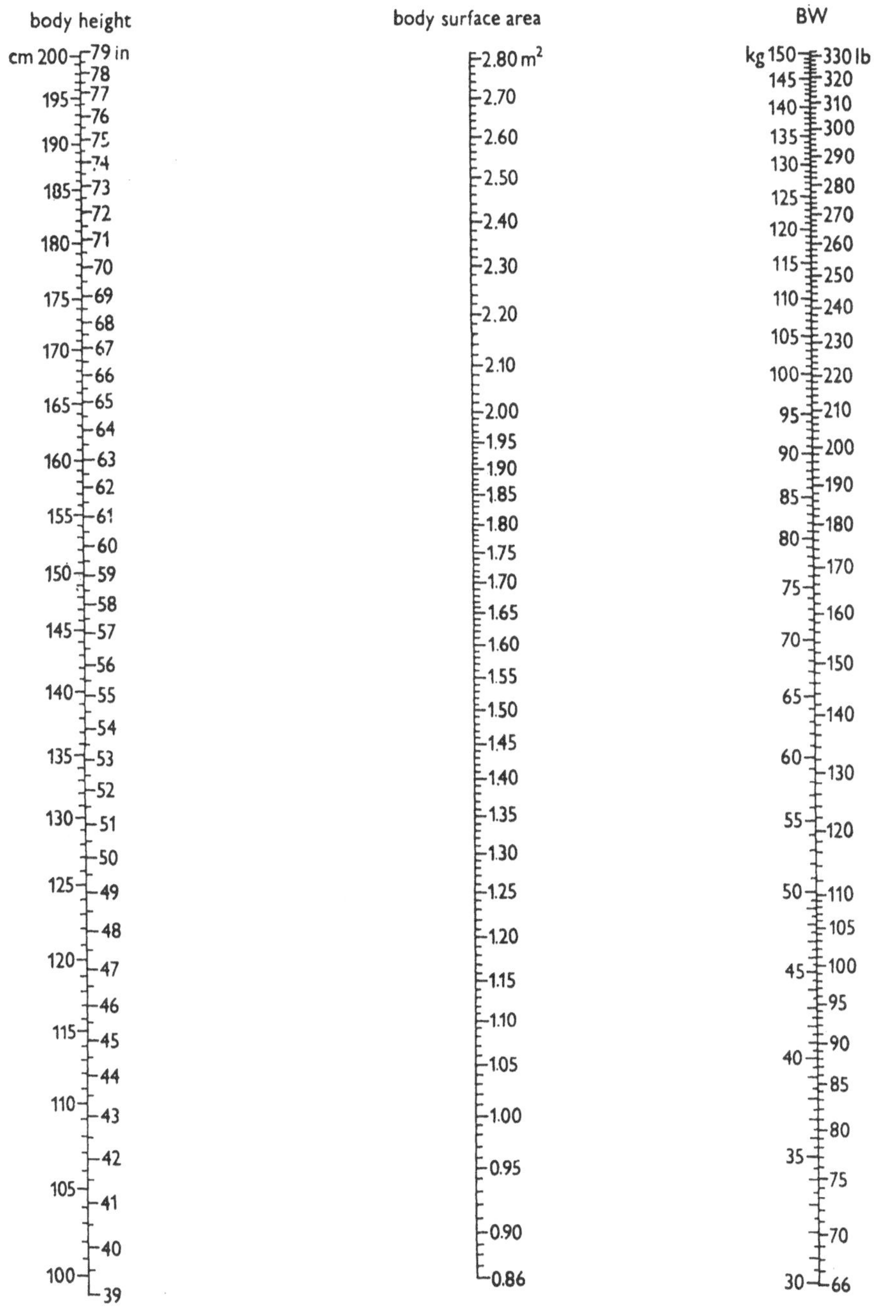

body height

cm 200 — 79 in
78
195 — 77
76
190 — 75
74
185 — 73
72
180 — 71
70
175 — 69
68
170 — 67
66
165 — 65
64
160 — 63
62
155 — 61
60
150 — 59
58
145 — 57
56
140 — 55
54
135 — 53
52
130 — 51
50
125 — 49
48
120 — 47
46
115 — 45
44
110 — 43
42
105 — 41
40
100 — 39

body surface area

2.80 m^2
2.70
2.60
2.50
2.40
2.30
2.20
2.10
2.00
1.95
1.90
1.85
1.80
1.75
1.70
1.65
1.60
1.55
1.50
1.45
1.40
1.35
1.30
1.25
1.20
1.15
1.10
1.05
1.00
0.95
0.90
0.86

BW

kg 150 — 330 lb
145 — 320
140 — 310
135 — 300
130 — 290
125 — 280
120 — 270
260
115 — 250
110 — 240
105 — 230
100 — 220
95 — 210
90 — 200
85 — 190
80 — 180
75 — 170
160
70 — 150
65 — 140
60 — 130
55 — 120
50 — 110
105
45 — 100
95
40 — 90
85
80
35 — 75
70
30 — 66

Fig. 5a: Nomogram for evaluation of body surface area in adults.

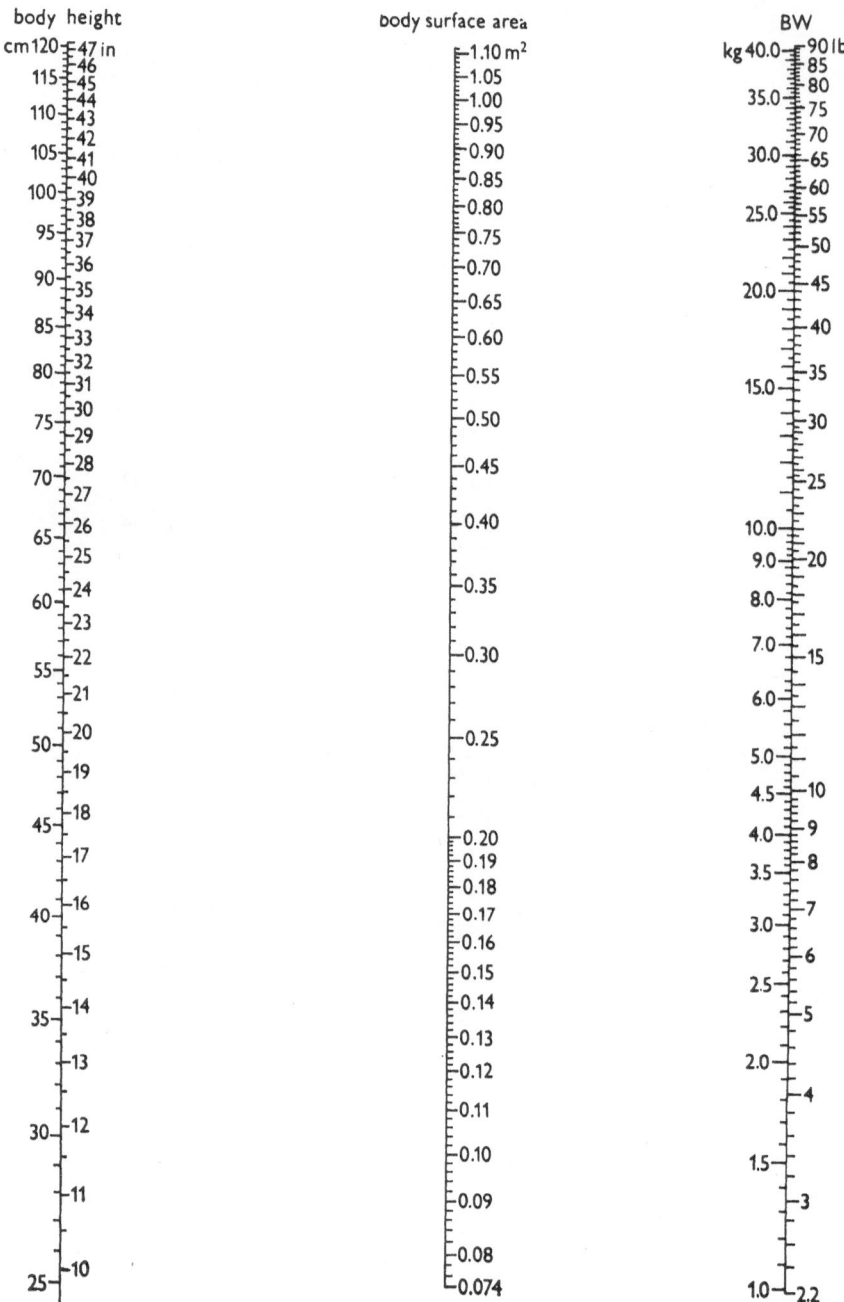

Fig. 5b: Nomogram for evaluation of body surface area in children.

20

Table 1

cm \\ kg	25	30	35	40	45	50	55	60	65	70	75	80	85	90	95	100	105
200							1.84	1.91	1.97	2.03	2.09	2.15	2.21	2.26	2.31	2.36	2.41
195						1.73	1.80	1.87	1.93	1.99	2.05	2.11	2.17	2.22	2.27	2.32	2.37
190				1.56	1.63	1.70	1.77	1.84	1.90	1.96	2.02	2.08	2.13	2.18	2.23	2.28	2.33
185				1.53	1.60	1.67	1.74	1.80	1.86	1.92	1.98	2.04	2.09	2.14	2.19	2.24	2.29
180				1.49	1.57	1.64	1.71	1.77	1.85	1.89	1.95	2.00	2.05	2.10	2.15	2.20	2.25
175	1.19	1.28	1.36	1.46	1.53	1.61	1.67	1.73	1.79	1.85	1.91	1.96	2.01	2.06	2.11	2.16	2.21
170	1.17	1.26	1.34	1.43	1.50	1.57	1.63	1.69	1.75	1.81	1.86	1.91	1.96	2.01	2.06	2.11	
165	1.14	1.23	1.31	1.40	1.47	1.54	1.60	1.66	1.72	1.78	1.83	1.88	1.93	1.98	2.03	2.07	
160	1.12	1.21	1.29	1.37	1.44	1.50	1.56	1.62	1.68	1.73	1.78	1.83	1.88	1.93	1.98		
155	1.09	1.18	1.26	1.33	1.40	1.46	1.52	1.58	1.64	1.69	1.74	1.79	1.84	1.89			
150	1.06	1.15	1.23	1.30	1.36	1.42	1.48	1.54	1.60	1.65	1.70	1.75	1.80				
145	1.03	1.12	1.20	1.27	1.33	1.39	1.45	1.51	1.56	1.61	1.66	1.71					
140	1.00	1,09	1.17	1.24	1.30	1.36	1.42	1.47	1.52	1.57							
135	0.97	1.06	1.14	1.20	1.26	1.32	1.38	1.43	1.48								
130	0.95	1.04	1.11	1.17	1.23	1.29	1.35	1.40									
125	0.93	1.01	1.08	1.14	1.20	1.26	1.31	1.36									
120	0.91	0.98	1.04	1.10	1.16	1.22	1.27										

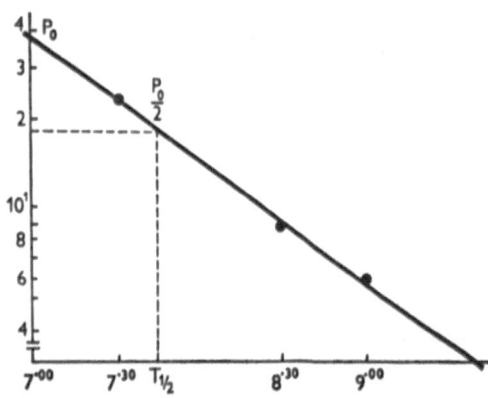

Fig. 6: Schematic presentation of exponential decrease of plasma concentrations and the evaluation of the biological half-life. P_0 indicates the extrapolated plasma concentration to the time of the injection of the test substance.

The renal clearance of polyfructosan S

Polyfructosan S is a polymer (of fructose) like inulin, but with a smaller dalton number (about 3500). The mechanism of renal excretion of polyfructosan S is the same as with inulin. Very good agreement has been reported for the clearance of both subtances. Mertz (1963) has reported a mean ratio of the clearances of polyfructosan S and inulin as 1.16 ± 0.099. Polyfructosan S has the advantage of being soluble in cold water.

Interpretation of findings

The value of C_{In} is dependent upon a number of factors. Those of particular relevance to clinical testing will be discussed in detail below.

Age and sex

According to Smith (1951), healthy normal controls investigated under baseline (AM) conditions give the following values:

Males 124 ± 5.8 ml/min/1.73 m²
Females 108 ± 13.5 ml/min/1.73 m²

A number of other studies have given the same results. Evaluation of these results shows that the mean C_{In} for adult males = 127 ml/min and for women = = 118 ml/min on the basis of 1.73 m² body surface area.

C_{In} changes, however, with age. Barnett (1940) reported that in the first days of life C $_{in}$ is about 20 ml/min/1.73 m². These values, in this age range, were highly variable. The latter appears to be related to the state of hydration. Low postnatal values were also reported by McCance and Young (1941), Young and McCance (1942), Barnett et al. (1942), Dean and McCance (1947) and Tudvad and Vesterdal (1949).

Premature children with body weight less than 2 kg show even lower C_{in} values than full term neonates (Tudvad and Vesterdal 1949, Vesterdal and Tudvad 1949).

Values corresponding to normal adult levels — per 1.73 m² body surface area — were attained at about age 1 year (West et al. 1948). After this point in time C_{in} remains stabilized at about 120 ml/min/1.73 m² up to 40 years of age. Following this there is a gradual decrease.

The relation between C_{in} and age is, according to Dean and McCance (1947) and Davies and Shock (1950) and collected by Watchinger (1964):

Age	C_{in} (ml/min/1.73 m²)
2–8 days	16.3–44.6
1 month	30–60
2–4 months	50–90
6–8 months	60–120
20–29 years	122.8 ± 16.4
30–39	115.0 ± 10.8
40–49	121.2 ± 23.3
50–59	99.3 ± 14.6
60–69	96.0 ± 22.5
70–79	89.0 ± 19.9
80–89	65.3 ± 20.4

The cause of this age-related decrease in C_{in} is not clear. According to Roessle and Roulet (1932) kidney weight decreases in the 80's to about 80–70% values determined in the age range 20–30 years. Oliver (1942) felt that regressive changes in the kidney are mainly the result of changes in the renal arteries. According to Bastai (1955) this decrease in C_{in} is probably related to gradual glomerular involution. In addition, Bush's pathological findings (1958) in a large group of elderly patients suggest that the main morphological substrate of renal regressive changes is arterio- and atherosclerosis.

The diurnal rhythm in C_{in}

Changes in C_{in} over 24 hr are not simple to measure since the investigation requires a continuous infusion. If the subject is reclining over the entire 24 hr, the results will be distorted by an absence of positional changes, and psychological effects can also play a role. The continuous infusion problem can be improved if a long cannula is used, enabling the subject to move about. Sirota et al. (1950) did not find significant differences in C_{in}, day vs. night. Brod and Fencl (1958) reported in healthy controls that the night values were lower than the daytime values.

Body position

Changes in renal haemodynamics vs body position are also manifest in measurement of GFR. Going from the horizontal to the vertical can moderately decrease GFR (Brun et al. 1945).

Diet and fluid intake

Jolliffe and Smith (1931), Shannon et al. (1935) and Moustgaard (1948) showed in dogs that protein-rich diet increases GFR.

The effect of protein intake on C_{in} is not so marked in man. Pullman et al. (1954) followed in a group of 10 subjects the effect of a high protein diet given over a fortnight on GFR and reported that in 8 there was an increase in GFR by a mean value of 29%. White and Rolf (1948) followed a single subject on a 220 g//day protein diet for one week and found that GFR increased by 31%.

Decreasing the NaCl content of the diet for 5–6 days results in a decrease in GFR (Leaf and Couter 1949, Black et al. 1942).

A clear decrease in GFR resulted when decreased NaCl intake was associated with increased salt losses in sweat (McCance and Widdowson 1937).

GFR depends upon fluid intake and dehydration decreases GFR (Black et al. 1942).

Increased water intake to the level of water diuresis does not result in significant changes in C_{in}. Thus the hydration which we apply during renal functional testing is innocuous to the validity of the results.

Psychological stress and pain

GFR changes can be part of the haemodynamic reactions to these stimuli. The changes are marked only when renal blood flow (RBF) is decreased significantly, since there is a simultaneous increase in filtration fraction (FF). (Smith 1939, 1940).

This should be kept in mind when measuring C_{in} in any subject. Pain stimuli should be avoided.

Pregnancy

In the first trimester, GFR is increased (by 20–30% or more) and this lasts up to delivery (Bucht 1951, Dignam et al. 1958, Sims 1958, Bonsnes and Lange 1950, Sohar et al. 1956). After delivery GFR decreases rapidly to the norm (Sims and Krantz 1958).

Measurement of C_{in} in a diseased kidney

The criteria which are valid for demonstration that inulin is an adequate substance to measure GFR (Smith 1951) were worked out on healthy controls. The question of the validity of these conditions in the presence of kidney pathology remains. In experimental acute renal failure, reabsorption of inulin from the tubules has been demonstrated (Bank et al. 1967, Tanner et al. 1973). Rosenbaum et al. (1979) assume that C_{in} is not an adequate marker of GFR in kidney donors and transplant recipients.

Although the problem of precision of measurements of GFR using C_{in} in various types of kidney pathology, and in various stages of the disease, has not yet been solved, measurement of C_{in} is at present generally assumed to be the adequate marker of GFR. The question of whether Bricker's "intact nephron hypothesis" (1965) can be applied to inulin excretion by residual nephrons remains to be answered.

Indications for investigation

Measurement of C_{in} is indicated in patients with chronic renal disease in whom it is necessary to know with precision the mass of functioning renal parenchyma. This includes the following:

a) Plasma concentration of endogenous creatinine is within normal limits or is a borderline value and C_{cr} is slightly decreased below normal.

As mentioned on p. 30, the P_{cr} value depends on the body size and the estimated C_{cr} can be affected by the incomplete urine collection, nevertheless, one cannot exclude a small decrease in GFR.

In such cases, C_{in} should be measured under conditions of adequate hydration, increased urine flow and precise urine collection (supervised by a technical assistant).

b) Evaluation of renal function before a planned nephrectomy.

Asymmetrical renal function in practice is usually diagnosed by i.v. urography or isotopic methods (cf. p. 79).

We often meet with patients in whom the kidney to remain after removing the more diseased organ, is not completely normal. It is necessary to determine the function of the better kidney, and whether it will suffice to maintain homeostasis of the milieu interieur.

In such cases we give preference to measurement of C_{in}. The total value of C_{in} does not tell us much about each organ separately. It does give us the maximal remaining GFR level with the better kidney.

c) Accurate measurement of GFR for research purposes.

LABORATORY METHODS

Several colorimetric methods can be used to determine inulin concentration in both plasma and urine. The methods are simple and do not require special instrumentation. The following can be recommended:
Resorcinol method (Roe et al. 1949, Schreiner 1950), fructose-specific resorcinol method adapted for autoanalyzer (Fjelbo and Stamey 1968), anthrone method (White and Samson 1954, Davidson and Sackner 1963), indolacetic acid method (Heyrovský 1956, Dawborn 1965), diphenylamine method (Harrison 1942) and the method utilizing the cysteine/tryptophane reaction (Waugh 1977).

CLEARANCE OF ENDOGENOUS CREATININE

As already metioned, measurement of C_{cr} is the most used method for measuring GFR in clinical practice. Creatinine (the anhydride of methylguanidinoacetic acid) is formed in muscle from creatine phosphate. The daily production is proportional to the total muscle mass and is relatively constant.

Creatinine is excreted in man mainly by glomerular filtration, but also to a small degree by tubular secretion (Jolliffe and Smith 1931, Shannon et al. 1932). The rate of tubular transport depends upon the plasma level.

Demonstration of the adequacy of the clearance of the endogenous creatinine (C_{cr}) to measure GFR in man was complicated by the variety of analytical methods employed.

The basis of these methods was that suggested by Folin and Wu. This has been variously modified. It was found, however, that alkaline picrate reacts to form an

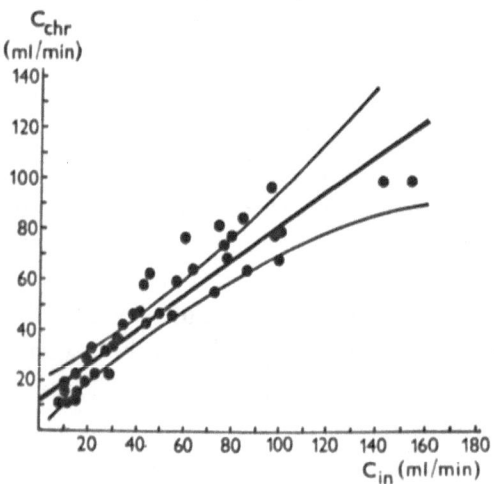

Fig. 7: Relationship between inulin clearance (C_{in}) and clearance of endogenous chromogen (C_{chr}) in patients with chronic renal diseases.

26

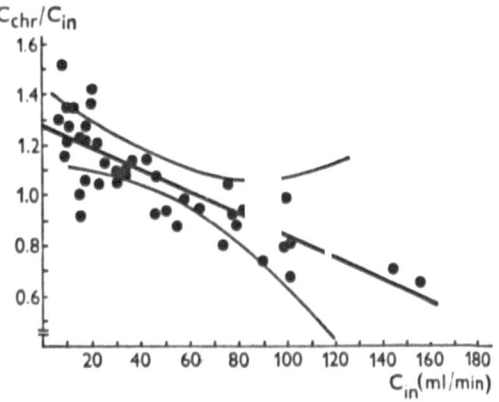

Fig. 8: Relationship between inulin clearance (C_{in}) and the ratio (C_{chr}/C_{in}) in patients with chronic renal diseases.

orange colour not only with creatinine, but also with other substances. The group of reacting substances is termed "Jaffé-positive chromogen". The non-creatinine components make up 10–20% of the total chromogen in plasma under normal conditions. In urine this fraction is negligible.

Some analytical methods determine the concentration of the entire complex. Other methods determine "true" creatinine. Thus, clearance results using different analytical methods gave a variety of numbers, with some scatter in the creatinine inulin clearance ratio.

The relation of the clearances of total chromogen (C_{chr}) to those of true endogenous creatinine (C_{cr}) and of inulin, is the subject of many reports (Doolan et al. 1962, Heaty 1968, Levander et al. 1969, Kim et al. 1969, Brod and Sirota 1948, Rapoport and Hudsan 1968, Mertz 1976).

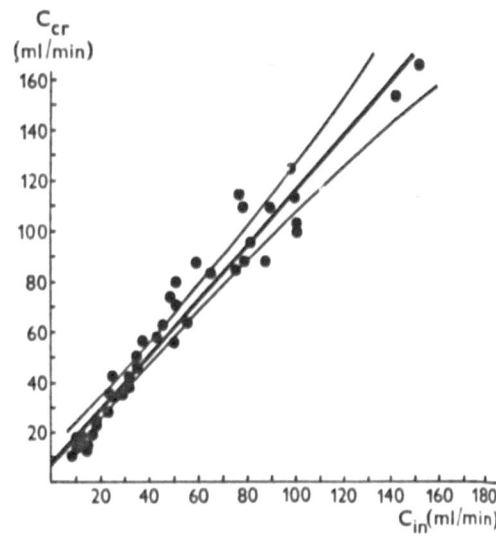

Fig. 9: Relationship between inulin clearance (C_{in}) and clearance of endogenous creatinine (C_{cr}) in patients with chronic renal diseases.

The relations between C_{chr}, C_{cr} and C_{in} in patients with various forms of chronic renal disease (mainly chronic glomerulonephritis, chronic pyelonephritis, vascular nephrosclerosis and polycystic kidneys) and in various stages of these diseases, found in our own laboratory (Schück et al. 1977) are as follows:

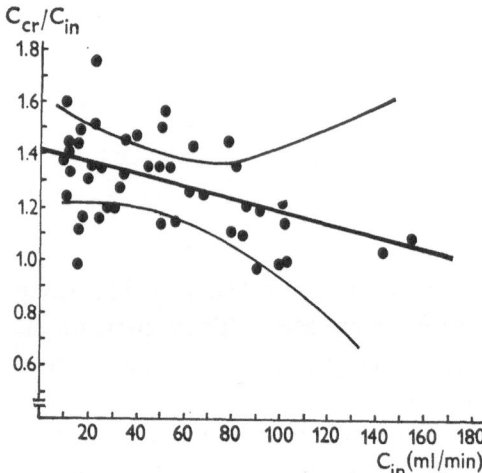

Fig. 10: Relationship between inulin clearance (C_{in}) and the ratio (C_{cr}/C_{in}) in patients with chronic renal diseases.

Fig. 7 shows data of C_{chr} vs C_{in}. There was a significant linear relation between the two values. The ratio C_{chr}/C_{in} increased with a decrease in C_{in} (Fig. 8). In subjects with a normal C_{in} the C_{chr}/C_{in} ratio could be significantly less than 1.0, so that the C_{chr} value could well give false information. On the other hand, in subjects with very low C_{in} values the C_{chr} values were usually larger than the former ones. The regression line crossed the ordinate at 1.28.

Fig. 9 shows data of C_{cr} vs C_{in}. Again we see a significant linear relation. In subjects with a normal C_{in} the C_{cr} value is slightly higher. In patients with very low C_{in} levels C_{cr} can give much higher values. In individual cases it was possible that C_{cr} is higher than C_{in} by 40–60% (Fig. 10).

The 24 – hour C_{cr}

The measurement involves a precise urine collection over 24 hr, with 1–2 venous blood samples. Some laboratories use only a single blood sample taken at the start or the end of the collection period. It is more precise to take one sample at the start and the second at the end of the period, and use the mean of the two values for the clearance calculation. The urine volume is precisely measured, and endogenous creatinine concentration is measured in a mixed urine sample and in the two plasma samples.

The clearance value is calculated according to the standard formula (see p. 13).

We recommend that during the collection period a fairly large fluid intake be allowed (if there is no contraindication) since urinary excretion of creatinine is decreased at low urine flow rates (Levinsky and Berliner 1959). No special diet is necessary. An increase in protein intake does not affect urinary excretion of creatinine significantly (Barret and Addis 1947). Heavy physical activity is not allowed since under these conditions GFR decreases (Merill and Cargill 1948, White and Rolf 1948, Wesson 1969).

The urine collection period must start by emptying the bladder and discarding the urine. In ambulant patients a well-sealed bottle can be carried about. Termination of the period, when the subject urinates into the bottle for the last time, must also be precise.

C_{cr} over several hr of urine collection

Usually 1–3 hr of urine collection gives us an opportunity to observe the precision of the collection procedure used by the subject. The test is usually carried out in the AM, 500 ml water is given as an oral load 30–60 min before the test begins.

The start and the end of the collection period are precisely recorded. A sample of venous blood is taken immediately after termination of the period. C_{cr} estimated in this manner need not be representative for the entire 24 hr, since there is a diurnal rhythm.

According to Brod (1973), C_{cr} in the early morning hours (6–9 AM) is relatively low, ranging from 80 to 100 ml/min. During the later morning hours this value increases, and in the afternoon (noon to 3:00 PM) reaches a maximum value about 150–180 ml/min. C_{cr} then gradually decreases and at night it is once again about 100 ml/min.

Richardson and Philbin (1971) have found a good correlation between C_{cr} values ascertained on the basis of a 1-hr urinary collection and a 24-hr collection period.

Interpretation of the results

The mean normal C_{cr} value in adult males is 130 ml/min/1.73 m^2 with and SD of $\pm 18\%$; in females 120 ml/min/1.73 m^2, SD = $\pm 14\%$ (Smith 1951, Wesson 1969). C_{cr} is also dependent on age. Brod (1973) has given the following data:

Age	Males	Females
21–40	133.2 ± 25.0	142.9 ± 27.3
41–60	122.1 ± 7.7	114.0 ± 16.1

The most detailed study in this respect is that of Rowe et al. (1976), who carried out both cross-sectional and longitudinal studies. The findings in the two groups were not significantly different one from the other. The following table gives the results of the cross-sectional study:

Age	C_{cr}(ml/min)	$U_{cr}V$(mg/day)
17–24	140.2 ± 3.7	1790 ± 52
25–34	140.1 ± 2.5	1862 ± 31
35–44	132.6 ± 1.8	1746 ± 24
45–54	126.8 ± 1.4	1689 ± 18
55–64	119.9 ± 1.7	1580 ± 22
65–74	109.5 ± 2.0	1409 ± 25
75–84	96.9 ± 2.9	1259 ± 45

The greatest problem associated with this test is the precision of the urine collection. Suspicion that urine collection was incomplete can arise when the clearance value calculated does not correspond to the plasma concentration. A low level of C_{cr} with normal P_{cr} suggests incomplete urine collection. Because of the problems of timed urine collection, glomerular function is usually assessed by measurement of the plasma creatinine concentration alone, in routine investigation. This simplification requires a more detailed analysis of the relation between P_{cr} and C_{cr}.

PLASMA CONCENTRATION OF ENDOGENOUS CREATININE

P_{cr} is a reflection of the amount of creatinine produced in muscle and the rate of excretion by the kidneys. The production of creatinine in muscle is minimally dependent on physical activity and protein intake (Barret and Addis 1947, Bleiler and Schedl 1962, Doolan et al. 1962). Endogenous creatinine is distributed throughout total body water (Edwards 1959) and is excreted from the organism only by the kidneys (Domingues and Pomerene 1945). P_{cr} is almost constant in the course of 24 hours. According to some authors (Rapoport and Hudsan 1968, Pasternack and Kuhlback 1971) the oscillation of P_{cr} can reach up to 30%, the highest values being reached at about 7 : 00 PM. P_{cr} varies with muscle volume. Values are lower in asthenic persons than in muscular individuals (Bleiler and Schedl 1962). The value of P_{cr} also depends on the age. In children under age 5 years, P_{cr} ranges from 0.3 to 0.5 mg%. From 5 years up it gradually increases (Kuhlback et al. 1968, Schwartz et al. 1976).

Normal values of P_{cr}

The plasma concentration of endogenous creatinine is expressed in mg% or in μmol/l. As mentioned above, it is necessary to consider which analytical method has been used.

30

The relation between the two concentration expressions is as follows:

$$P_{cr} (\mu mol/l) = \frac{P_{cr} (mg\%)\ 10000}{113}$$

(113 is the molecular weight of creatinine). For total chromogen (P_{chr}) (mg%) the following values are given:

	Males	Felmaes
Addis et al. (1951)	1.03 ± 0.8	0.79 ± 0.17
Hopper (1951)	1.27 ± 0.12	1.09 ± 0.15
Doolan et al. (1962)	1.17 ± 0.13	0.98 ± 0.05

Schirmeister et al. (1964) give the following values for different age categories:

Age	Males	Females
10–20	0.74 (±0.17)	0.70 (±0.12)
20–30	0.92 (±0.09)	0.76 (±0.08)
30–40	0.92 (±0.11)	0.77 (±0.11)
40–50	0.93 (±0.15)	0.75 (±0.08)
50–60	0.88 (±0.16)	0.71 (±0.11)

For P_{cr} the following values are given:

	Males	Females
Edwards and Whyte (1959)	0.93 (±0.14)	0.73 (±0.15)
Doolan et al. (1962)	1.01 (±0.11)	0.82 (±0.09)

Rowe et al. (1976) give the following values with respect to age:

Age	P_{cr}(mg%)
17–24	0.808 ± 0.026
25–34	0.808 ± 0.100
35–44	0.813 ± 0.009
45–54	0.829 ± 0.008
55–64	0.837 ± 0.012
65–74	0.825 ± 0.012
75–84	0.843 ± 0.019

Kassirer (1971) gives the normal range of P_{cr} as follows: males: 0.8–1.3 mg%, females: 0.6–1.0 mg%.

Roberts (1967) gives normal P_{cr} values found by the Auto Technicon Analyzer for males 71–124 μmol/l and for females 62–106 μmol/l.

The total chromogen methods give higher concentrations. The differences between P_{cr} and P_{chr} values manifest themselves especially when these values are within normal limits, or slightly elevated. The participation of the non-creatinine chromogen on the total chromogen concentration becomes insignificant with increase of P_{cr}. The increase of P_{chr} in patients with chronic renal diseases is conditioned by the increase of P_{cr}.

RELATION BETWEEN P_{cr} AND GFR IN PATIENTS WITH CHRONIC RENAL DISEASES

It has been demonstrated by many authors that P_{cr} increases in hyperbolic relation with GFR decrease. A typical example of this relation in patients with various forms of chronic renal diseases shows Fig. 11.

The relationship between P_{cr} and GFR can be demonstrated, however, only under conditions of a balanced state. If there are acute changes in GFR, the relation between P_{cr} and GFR disappears until a new balanced state is established.

Fig. 11 shows that a decrease of C_{in} to about 50% of the normal value is associated with a small increase in P_{cr}. On the other hand, if C_{in} decreases to very low values, the rise in P_{cr} becomes quite striking. Thus, changes in P_{cr} are not a sensitive reflection of a decrease in renal function in the initial stages of kidney disease. In advanced stages with a low GFR, even small changes in GFR have a clear and measurable effect on P_{cr}.

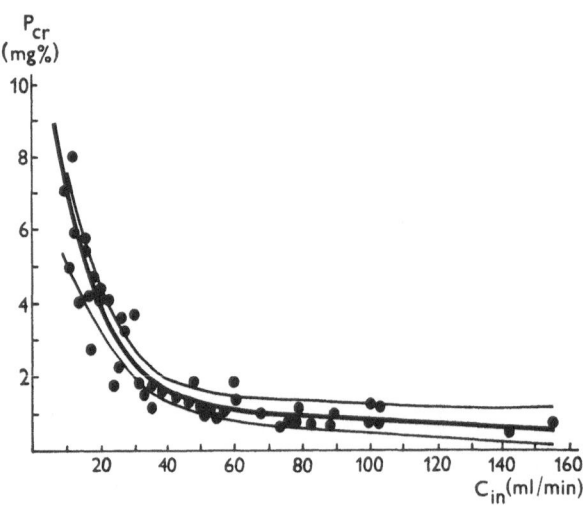

Fig. 11: Relationship between inulin clearance (C_{in}) and plasma concentration of endogenous creatinine (P_{cr}) in patients with chronic renal diseases.

Clinical observations indicate that the urinary excretion of creatinine ($U_{cr}V$) does not change with a decrease of GFR since the latter is compensated by the increase of P_{cr} (under conditions of a balanced state). Only in patients with advanced renal failure does $U_{cr}V$ decrease (Goldman et al. 1954, 1959, Effersoe 1957, Enger 1964).

If $U_{cr}V$ does not change significantly, then — under conditions of a balanced state — the following simple relation between pathological (path) and normal (norm) values of P_{cr} and C_{cr} should hold:

$$\frac{(C_{cr})_{path}}{(C_{cr})_{norm}} = \frac{(P_{cr})_{norm}}{(P_{cr})_{path}} \qquad (10)$$

In this equation $(P_{cr})_{norm}$ represents the normal value of P_{cr} with respect to sex, age and even body size.

The coefficient of variation of the most widely used analytical methods is about 10% (Kassirer and Gennari 1979). For instance, if, in a person suffering from chronic renal disease, P_{cr} is stabilized at 4 mg% and the normal P_{cr} corresponding to sex, age and body size is 0.8 (± 0.08) mg%, then according to equation (10) it can be assumed that the residual C_{cr} amounts to 20% of its normal value. With respect to the SD of $(P_{cr})_{norm}$, it can therefore be assumed that, with 95% probability, the true value of $(C_{cr})_{path}/(C_{cr})_{norm} \times 100$ in the investigated subject is not lower than 16% and does not exceed 24%.

Actually, this calculation expresses the C_{cr} of the investigated subject as a percentage of the value that would, theoretically, exist if he were healthy at the time of examination (provided the disease was not associated with muscle atrophy and the renal disease had not reached the advanced stage of chronic renal failure).

A number of published reports deal with attempts at estimating C_{cr} from P_{cr}.

Sierbaek and Nielsen (1971) recommended the use of a nomogram for this purpose. C_{cr} values here are given per 70 kg body weight.

Jelliffe (1973) recommended the following formula to calculate C_{cr}:

$$C_{cr} \text{ (ml/min/1.73 m}^2) = \frac{98 - 0.8(\text{age in years} - 20)}{P_{cr} \text{ (mg\%)}} \qquad (11)$$

This equation was used in males from 20 to 80 years. C_{cr} values in women were calculated as 90% of the male value for the same age.

Cockroft and Gault (1976) have used another equation:

$$C_{cr} \text{ (ml/min)} = \frac{(140 - \text{age in years})(\text{wt kg})}{72 P_{cr} \text{ (mg\%)}} \qquad (12)$$

Values calculated from the latter equation are valid for males in the age range 18–92 years. In women, according to these investigators, we use a factor of 0.85 times the value calculated for males.

33

Edwards and Whyte (1959) proposed the following formula for C_{cr} estimation:

$$C_{cr}\,(\text{ml/min/1.73 m}^2) = \frac{94.3}{P_{cr}} - 1.8 \qquad (13)$$

Schwartz et al. (1976) used the following formula for calculation of C_{cr} in children:

$$C_{cr}\,(\text{ml/min/1.73 m}^2) = \frac{0.55\;\text{body length}}{P_{cr}} \qquad (14)$$

Interestingly, various proposed formulae for the estimation of C_{cr} from P_{cr} can be transformed in the simple form of formula (10).

For example, if formula (12) is used for the normal and pathological state of the investigated subject, the following adaptation can be made:

$$\frac{(C_{cr})_{\text{path}}}{(C_{cr})_{\text{norm}}} = \frac{\dfrac{(140 - \text{age})\,(\text{wt kg})}{72\,(P_{cr})_{\text{path}}}}{\dfrac{(140 - \text{age})\,(\text{wt kg})}{72\,(P_{cr})_{\text{norm}}}} = \frac{(P_{cr})_{\text{norm}}}{(P_{cr})_{\text{path}}}$$

In an analogous manner, the formulae proposed by Jellife (1973) and Schwartz et eal. (1976) can also be simplified.

With respect to equation (13) the following transformation can be made:

$$\frac{(C_{cr})_{\text{path}}}{(C_{cr})_{\text{norm}}} = \frac{\dfrac{94.3}{(P_{cr})_{\text{path}}} - 1.8}{\dfrac{94.3}{(P_{cr})_{\text{norm}}} - 1.8}$$

Since the constant 1.8 is usually negligible in comparison with the value of the ratio $94.3/P_{cr}$, the results given by this formula are also close to the results obtained by equation (10).

The interpretation of P_{cr} as an indicator of GFR is easier if P_{cr} is followed over time in the same individual, since the effects of sex, age and body size on GFR and P_{cr} are excluded (if the body weight does not change significantly and if there is no significant change in muscle metabolism).

As stated above, P_{cr} values should be compared under conditions of a balanced state.

Changes in P_{cr} with sudden changes in renal function

If there is a sudden collapse of renal function and, for example, 1000 mg cr are retained in 24 hr, then with distribution of this amount throughout body water (about 60% of body wt) a 70 kg man will experience an increase in P_{cr} by $1000/42 = 24$ mg/l $= 2.4$ mg%.

If ΔP_{cr} is greater than 3.0 mg%/24 hr, it is probable that more creatinine is being produced in tissue (e.g. in crush syndrome). These figures are only for orientational purposes.

34

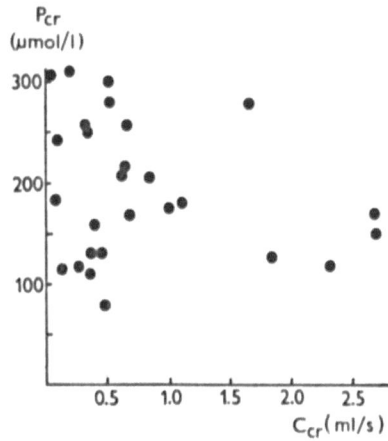

Fig. 12: Relationship between endogenous creatinine clearance (C_{cr}) and plasma concentration of endogenous creatinine (P_{cr}) in patients with brain death.

Since the retained creatinine is distributed throughout total body water, an increase in P_{cr} is delayed with respect to a decrease in GFR. For instance, in patients with brain death caused by cranial trauma there is no correlation between P_{cr} and C_{cr} (Fig. 12) and P_{cr} alone does not express the actual state of kidney function. Similarly, Wilson et al. (1979) have ascertained that in critically ill surgical patients P_{cr} is not a true reflection of C_{cr}.

Indications for investigation

Measurement of P_{cr} is a necessary part of any nephrological workup. On the other hand, this value cannot substitute for precise clinical examination of the kidneys. P_{cr} gives only a **semiquantitative** estimate of GFR.

If P_{cr} is a borderline value, mild impairment of GFR cannot be excluded. In these cases measurement of C_{cr} (or C_{in}) is necessary.

If the value of the patient's GFR is known, further follow-up measurements can be based on P_{cr} estimation. Measurement of C_{cr} can then be repeated after a longer time interval. Repetitive measurements of P_{cr} and C_{cr} in patients with chronic renal disease is useful in evaluating the time-course of the disease and can help construct a "prognostic" curve in the individual case. An example of such a "prognostic" curve or line is shown in Fig. 13. On the basis of such a graphic presentation of the changes in C_{cr} in the course of time, the "activity" of the disease can be evaluated. Progression of chronice renal disease can be estimated on the basis of values of $1/P_{cr}$ (Mitch et al. 1976).

35

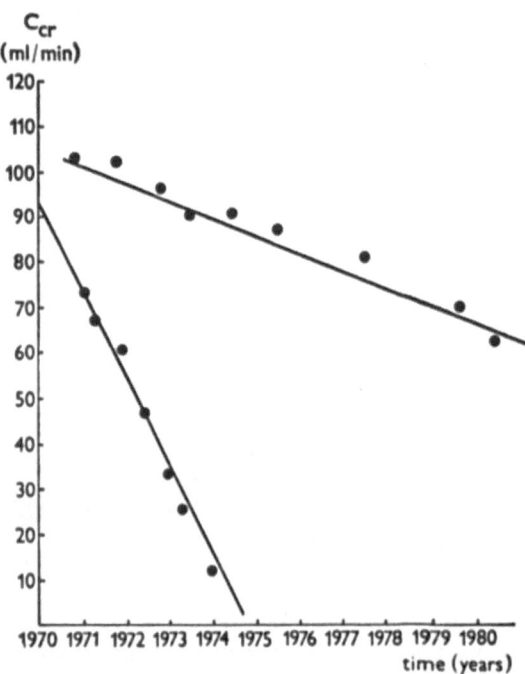

C_{cr}
(ml/min)

time (years)

Fig. 13: The decrease of endogenous creatinine clearance (C_{cr}) during the long term observation of patients with different activity of the renal diseases progression.

Laboratory methods

At present, large laboratories usually measure creatinine concentration using an Auto-Analyzer. For estimation of total chromogen the method of Bonsnes and Taussky (1945) can be recommended. The error of this method does not exceed 5%. For estimation of "true" creatinine the method described by Hare (1950) is adequate; it consists of separating the non-creatinine chromogen and creatinine by means of Lloyd's reagent. Recovery of creatinine added to serum is $100 \pm 1.7\%$ (Rowe et al. 1976).

The concentration of creatinine can be determined by a rate-dependent modification of the Jaffé reaction, employing a Beckman creatinine analyzer (Fabiny and Ertinghausen 1971, Heinegard and Tidestrom 1973). This method minimizes the influence of slow-reacting, noncreatinine plasma chromogens and thus provides an estimate of true creatinine concentration.

MEASUREMENT OF GFR BY MEANS OF RADIONUCLIDES

In recent years measurement of GFR in clinical practice has been also carried out by following the kinetics of substances, labelled with radionuclides, which are excreted by glomerular filtration only.

These methods consist of a single intravenous application of the labelled substance and measurement of the decrease of activity in plasma. An external detector is also used (for details see p. 73). These methods are advantageous since they do not require the quantitative urine collection. The following radio-labelled ubstances are in use at present:

^{51}Cr — EDTA (ethylenediaminetetracetic acid)
    (Garnett et al. 1967, Chantler et al. 1969, Brochner — Mortensen 1980)
^{131}I — Iothalamate (Cohen et al. 1969)
$^{99m}T_c$ — DTPA (diethylenetriaminepentaacetic acid)
    (Klopper et al. 1972)

Labels other than Tc can also be bound to DTPA, such as Chromium, Yttebrium and Indium. These chelates are excreted by the kidneys in a fashion similar to inulin (Bianchi 1972, Sziklas et al. 1971). The most frequently used is ^{99m}Tc — DTPA.

DTPA chelates are stable in vivo, are only slightly bound to serum proteins (4 to 10%), negligibly bound to erythrocytes and their distribution volume is identical with the extracellular fluid volume.

The examination is carried out as follows: After a single intravenous injection of the labelled substance blood samples are taken from the contralateral antecubital vein at intervals of two to six hours. The decrease of activity in the blood samples over this time interval can be expressed as a single exponential curve. On semi-log paper the decrease of plasma activity forms a straight line.

The more depressed the GFR, the slower the decrease in blood activity. The decrease in plasma activity can be expressed as an elimination constant or a biological half-life (calculation of these parameters is given on p. 75).

On the basis of the half-life or elimination constant, and the administered amount of activity, the total plasma clearance of the labelled substance can be evaluated. If the substance is eliminated by glomerular filtration only — the clearance should be identical with GFR.

The above investigation procedure can be combined with measurement of the urinary excretion of the indicator.

When ^{99m}Tc — DTPA is used, 20–40% is excreted during the first hour after application, 55–75% over four hours and 65–85% over six hours. In 24 hours more than 90% of the applied substance is excreted (Strauss et al. 1979).

For interpretation of clearance values calculated on the basis of the slope method see p. 77.

NON-ROUTINE METHODS OF MEASUREMENT OF GFR UNDER SPECIAL CONDITIONS

Under certain circumstances GFR can also be evaluated on the basis of substances that are reabsorbed or secreted by the tubules. This can occur under the condition that tubular transport of such a substance has achieved its maximum value (Tm). Under this circumstance the urinary excretion of the substance (which is reabsorbed in the tubules) can be expressed as follows:

$$UV = GFR \times P - Tm \tag{15}$$

For two levels of P, P_1 and P_2 — both greater than the maximal threshold (the P level at which Tm is achieved) — we will have:

$Tm = GFR \times P_1 - (UV)_1$

$Tm = GFR \times P_2 - (UV)_2$

If we collect both equations we have:

$$\Delta UV/\Delta P = GFR \tag{16}$$

It would appear from equation (15) that under these conditions the relation between UV and P is linear, and further, that the slope of the straight line $=$ GFR. Measurement of GFR in this way is usually a very useful "byproduct" of the investigation of maximal reabsorption of glucose (cf.p. 239), phosphates (cf.p. 210) and bicarbonates (cf.p. 229).

Simultaneous measurement of GFR with this approach and with C_{in} or with radioactively labelled EDTA (Stamp and Stacey 1970) gives very close results.

The same relation can also be derived for a substance with a secretion Tm like para-aminohippuric acid.

The relationship between UV and P for substances with various mechanisms of tubular handling is shown in Fig. 14.

The possibility of measuring GFR on the basis of urea clearance is explained on p. 54.

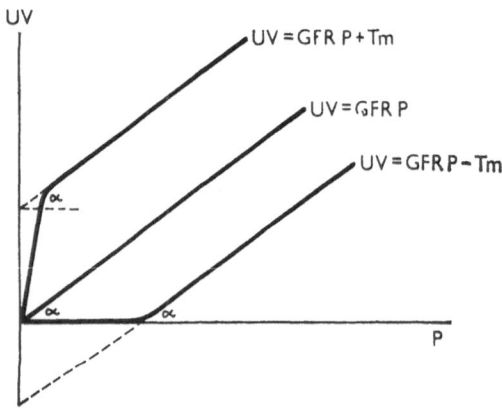

Fig. 14: Schematic presentation of the relationship between plasma concentration (P) and urinary excretion (UV) of substances with different mechanism of renal excretion.

REFERENCES

Addis, T., Barrett, E., Poo, L. J., et al.: The relation between protein consumption and diurnal variations of endogenous creatinine clearance in normal individuals. J. clin. Invest. *30*: 206, 1951

Auto Technicon (1963). Autoanalyser Methodology. File N-11 a. Chauncey New York. Technicon Instruments Corporation.

Bank, N., Aynedjian, H. S.: Individual nephron function in experimental bilateral pyelonephritis I. Glomerular filtration rate and proximal tubular sodium, potassium and water reabsorption. J. lab. clin. Med. *68*: 713, 1966

Barret, E., Addis, T.: The serum creatinine concentration of normal individuals. J. clin. Invest. *26*: 875, 1947

Barnett, H. L.: Renal physiology in infants and children: method for estimation of glomerular filtration rate. Proc. Soc. exp. Biol. N. Y. *44*: 654, 1940

Barnett, H. L., Perley, A. M., McGinnis, H. G.: Renal physiology in infants and children: inulin clearances in newborn infant with extrophy of bladder. Proc. Soc. exp. Biol. N. Y. *49*: 90, 1942

Bastai, P.: Die biologischen Grundlagen des Alterns. Zschr. Altersforsch. *9:* 193, 1955

Baylis, C., Deen, W. M., Myers, B. D., Brenner, B. M.0: Effect of some vasodilator drugs on transcapillary fluid exchange in the renal cortex. Am. J. Physiol. *230*: 1148, 1976

Black, D. A. K., McCance, R. A., Young, W. F.: Function of the kidney in dehydration. Nature (London) *150*: 461, 1942

Bleieter, R. E., Schedl, H. P.: Creatinine excretion: variability and relationships to diet and body size. J. lab. clin. Med. *59*: 945, 1962

Bianchi, C.: Measurement of the glomerular filtration rate. Prog. Nucl. Med. *2*: 21, 1972

Bonsnes, R. W., Lange, W. A.: Inulin clearance during pregnancy. Fed. Proc. *9*: 154, 1950

Bonsnes, R. W., Taussky, H.: On the colorimetric determination of creatinine by the Jaffé reaction. J. biol. Chem. *158*: 581, 1945

Brenner, B. M., Troy, J. L., Daugharty, T. M., Deen, W. M., Robertson, C. R.: Dynamics of glomerular ultrafiltration in the rat II. Plasma-flow dependence of GFR. Am. J. Physiol. *223*: 1184, 1972

Brenner, B. M., Troy, J. L., Daugharty, T. M.: The dynamics of glomerular ultrafiltration in the rat. J. clin. Invest. *50*: 1776, 1971

Brenner, B. M., Troy, J. L., Daugharty, T. M.: The dynamics of glomerular ultrafiltration in the rat. J. clin. Invest. *50:* 1776, 1971

Bricker, N. S., Klahr, S., Parkerson, M., Schultze, R. G.: Renal function in chronic renal disease. Medicine *44*: 263, 1965

Brochner-Mortensen, J.: A simple single injection method for determination of the extracelullar fluid volume. Scand. clin. lab. Invest. *40:* 567, 1980

Brod, J.: The kidney. London, Butterworths, 1973

Brod, J., Fencl, V.: Mechanismus celkových a ledvinových hemodynamických změn průběhu dne a noci. I. Chování zdravých lidí. Čas. Lék. čes. *97*: 33, 1958

Brod, J., Sirota, J. H.: Renal clearance of endogenous creatinine in man. J. clin. Invest. *27*: 645, 1948

Brun, C., Knudsen, E. O. E. Raaschou, F.: On the cause of postsyncopal oliguria. Acta med. Scand. *122*: 486, 1945

Bucht, H.: Studies on renal function in man with special reference to glomerular filtration and renal plasma flow in pregnancy. Scand. J. clin. lab. Invest. *3*, suppl. 3, 1951

Busch, W.: Pathologisch-anatomische Beobachtungen bei Angehörigen des hohen Greisenalters Z. Altersforsch. *12*: 103, 1958

Chantler, C., Garnett, E. S., Parsons, V., Veall, N.: Glomerular filtration rate measurement in man by single injection method using ^{51}Cr EDTA. Clin. Sci. *37:* 169, 1969

Chasson, A. L., Grady, H. T., Stanley, M. A.: Determination of creatinine by means of automatic chemical analysis. Am. J. clin. Pathol. *35:* 83, 1961

Chinard, F. P.: Possible mechanism of formation of glomerular fluid. Trans. third Josiah Macy, Jr. Conference on renal function. New York Josiah Macy Foundation, 1952.

Cockcroft, D. W., Gault, M. H.: Prediction of creatinine clearance from serum creatinine. Nephron *16:* 31, 1976

Cohen, M. L., Smith, F. G., Mindell, R. S., Vernier, R. L.: A simple reliable method of measuring glomerular filtration using single, low dose sodium iothalamate ^{131}I. Pediatrics *43:* 407, 1969

Davidson, W. D., Sackner, M. A.: Simplification of anthrone method for determination of inulin in clearance studies. J. lab. clin. Med. *62:* 351, 1963

Davies, D. F., Shock, N. W.: Age changes in glomerular filtration rate, effective renal plasma flow and tubular excretory capacity in adult males. J. clin. Invest. *29:* 496, 1950

Dawborn, J. K. Application of Heyrovský's inulin method to automatic analysis. Clin. Chim. Acta *52:* 63, 1956

Dean, R. F., McCance, R. A.: Inulin, diodine, creatinine and urea clearances in newborn infants. J. Physiol. (London) *106:* 431, 1947

Deen, W. M., Troy, J. L., Robertson, C. R., Brenner, B. M.: Dynamics of glomerular ultrafiltration in the rat IV. Determination of the ultrafiltration coefficient. J. clin. Invest. *52:* 1500, 1973

Dignam, W. J., Titus, P., Assali, N. S.: Renal function in human pregnancy I. Changes in glomerular filtration rate and renal plasma flow. Proc. Soc. exp. Biol. N. Y. *97:* 512, 1958

Doolan, P. D., Alpen, E. L., Theil, G. B.: A clinical appraisal of the plasma concentration and endogenous clearance of creatinine. Am. J. Med. *32:* 65, 1962

Dominguez, R., Pomerene, E.: Recovery of creatinine after ingestion and after intravenous injection in man. Proc. Soc. exp. Biol. Med. 58: 26, 1945

Edwards, K. D. G., Whyte, H. M.: Plasma creatinine level and creatinine clearance as tests of renal function. Aust. Ann. Med. *8:* 218, 1959

Effersoe, P.: Relationship between endogenous 24-hour creatinine clearance and serum creatinine concentration in patients with chronic renal disease. Acta med. Scand. *156:* 429, 1957

Enger, E., Blegen, E. M.: The relationship between endogenous creatinine clearance and serum creatinine in renal failure. Scand. J. clin. lab. Invest. *16:* 273, 1964

Fabiny, D. L., Ertinghausen, G.: Automated reaction-rate method for determination of serum creatinine with Centrifichem. Clin. Chem. *17:* 696, 1971

Fjeldbo, W., Stamey, T. A.: Adapted method for determination of inulin in serum and urine with an autoanalyzer. J. lab. clin. Med. *72:* 353, 1968

Garnett, E. S., Parsons, V., Veall, N.: Measurement of glomerular filtration rate in man using a ^{51}Cr Edetic-acid complex. Lancet *1:* 818, 1967

Goldman, R.: Creatinine excretion in renal failure. Proc. Soc. exp. Biol. Med. *85:* 446, 1954

Goldman, R., Moss, J. X.: Synthesis of creatinine in nephrectomized rats. Am. J. Physiol. *197:* 865, 1959

Gutman, Y., Gottschalk, C. W., Lassiter, W. E.: Micropuncture study of inulin absorption in the rat kidney. Science *147:* 753, 1965

Hare, R. S.: Endogenous creatinine in serum and urine. Proc. Soc. exp. Biol. Med. *74:* 148, 1950

Harris, C. A., Baer, P. G., Chirits, E. Dirks, J. H.: Composition of mammalian glomerular filtrate. Am. J. Physiol. *227:* 972, 1974

Harrison, H. E.: Modification of diphenylamine method for determination of inulin. Proc. Soc. exp. Biol. Med. *49:* 111, 1942

Hayslett, J. P., Kashgarian, M., Epstein, F. H.: Functional correlates of compensatory renal hyper-trophy. J. clin. Invest. *47*: 774, 1968

Healy, J. K.: Clinical assessment of glomerular filtration rate by different forms of creatinine clearance and a modified urinary phenolsulphonphthalein excretion test. Am. J. Med. *44*: 348, 1968

Heinegard, D., Tidestrom, G.: Determination of serum creatinine by a direct colorimetric method. Clin. chim. Acta *43*: 305, 1973

Heyrovsky, A. A.: A new method for determination of inulin in plasma and urine. Clin. chim. Acta *1*: 470, 1956

Hopper, J. Jr.: Creatinine clearance: A simple way of measuring kidney function. Bull. Univ. Calif. Med. Center 2: 315, 1951.

Jelliffe, R. W.: Estimation of creatinine clearance when urine cannot be collected. Lancet *1*: 975, 1971

Jelliffe, R. W.: Creatinine clearance. Bedside estimate. Ann. intern. Med. *79*: 604, 1973

Jollife, N. Smith, H. W.: The excretion of urine in the dog II. The urea and creatinine clearance on cracker meal diet. Am. J. Physiol. *99*: 101, 1931

Kassirer, J. P.: Clinical evaluation of kidney function — glomerular function. New Engl. J. Med. *285*: 385, 1971

Kassirer, J. P., Gennari, F. J.: Laboratory evaluation of renal function. In: Strauss and Welt's Diseases of the Kidney. Third edition (Eds. L. E. Earley and C. W. Gottschalk) Vol. I. Boston Little, Brown Co. 41—91, 1979

Kim. K. E., Onseti, G., Ramirez, O., Brest, A. N., Swartz, C.: Creatinine clearance in renal disease. A reappraisal. Brit. med. J. *4*: 11, 1969

Klopper, J. F., Hauser, W., Atkins, H. L., Eckelmann, W. C., Richards, P.: Evaluation of ^{90m}Tc-DTPA for the measurement of glomerular filtration rate. J. Nucl. Med. *13*: 107, 1972

Kuhlback, B., Pasternack, A., Launiala, K., Stenberg, M.: Serum creatine and creatinine in children and adolescents. Scand. J. clin. lab. Invest. *22*: 37, 1968

Leaf, A. Couter, W. T.: Evidence that the renal sodium excretion by normal human subjects is regulated by adrenal cortical activity. J. clin. Invest. *28*: 1067, 1949

Levender, S., Hilton, P. J., Jones, N. F.: The measurement of glomerular filtration in renal disease. Lancet *2*: 1216, 1969

Levinsky, N. G., Berliner, R. W.: The role of urea in the concentrating mechanism. J. clin. Invest. *38*: 741, 1958

Maude, D. L., Scott, W. N., Shebadeh, I., Solomon, A. K.: Further studies on the behavior of inulin and serum albumin in rat kidney tubule. Pflüger's. Arch. ges. Physiol. *285*: 313, 1965

McCance, R. A., Widdowson, E. M.: The secretion of urine in man during experimental salt deficiency. J. Physiol. (London) *91*: 222, 1937

McCance, R. A., Young, W. F.: Secretion of urine by newborn infants. J. Physiol. (London) *99*: 265, 1941

Merill, J. A., Cargill, W. H.: The effect of exercise on the renal plasma flow and filtration rate of normal and cardiac subjects. J. clin. Invest. *27*: 272, 1948

Mertz, D. P.: Observations on the renal clearance and the volume of distribution of polyfructosan-S, a new inulin-like substance. Experientia *19*: 248, 1963

Mertz, D. P.: Quantitative Nierenfunktionsproben. In: H. Sarre: Nierenkrankheiten. Stuttgart, Thieme 1976, p. 115

Miles, B. E., De Wardener, H. E., Mc Swiney, R. R.: Renal function during emotional diuresis. Am. J. Med. *12*: 659, 1952

Mitch, W. E., Walser, M., Buffington, G. A., Leman, J.: A simple method of estimating progression of chronic renal failure. Lancet II: 1326, 1976.

Möller, E., McIntosh, J. R., Van Slyke, D. D.: Studies of urea excretion II. Relationship between urine volume and rate of urea excretion by normal adults. J. clin. Invest. *6:* 427, 1929

Moustgaard, J.: Om proteinstoffernes inflydelese paa nyrefunktionen hos hund. Kopenhavn, Ejoiud Christensen Forlag, 1948

Newman, E. V., Bordley, J., Winternitz, J.: The interrelationship of glomerular filtration rate (mannitol clearance), extracellular fluid volume, surface area of the body and plasma concentration of mannitol. A definition of extracellular fluid clearance determined by following plasma concentration after a single injection of mannitol. Bull. Johns Hopk. Hosp. *75:* 253, 1944

Oliver, J.: Problems of aging. 2nd ed. E.E.V. Lowdry Williams and Wilkins, Baltimore 1942

Pappenheimer, J. R.: Passage of molecules through capillary walls. Physiol. Rev. *33:* 387, 1953

Pappenheimer, J. R., Renkin, E. M., Borero, L. M.: Filtration, diffusion and molecular sieving through peripheral capillary membranes: A contribution to the pore theory of capillary permeability. Am. J. Physiol. *167:* 13, 1951

Pasternack, A., Kuhback, B.: Diurnal variations of serum and urine creatine. Scand. J. lab. Invest. *27:* 1, 1971

Pullman, T. N., Alving, A. S., Dern, R. J., Landowne, M.: The influence of dietary protein intake on specific renal functions in normal man. J. lab. clin. Med. *44:* 320, 1954

Rapoport, A., Hudsan, H.: Endogenous creatinine clearance and serum creatinine in the clinical assessment of kidney function. Can. Med. Assoc. J. *99:* 149, 1968

Richards, A. N., Westfall, B. B., Bott, P. A.: Renal excretion of inulin, creatinine and xylose in normal dogs. Proc. Soc. exp. Biol. N. Y. *32:* 73, 1934

Richardson, J. A., Philbin, P. E.: The one-hour creatinine clearance rate in healthy men. J. Am. med. Assoc. *216:* 987, 1971

Roberts, L. B.: The normal ranges, with statistical analysis, for seventeen blood constituents Clin. chim. Acta *16:* 69, 1967

Roe, J. H., Epstein, J. H., Goldstein, N. P. A.: A photometric method for determination of inulin in plasma and urine. J. biol. Chem. *178:* 839, 1949

Rosenbaum, R. W., Hruska, K. A., Anderson, Ch., Robson, A. M., Slapotolsky, E., Klahr, S.: Inulin: An inadequate marker of glomerular filtration rate in kidney donors and transplant recipients? Kidney int. *16:* 179, 1979

Roessle, R., Roulet, F.: Mass and Zahl in der Pathologie. Berlin, Springer, 1932

Rowe, J. W., Andres, R., Tobian, J. D., Norris, A. H., Shock, N. W.: The effect of age on creatinine clearance in men: a cross-sectional and longitudinal study. J. Gerong. *31:* 155, 1976

Schreiner, G. E.: Determination of inulin by means of resorcinol. Proc. Soc. exp. Biol. Med. *74:* 117, 1950

Schirmeister, J., Willmann, H., Kiefer, H.: Plasmakreatinin als grober Indikator der Nierenfunktion. Dtsch. med. Wschr. *89:* 1018, 1964

Schück, O., Nádvorniková, H., Prát, V.: The problem of drug dosage in patients with chronic renal impairment. Zbl. Pharm. *116:* 601, 1977

Schück, O., Stříbrná, J., Kotátko, J., Pacovský, V., Fabian, F.: Změny ledvinných funkcí při cévkování močového měchýře. Čas. Lék. čes. *97:* 1217, 1958

Schwartz, G. J., Haycock, G. B., Edelman, C. M., Spitzer, A.: A simple estimate of glomerular filtration rate in children derived from body length and plasma creatinine. Pediatrics *58:* 259, 1976

Schwartz, G. J., Haycock, G. B., Spitzer, A.: Plasma creatinine and urea concentration in children: normal values for age and sex. J. Pediatr. *88:* 828, 1976

Shannon, J. A., Joliffe, N., Smith, H. W.: The excretion of urine in the dog VI. The filtration and secretion of exogenous creatinine. Am. J. Physiol. *102:* 534, 1932

42

Shannon, J. A., Smith, H. W.: The excretion of inulin, xytose and urea by normal and phlorinized man. J. clin. Invest. *14*: 393, 1935

Sierbaek-Nielsen, K., Hansen, J. M., Kampmann, J., Kristensen, M.: Rapid evaluation of creatinine clearance. Lancet *1*: 1133, 1971

Sims, E. A. H., Krantz, K. E.: Serial studies of renal function during pregnancy and the puerperium in normal woman. J. clin. Invest. *37*: 1764, 1958

Sirota, J. H., Baldwin, D. S., Villareal, H.: Diurnal variations of renal function in man. J. clin. Invest. *29*: 187, 1950

Smith, H. W.: The physiology of renal circulation. Harvey Lect. *35*: 166, 1940

Smith, H. W.: The kidney, structure and function in health and disease. New York, Oxford Univ. Press 1951

Smith, H. W.: Principles of renal physiology. Oxford Univ. Press New York 1956

Sohar, E., Scadron, E., Levitt, M. F.: Changes in renal hemodynamics during normal pregnancy. Clin. Res. Proc. (Abstract) *4*: 142, 1956

Stamp, T. C. B., Stacey, T. E.: Evaluation of theoretical renal phosphorus threshold as an index of renal phosphorus handling. Clin. Sci., *39*: 505, 1970.

Strauss, H. W., Kirschner, P. T., Wagner, H. N. Jr.: Nuclear medicine in the evaluation of renal disease. In: Strauss and Welt's Diseases of the Kidney, 3. ed. (Eds. L. E. Earley and C. W. Gottschalk) Vol. I., Boston Little, Brown Co. 1979 pp. 149—164

Stříbrná, J.: Über die Bestimmung der Menge des Residualharnes. Urol. int. *20*: 117, 1965

Sziklas, J. J., Hosian, F., Reba, R. C., Wagner, H. N. Jr.: Comparison of 169 ytterbium-DTPA 113 m indiumDTPA, C^{14} inulin, and endogenous creatinine to estimate glomerular filtration. J. nucl. Biol. Med. *15*: 122, 1971

Tanner, G. A., Sloan, K. L., Sophasan, S.: Effects of renal artery occlusion on kidney function in the rat. Kidney int. *4*: 377, 1973

Tudvad, F., Vesterdal, J.: Inulin and PAH clearances in newborn infants. Scand. J. clin. Lab. Invest. *1*: 345, 1949

Vesterdal, J., Tudvad, F.: Studies on the kidney function in premature and fullterm infants by estimation of the inulin and paraaminohippurate clearances. Acta paediat. (Upsalla) *37*: 429, 1949

Watchinger, B., Kobinger, I.: Clearancebestimmung mit Polyfructosan S (Inutest) Wien. Zschr. inn. Med. *45*: 219, 1964

Waugh, W. H.: Photometry of inulin and polyfructosan by use of a cysteine/tryptophan reaction. Clin. Chem. *23*: 639, 1977

Wesson, L. G. Jr.: Physiology of the human kidney. New York Grune and Stratton, 1969

West, J. R., Smith, H. W., Chasis, H.: Glomerular filtration rate, effective renal plasma flow, and maximal tubular excretory capacity in infancy. J. Pediat. *32*: 10, 1948

White, H. L., Rolf, D.: Effects of exercise and some other influences on the renal circulation in man. Am. J. Physiol. *152*: 505, 1948

White, R. P., Samson, F. E.: Determination of inulin in plasma and urine by use of anthrone. J. lab. clin. Med. *43*: 475, 1954

Wilson, E. F., Soullier, G., Antonenko, D.: Creatinine clearance in criticially ill surgical patients. Arch. Surg. *114*: 461, 1979

Young, W. F., McCanse, R. A.: Secretion of urine by dehydrated and normal infants. Arch. Dis. Child. *17*: 65, 1942

UREA

Historical remarks

The first observation that diseased kidneys retain urea in the blood was made by Bright at the start of the 19th century. Richard Bright (1827, 1836) described cases in which anatomical evidence of kidney disease (at post mortem) was associated during the life of the patients with oedema, cardiac hypertrophy, proteinuria and increased levels of urea in the blood.

Increased blood levels of urea were termed uremia. Since these patients had low urea concentrations in the urine, the origin of uremia was explained as an inability of the diseased kidneys to excrete urea. This observation was then repeatedly confirmed by others. With the development of biochemical methods, determination of blood urea — or determination of non-protein nitrogen (mostly urea) — became a method of clinical diagnosis (Strauss 1916).

At the start of the 20th century a number of investigators followed in detail the relation between urinary urea excretion and blood levels.

In 1912 Ambard and Weill presented a complex equation describing the relation between urinary urea excretion and blood levels under conditions of low urine flow rate. This equation was called the "Ambard constant".

Addis, in rabbit experiments, observed that urinary urea excretion depended to a large degree on the rate of urine flow. If urine flow rate was high, urinary urea excretion ($U_U V$) was directly related to the blood concentration (B_U). The ratio $U_U V / B_U$ was called the Addis "urea excretion ratio" and it was recommended as a rough index of the mass of active renal parenchyma (Addis 1917, 1928). In 1921 Austin, Stillman and van Slyke confirmed that in man with high urine flow rate $U_U V$ is linearly related to B. This was found to be the case if urine flow rate was 2 ml/min/1.73 m^2 or higher. The latter critical value was called the "augmentation limit".

Moeller, McIntosh and van Slyke (1929) studied in detail the relation between $U_U V$ and B_U at various urine flow rates in healthy controls and patients with Bright's disease. They found that if urine flow rate was less than the augmentation limit, the ratio $U_U | V / B_U$ was constant. The ratio $U_U V / B_U$ was termed the maximal clearance of urea, and $U_U\sqrt{V}/B_U$ was called the standard urea clearance. These terms were quickly accepted, but the double mathematical expression (for standard and maximal values) caused complications.

The term "clearance" very clearly expresses one of the basic functions of the kidneys, to "clear" or "cleanse" blood of metabolic products. In ensuing years the concept of clearance was made more precise, as the value of a virtual plasma volume completely "cleared" or "cleansed" per unit time (usually, 1 min). The precise definition of clearance is: the volume of plasma which contains that amount of the substance in question excreted into the urine per unit time.

Renal clearances (C) are always calculated according to:

$$C = \frac{UV}{P} \qquad (1)$$

The concentration of the substance in question must be related to plasma volume and not blood volume.

Measurement of plasma urea concentration is to this day one of the basic criteria of renal function. Little has changed in the evaluation of Bright's classical discovery — time has improved the analytical methods, and interpretation of changes in plasma urea concentration has become more detailed in patients with chronic renal disease.

PHYSIOLOGY AND PATHOPHYSIOLOGY

Urea is the main nitrogenous substance derived from protein metabolism. It is formed in the Krebs-Henseleit cycle.

Under normal conditions, metabolism of 100 g protein gives rise to the formation of 33 g urea. In other words, in a healthy adult on a normal diet containing about 70 g protein/day, about 23 g urea is formed. 70–80% of the urea formed is excreted by the kidneys.

In patients in the more advanced stages of chronic renal failure, there can be changes in protein metabolism. N freed up during metabolism need not be completely utilized for synthesis of urea. Part of the freed N can be attached to short-chain fatty acids. Freed N can also appear attached to other amino acids, with the formation of guanidino compounds (Cohen 1972). Part of the urea pool can be degraded in the gut lumen by microbial urease. Ammonia formed in the gut is absorbed by the portal system into the liver, where it is used for resynthesis of amino acids (Giordano et al. 1963, 1968). For the above reasons, the amount of urea formed by metabolism of protein in patients with chronic renal failure can be less than in normals. Metabolism of protein and the formation of urea in chronic renal failure is influenced by a number of factors, among which belongs a lower protein intake (Giovanetti and Maggiore 1964, Kluthe et al. 1972, Bergstrom et al. 1972). It is therefore clear that in patients with chronic renal disease, particularly the advanced stage, P_U is determined not only by renal function but by metabolic processes as well.

The mechanism of renal urea excretion is not yet completely clear. The first important observations here followed shortly after the measurement of GFR became possible. The renal urea clearance is lower than GFR. This finding showed that part of the filtered urea load is reabsorbed by the tubules.

The rate of this reabsorption depends upon the rate of tubular water reabsorption. A decrease in the latter results in a decrease in urea reabsorption (Shannon 1938, Chasis and Smith 1938). This finding agrees with the view that diffusion plays a large role in trans-tubular urea movement.

A decrease in tubular water reabsorption and an increase in urine flow rate can involve processes which take place at different intensities at different tubular sites. A water load results in a diuresis because of the decrease in water reabsorption in the distal segment of the nephron. Since the diuresis in this case also results in an increase in urea excretion, it would appear that diffusion of urea across the tubular wall occurs in the distal nephron. After attaining a maximal water diuresis (at which point distal water reabsorption falls to its minimum), a further increase in urine flow rate can only occur if the filtered load increases for osmotically active solute (a hypertonic infusion). Unreabsorbed osmotically active solute can decrease water reabsorption in the proximal nephron since water is "bound" to the solute in the lumen. Under these conditions, there is a further increase in urea excretion, which suggests that this substance is also diffusable in the proximal nephron as well. The relation between the rate of water reabsorption (as expressed by the concentration index of inulin) and the rate of urea excretion (as expressed by the ratio C_U/C_{in}) is shown in Fig. 15.

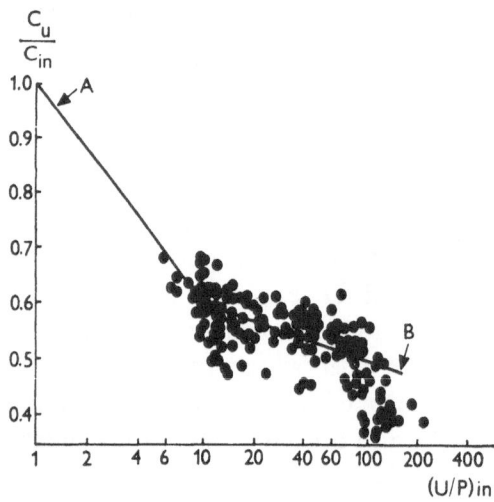

Fig. 15: Relationship between concentration index of inulin (U/P) in and the ratio of clearance of urea and inulin (C_u/C_{in}) under conditions of various diuretic states (Chassis and Smith 1938).

This last Fig. shows that the relation between these parameters has a different nature in the U_{in}/P_{in} region of pure water diuresis (in the range 8 to 200) than in the region of osmotic diuresis superimposed on water diuresis (i.e. ratio less than 8). This finding indirectly suggests that the permeabilities of the proximal and distal tubules for urea are not equivalent. The proximal segment is more permeable to urea than the distal.

Micropuncture data in recent years has complemented the above data based upon clearance experiments. It was confirmed that urea freely penetrates the glomerular membrane, so that its concentration in the glomerular filtrate is the same as in plasma. In the proximal tubule about 50% of the filtered load is reabsorbed (Lassiter et al. 1961). At the start of the distal tubule, the total amount of urea in the luminal fluid is again the same as in the filtered load, or even exceeds it. This finding shows that in the medulla there must have been urea transport from the interstitial fluid into the lumen of the loop of Henle.

Measurement of urea in different parts of the medulla (Ullrich and Jarausch 1956) showed that there is a rise from the cortico-medullary boundary to the tip of the papilla. (This concentration gradient is called the urea medullary-concentration gradient).

The medullary urea concentration gradient results from a recycling of urea. The condition for its formation is penetration from collecting ducts into the medullary interstitium. This process was demonstrated by microcatheterization of the collecting ducts (Hilger et al. 1958). Urea from the medullary interstitium diffuses into the lumen of the loops of Henle and vasa recta. Since the blood and urine flowing into the medulla contain less urea than is present in the interstitium, conditions favour the function of the counter-current mechanism.

Diffusion of urea from the collecting ducts into the medulla is made possible by the fact that into the distal parts of the former there is a flow of luminal fluid of high urea content. Attainment of a high urea concentration in the distal part of the collecting ducts is made possible by the fact that the walls of the distal tubule and the proximal part of the collecting ducts are relatively impermeable to urea diffusion.

The degree of the medullary urea gradient depends in large measure on the rate of urine flow. When the latter is low, urea forms 40–50% of the total osmotic gradient of the medulla, whereas in water diuresis urea is only 10% of the total.

Renal urea excretion is significantly changed with various pathologies of the kidney.

A decrease in GFR is associated with a decrease in C_U. The latter decrease need not, however, be associated with a decrease in $U_U V$. The equation for the calculation of C_U shows that $U_U V = C_U P_U$. In other words, if the decrease in C_U is associated with a rise in P_U there need not be a decrease in $U_U V$. The external N balance can be 0 with varying levels of P_U. As has been explained, C_U depends on fractional water reabsorption (FR_{H2O}). Since with a gradual decrease in the number of functional nephrons (in chronic renal disease) there is a situation of osmotic diuresis in the residual nephrons (cf.p. 162), it is clear that also FR_U in the residual nephrons is decreased. Chasis and Smith (1938) showed that the relation between C_U/C_{in} and U_{in}/P_{in} in various states of urine flow in patients with chronic glomerulonephritis has the same nature as in healthy controls.

At present there is too little information on whether in some renal pathologies the tubular permeability for urea is changed overall or even in tubular segments. Goaverts (1948) observed a decrease in C_U/C_{in} during the rising phase of diuresis in toxic renal damage. This finding might be due to a rise in urea permeability of some nephron segments.

Anatomical changes in the kidney which deform the medullary counter-current system, or serous and cellular infiltrates in the medulla, can alter the recycling of urea, the formation of an adequate gradient and, thus, the ability of the kidney to form a concentrated urine (cf.p. 111).

METHODS OF INVESTIGATION

PLASMA UREA CONCENTRATION (P_U) AND BLOOD UREA NITROGEN (BUN)

Under normal conditions P_U varies between 20 and 40 mg %. Since urea has a Dalton number 60, and each molecule of urea contains 2 N atoms (28) the relation between P_U and BUN is as follows:

$$P_U = \frac{60}{28} BUN = 2.14 BUN$$

Approximately $P_U \doteq 2 BUN$. That means that under normal conditions BUN varies between 10 and 20 mg %.

If the plasma concentration of urea is expressed in mmol/l the normal interval of P_{urea} is: 3,4 to 6,7. For expression of P_{urea} in mmol/l the following formula is used:

$$P(mmol/l) = \frac{P(mg\%)\, 10}{60}$$

P increases as renal function is destroyed, but is heavily under the influence of a number of extrarenal factors.

The relation between P and the most important factors which influence this value can be derived as follows:

Under conditions of a balanced external state of N exchange, the amount of N

48

taken orally (I_N) equals the sum of urinary N excretion (U_NV) and fecal N excretion (F_N).

$$I_N = U_NV + F_N \tag{2}$$

If the fecal excretion of N is small in comparison with N taken orally and this value is neglected and if I_{Pr} (protein intake) is expressed in g/day the following simplification can be made:

$$P_U \, (mg\%) = \frac{23 \, I_{Pr}}{C_U} \, \frac{(g/day)}{(ml/min)} \tag{3}$$

For example, if a patient has an intake of 60 g protein/day and $C_U = 20$ ml/min, then if external N balance is 0, P_U will be maximally 69 mg%.

Equation (3) is of practical importance. Fig. 16 shows the relationship between P_U, I_{Pr} and C_U (expressed by equation /3/) graphically.

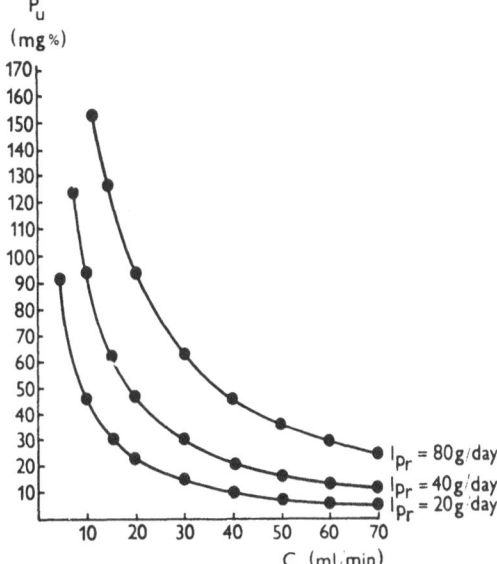

Fig. 16: Relationship between urea clearance (C_u) and plasma urea concentration (P_u) under conditions of different protein intake (I_{Pr}).

Since in patients with chronic renal insufficiency C_U approximates C_{cr}, the latter can be used for calculation of P_U.

Fig. 16 shows the known hyperbolic relation between C_U and P_U. Since the position of the hyperbola depends very much on the protein intake, the estimate of C_U (or in general, kidney function) on the basis of P_U carries a large degree of error. It would also appear from the various hyperbolic relations shown that with a decrease in C_U from the normal range to moderately decreased values, the increase in P_U is relatively small, especially in cases with low protein intake.

On the other hand, if C_U decreases to very low values, the rise in P_U becomes quite striking. Thus the changes in P_U are not a sensitive reflection of a decrease in renal function in the initial stages of kidney disease — in advanced stages even

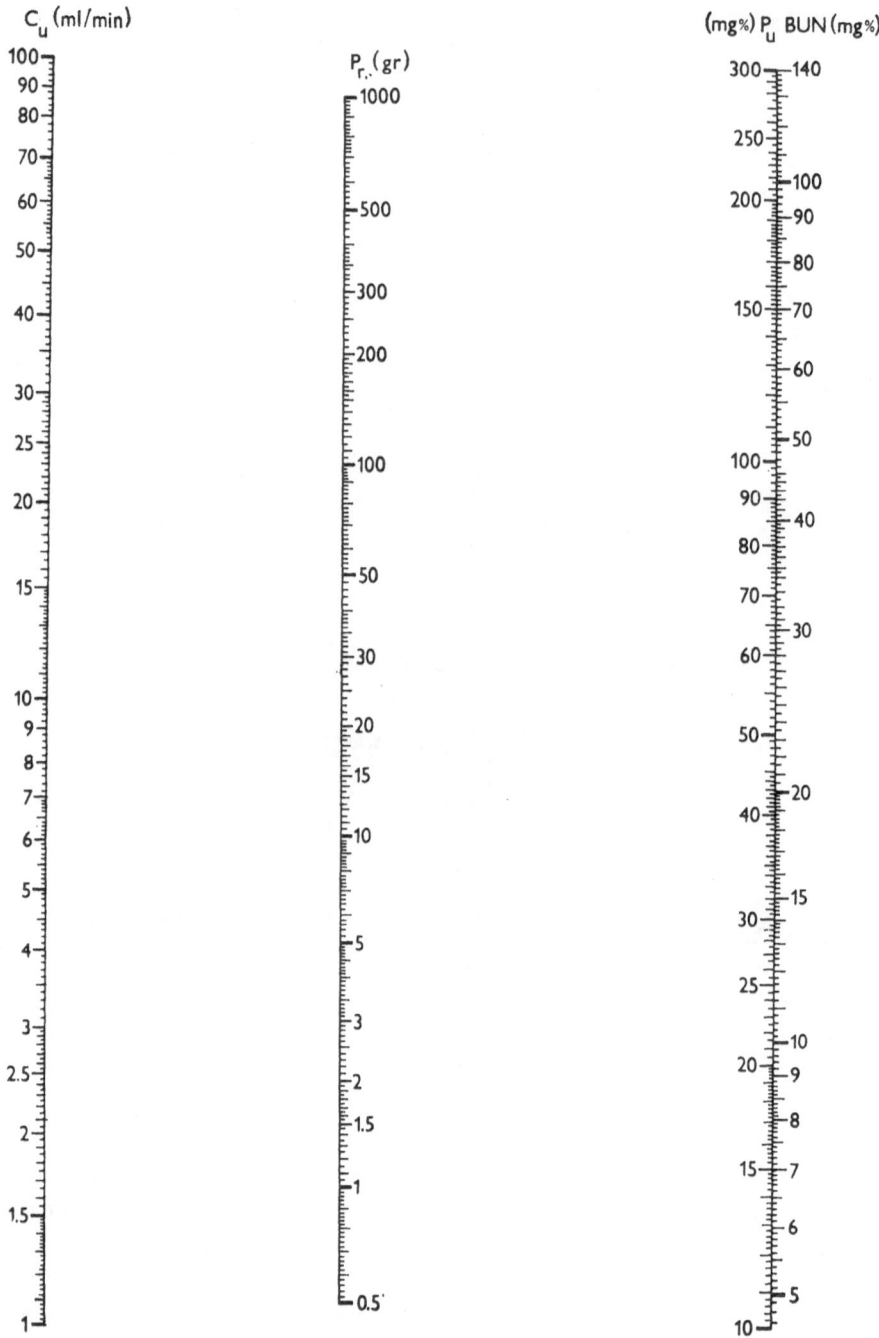

Fig. 17: Nomogram for evaluation of plasma urea concentration (P_u) and blood urea nitrogen (BUN) on the basis of urea clearance (C_u) and daily protein intake (Pr).

small changes in kidney function will have a clear and measurable effect on P_U.

Since evaluation of kidney function on the basis of P_U must take into account the protein intake, we have constructed a nomogram (Fig. 17) which is another form of expression of equation (3). It should be stressed again that equation (3) and the nomogram can help in the interpretation of P_U only under conditions of a balanced state. Furthermore it should be born in mind that in patients with advanced chronic renal failure on a low protein intake, the amount of urea produced by the metabolism of protein can be lower than $0.33 \, I_{Pr}$, and that extrarenal elimination of urea becomes not at all negligible with respect to its metabolic production.

In patients with a sudden decrease of renal function the retained urea is distributed throughout the total body water. The production of urea may be increased by excessive catabolism of protein, absorption of blood from the gastrointestinal tract or by steroid therapy.

THE UREA CONCENTRATION IN THE URINE (U_U)

This value depends on the rate of urine flow and the total urea quantity to be excreted in the urine.

Table 1 gives the mean values of U_U ($\pm$SD) in healthy adult controls after varying periods of fluid withdrawal. NaCl intake was normal.

Table 1

	12–16	16–20	20–24	24–28	28–32	32–36 (hr without fluids)
U_U (mmol/l)	419	430	470	547	645	639
$\pm$ SD	(151)	(97)	(93)	(109)	(118)	(128)

This table shows that withdrawal of oral fluids causes a rise in U_U which after 28hr reaches a value in excess of 600 mmol/l. If Na excretion is low, U_U can be even higher. If U_{Na} is extremely low, and fluid restriction has lasted some time, U_U can reach 800–1000 mmol/l. The same levels can be found in patients with severe NaCl and water retention because of secondary hyperaldosteronism.

At the height of a water diuresis, U_U decreases to levels about 30 mmol/l. In patients with isosthenuria, U_U ranges about 150 mmol/l and urea forms about 50% of total urine osmolality. Under normal conditions U_U/P_U ranges most frequently between 50 and 100 depending on urine flow rate.

URINARY UREA EXCRETION (U_UV)

This measure is part of any investigation of the external N balance. It requires careful collection of urine over 24 hr and determination of U_U in the mixed sample. Any action of bacterial urease on the urine must be prevented. The urine should be subjected to bacteriological examination (in patients with infections of the urinary passages and pyelonephritis). Samples in women may be contaminated by gynecological infections. The urine can also be exogenously contaminated.

U_UV depends on protein intake. With a normal protein intake in normal adults, U_UV ranges from 15 to 30 g/day, i.e. 250–500 mmol/day.

Precise measurements of N balance require collection of feces for analysis. N intake is read off from tables. Many institutions have prepared diets on hand with known protein content. The balance measurements must be carried out for several days (usually 3 weeks) so that a balanced metabolic state can be achieved.

U_UV on its own does not assist us to evaluate renal function.

RENAL UREA CLEARANCE (C_U)

This parameter is usually measured in 1–2 one hour collection periods in the A.M. The subject has an empty stomach and drinks 500–1000 ml water 1 hr before the onset. Measurement of C_U requires a high urine flow rate, at least higher than the augmentation limit (2 ml/min, with adults of normal proportions).

In patients with chronic renal disease and a low GFR, FE_{H_2O} is usually sufficiently high because of the spontaneous osmotic diuretic state. Despite this, even such cases should receive an oral water load so that the change in urea diffusion

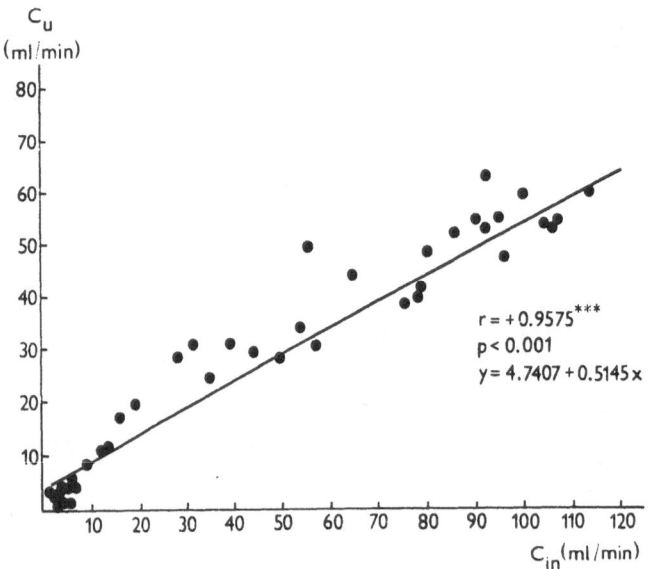

$r = +0.9575^{***}$
$p < 0.001$
$y = 4.7407 + 0.5145x$

Fig. 18: Relationship between inulin clearance (C_{in}) and urea clearance (C_u) in patients with chronic renal diseases.

in the distal nephron should be constant if the C_U values are to be relied upon.

Measurement of C_U under conditions of induced water diuresis should make allowance for the transitional increase in urea excretion at the start of the diuresis (because of a "washout" of the medullary urea gradient). C_U should be measured during diuresis, but better if the subject is in the descending phase of the induced diuresis or during a maintained diuresis after some time has elapsed. The washout reaction should be gone within 30 min of the start of a water diuretic state.

The actual measurement starts with spontaneous bladder emptying. The time of termination of this flow is recorded (the subject's watch should be synchronized with the investigator's). The urine volume is measured exactly. The collection period is 60 min and is terminated with spontaneous voiding.

At 30 min blood is sampled from the antecubital vein. C_U is calculated from U_U, the mean rate of urine flow/min and P_U in the usual manner according to equation 1). Normal values of C_U in 20 healthy adults on a normal diet under conditions of varying water diuresis are given in Table 2.

Table 2

V ml/min	$\dfrac{V}{C_{in}} 100$ %	C_U ml/min	$\dfrac{C_U}{C_{in}} 100$ %
3.2 ± 1.8	2.9 ± 1.2	71.8 ± 6.9	63.9 ± 11.6
14.7 ± 4.9	13.7 ± 2.4	78.2 ± 9.6	75.2 ± 12.6

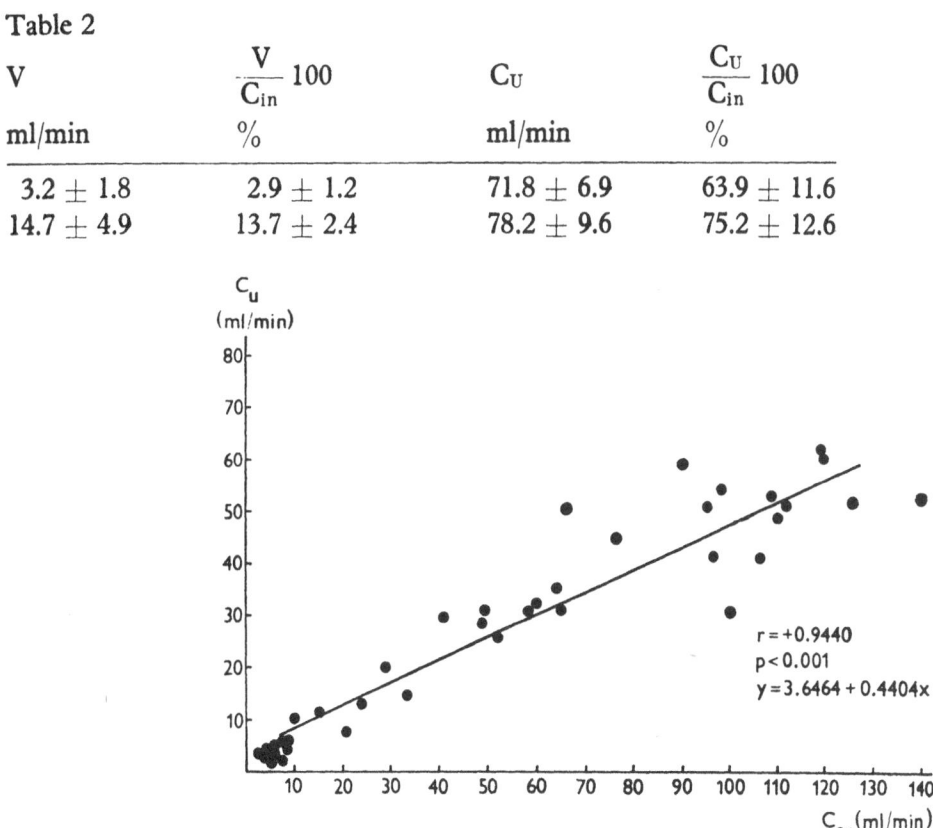

Fig. 19: Relationship between clearance of endogenous creatinine (C_{cr}) and urea clearance (C_u) in patients with chronic renal diseases.

The above data suggest that in healthy subjects with diuresis at the augmentation limit, C_U reaches at least 60 ml/min. It is sufficient if the urine flow rate is only slightly above the augmentation limit. C_U values at the height of water diuresis are only slightly higher than with sub-maximal diuresis.

C_U is age dependent. Lewis and Alving (1938) found that in subjects aged 89, C_U was on the average only 55% of those values found in 40-year olds. C_U decreases in patients with chronic renal disease in relation to the decrease in C_{in}. The relation of these two parameters in patients in various stages of chronic renal disease (mainly glomerulonephritis and interstitial nephritis) is shown in Fig. 18.

Fig. No. 19 shows that C_U decreases in linear relation also to the decrease in C_{cr} in the course of chronic renal disease. The slope of the regression line is lower than the diagonal. If C_{cr} is very low, C_U approximates C_{cr} in absolute value.

FRACTIONAL UREA EXCRETION (FE$_U$)

FE$_U$ gives the relation of urea excretion to the filtered load (for calculation of FE$_U$ see p. 262). Estimation of FE$_U$ requires simultaneous measurements from urine and plasma of urea and endogenous creatinine.

Measurement of FE$_U$ is carried out at the same time as that of C_U, and the

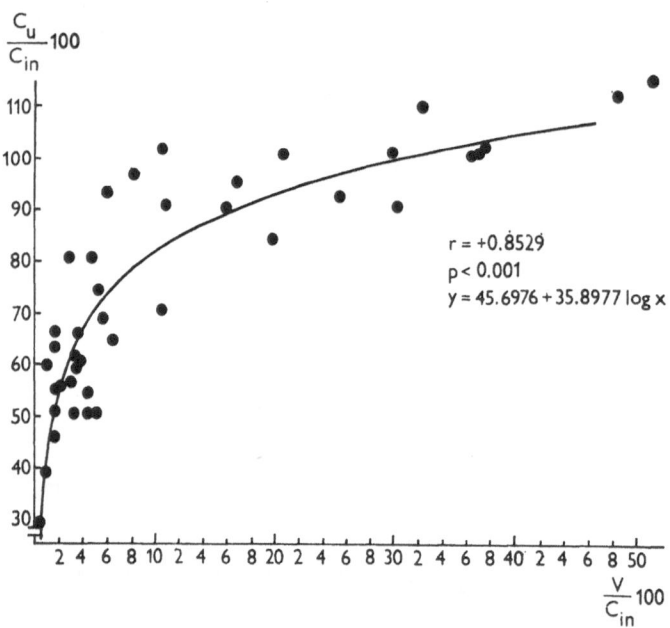

Fig. 20: Relationship between fractional water excretion (calculated as V/C_{in} 100) and the ratio (C_u/C_{in}) 100 in patients with chronic renal disesases.

procedure is unchanged from the above. Normal values of FE_U calculated from C_{in} in healthy adults with sub-maximal and maximal water diuresis are given in Table 2. These data show that under the given conditions, the mean $- 2 \times SD =$ = about 45%. FE_U calculated from C_{cr} in healthy controls (n = 91) at high levels of water diuresis is given in Table 3.

Table 3

$\dfrac{V}{C_{cr}} 100 \,(\%)$	$\dfrac{C_U}{C_{cr}} 100 \,(\%)$
10.5 ± 2.4	61.7 ± 12.4

In patients with chronic renal disease, FE_U increases in relation to the decrease in GFR. If GFR is very low, FE_U approximates 100%. These findings can be interpreted as showing that with a decreasing number of functional nephrons because of chronic renal disease, there is a decrease in FR_U in residual nephrons.

A decrease in FR_U in residual nephrons is the result of a decrease in FR_{H_2O} because of an osmotic diuretic state. The relation between (V/C_{in}) 100 and (C_U/C_{in}) 100 is shown in Fig. 20. As in healthy subjects, this latter relation does not have a simple linear nature. In the region of low values, a relatively small increase in FE_{H_2O} is associated with a relatively large change in FE_U. If values are high, FE_{H_2O} changes cause smaller changes in FE_U.

A similar relation can be seen between (V/C_{cr}) 100 and (C_U/C_{cr}) 100, as shown in Fig. 21.

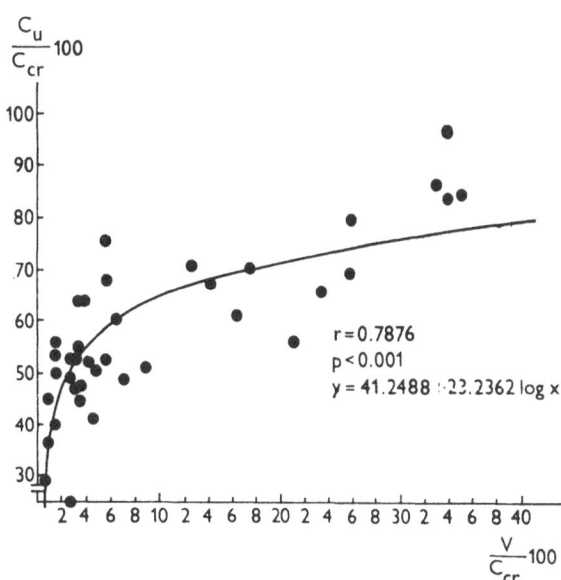

Fig. 21: Relationship between fractional water excretion (calculated as V/C_{cr} 100) and the ratio (C_u/C_{cr}) 100 in patients with chronic renal diseases.

Indications for investigation

Measurement of P_U is a basic criterion to be determined in all patients with renal disease.

In patients with acute disease, P_U is measured frequently. The dynamics of change in P_U can assist in evaluating changes in renal function. At the same time one must keep in mind that all the other factors (cf. above) play their roles.

In patients with chronic disease, P_U is measured less frequently. This measurement also allows us to judge the effect of dietary therapy.

Measurement of U_U/P_U can assist in the differential diagnosis of **acute renal failure.** In acute oliguric renal failure U_U/P_U average values have been found to vary between 2.0 and 3.4. On the other hand in acute non-oliguric acute tubular necrosis U_U/P_U values have been found between 6 and 7 (Bull et al. 1950, Luke et al. 1970, Perlmutter et al. 1959).

The comparison of individual values for U_U/P_U in patients with prerenal azotaemia and with acute tubular necrosis shows a great deal of overlap. Values less than 3, however, are virtually never found in prerenal azotaemia, values greater than 8 are relatively uncommon in acute tubular necrosis whether oliguric or non--oliguric (Bastl et al. 1980).

The ratio BUN/P_{cr} is increased in prerenal azotaemia. In cases with urinary tract obstruction the BUN/P_{cr} ratio can be increased since C_U is more depressed than C_{cr} because of increased urea diffusion and because the distal urine flow slows down. Thus a high BUN/P_{cr} ratio in a patient who is not hypercatabolic suggests either prerenal or postrenal azotaemia (Bastl et al. 1980).

In patients with **chronic renal failure**, the measurement of C_U can help in the prediction of the effect of low protein intake on P_U (on the basis of equation (3) or the nomogram).

Laboratory methods

Plasma and urine urea levels are best determined by autoanalyzer techniques (Marsh et al. 1965).

REFERENCES

Addis, T.: The ratio between the urea content of the urine and of the blood after the administration of large quantities of urea. An approximate index of the quantity of actively functioning kidney tissue. J. Urol. *1*: 263, 1917

Addis, T.: The renal lesion in Bright's disease. J. Am. med. Assoc. *85*: 163, 1928

Ambard, L.: Physiologie normale et pathologique des reins. Paris, Masson, 1931

Ambard, L., Weill, A.: Les lois numeriques de la sécrétion rénale de l'urée et du chlorure de sodium. J. Physiol. Path. gén. *14*: 753, 1912

Bergström, J., Fürst, P., Josephson, B., Norée, L. O.: Factors affecting the nitrogen balance in chronic uremic patients receiving essential aminoacids intravenously or by mouth. Nutr. Metabol. *14* suppl.: 162, 1972

Bastl, C. P., Rudnick, M. R., Narins, R. G.: Diagnostic approaches to acute renal failure. (Eds. B. M. Brenner and J. H. Stein) Edinburgh Churchill Livingstone 1980

Bright, R.: Reports of medical cases selected with a view of illustrating the symptoms and cure of disease by reference to morbid anatomy. London, Longman, Rees, Orne, Brown and Green 1827

Bright, R.: Cases and observations illustrative of renal disease accompanied with the secretion of albuninous urine. Guy's Hosp. Rep. *1*: 338, 1836

Bull, G. M., Jokes, A. M., Lowe, K. G.: Renal function studies in acute tubular necrosis. Clin. Sci. *9*: 379, 1950

Chasis, H., Smith, H. W.: The excretion of urea in normal man and in subjects with glomerulo-nephritis. J. clin. Invest. *17*: 347, 1938

Cohen, B. D.: Aberrations of the urea cycle in uremia. In: Uremia (ed. R. Kluthe et al.) Stuttgart, Thieme, 1972, 1–7

Giordano, C.: Use of exogenous and endogenous urea for protein synthesis in normal and uremic subjects. J. lab. clin. Med, *62*: 231, 1963

Giordano, C., Pascale, D., Balestrieri, C., Cittadini, D. Crescenai, A.: Incorporation of urea 15-N in amino-acids of patients with chronic renal failure on low nitrogen diet. Am. J. clin. Nutr. *24*: 394, 1968

Giovannetti, S., Maggiore, Q.: A low-nitrogen diet with proteins of high biological value for severe chronic uraemia. Lancet *1*: 1000, 1964

Goaverts, P.: The ratio of creatinine clearance to urea clearance in toxic nephropathies. Festschrift for Thomas Addis Standford M. Bull. *6*: 71, 1948

Hilger, H. H., Klümper, J. D., Ullrich, K. J.: Wasserrückresorption und Ionentransport durch die Sammelrohrzellen der Saugetierniere. Pflüger's Arch. ges. Physiol. *267*: 218, 1958

Kluthe, R., Quirin, H., Jezdinsky, H. J.: Six years, experience with a special low-protein diet. In: Uremia (ed. R. Kluthe et al.) Stuttgart, Thieme 1972, 250—256

Lassiter, W. E., Gottschalk, C. W., Mylle, M.: Micropuncture study of net transtubular movement of water and urea in nondiuretic mammalian kidney. Am. J. Physiol. *200*: 214, 1961.

Lewis, W. H. Jr., Alving, A. S.: Changes with age in the renal function in adult men I. Clearance of urea, II. Amount of urea nitrogen in the blood, III. Concentrating ability of the kidneys. Am. J. Physiol. *123*: 500, 1938

Luke, R. G., Briggs, J. D., Allison, M. E. M., Kennedy, A. C.: Factors determining response to mannitol in acute renal failure. Am. J. med. Sci. *259*: 168, 1970

Marsch, W. H., Fingerhut, B., Miller, H.: Automated and manual direct methods for the determination of blood urea. Clin. Chem. *11*: 624, 1965

Möller, E., McIntosh, J. R., Van Slyke, D. D.: Studies of urea excretion II. Relationship between urine volume and rate of urea excretion by normal adults. J. clin. Invest. *6*: 927, 1929

Perlmutter, M., Grossman, S. L., Rothenberg, S., Doblan, G.: Urine-serum urea nitrogen ratio: simple test of renal function in acute azotemia and oliguria. J. Am. med. Assoc. *170*: 1533, 1959

Shannon, J. A.: The urea reabsorption and excretion of urea under conditions of extreme diuresis. Am. J. Physiol. *123*: 182, 1938

Strauss, H.: Die Nephritiden. Abriss ihrer Diagnostik und Therapie auf Grund der neueren Forschungsergebnisse. Wien, Urban und Schwarzenberg 1916

Ullrich, J. K., Jarausch, K. H.: Untersuchungen zum Problem der Harnkonzentrierung und Harnverdünnung. Pflüger's Arch. ges. Physiol. *267*: 207, 1956

RENAL PLASMA AND BLOOD FLOW

Measurement of renal plasma and blood flows do not belong to the category of routine investigatory methods. In indicated cases these parameters can be measured using the "classical" method [renal clearance of paraaminohippuric acid(PAH)] or radionuclide methods.

Radionuclide diagnostic methods are applicable in the measurement of renal blood flow since some compounds (^{131}I-Hippuran) are excreted by the same mechanism as PAH, and its handling can be followed by external counting techniques.

From the clinical point of view it is very important that relative renal blood flow can be estimated noninvasively using a scintillation camera and initial transit of tracers through the kidney.

Measurement of separate kidney function is important in the differential diagnosis of arterial hypertension and in cases where surgical reduction of renal parenchyma is considered. Another useful area of the investigation of renal blood flow is the evaluation of renal transplant.

At present there are a number of methods to measure RBF which can be used clinically. There have also been attempts to work out methods to evaluate RBF in different portions of the renal parenchyma (i.e. cortical and medullary flows) but it is doubtful whether these methods have any degree of accuracy in man.

PHYSIOLOGY AND PATHOPHYSIOLOGY

Renal blood flow is a large proportion of cardiac output. In normal adults at rest, both kidneys have a blood flow of 1200 ml/min, i.e. 20–25% of cardiac output. This high blood flow is not, evidently, necessary to supply O_2 to the organ, since the renal A-V O_2 difference is only about 1.7 ml O_2/100 ml blood. This value is significantly smaller than A-V differences in general (arterial blood — mixed venous blood) which vary about 4–6 ml O_2/100 ml blood. Despite the small renal A-V O_2 difference, the total uptake of O_2 by the kidney (because of the high blood flow) is also large. It is estimated that under resting conditions, the kidneys take 8% of the total body O_2 uptake.

It is striking that the renal A-V O_2 difference is relatively constant even with changes in RBF. As a result of this, renal O_2 utilization changes more or less as a function of RBF. The latter (RBF) is regulated by the tone of the renal arterioles, which determines the lumen size of the renal vascular resistance. Interplay of tone between the afferent and efferent arterioles maintains a sufficiently high intraglomerular pressure so that ultrafiltration continues. At present it would appear that the afferent arteriolar tone regulates RBF, whereas efferent arteriolar tone changes

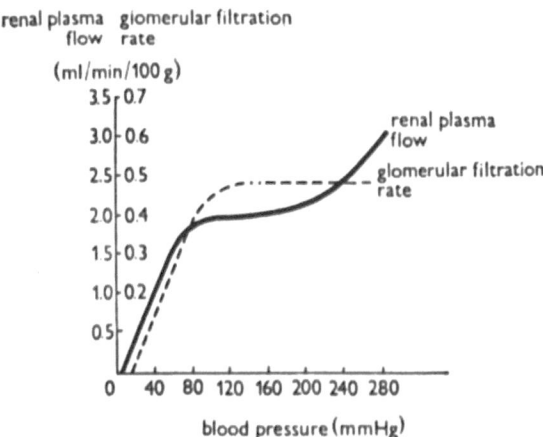

Fig. 22: Influence of changes in renal arterial pressure on renal plasma flow andglomerular filtration rate (Shipley and Study 1951).

to maintain glomerular filtration pressure with respect to changes in afferent arteriolar tone. As was discussed in the chapter on glomerular filtration, it is not clear whether in man this interplay enables the establishment of a pressure equilibrium in the glomerulus (with respect to the level of oncotic pressure).

Measurements of pressure in separate parts of the renal vascular bed have shown that the largest pressure gradient is determined by the afferent-efferent arteriolar gradient. The pressure drop over the course of the glomerular capillaries is minimal, and also in the peritubular capillaries there are few pressure changes.

Values of RBF are maintained relatively constant over a large range of values of arterial BP (from 80 to 180 torr) (Fig. 22). This effect is called renal blood flow autoregulation, since it can be demonstrated in denervated and isolated organs (Forster and Maes 1947; Selkurt, 1949; Shipley and Stady, 1951). Thanks to autoregulation of RBF, GFR can also be maintained relatively constant over the same large range of BP values (Forster and Maes, 1947; Selkurt et al. 1949; Gomez, 1951; Shipley and Stady 1951; Smith 1951; Thurau, 1964; Robertson et al. 1972).

The mechanism of autoregulation of RBF is not yet clear. RBF values can be characterized by their relation to mean arterial pressure values ($\overline{AP}$) and renal vascular resistance (RVR) by the following equation:

$$RVR = \frac{\bar{AP}}{RBF} \tag{1}$$

This equation can be altered thus:

$$RBF = \frac{\bar{AP}}{RVR}$$

This equation shows that RBF does not change in relation to $\bar{AP}$ if changes in the latter are associated with proportional changes in RViR

At present it would appear that RVR is determined by the renal arterioles. The view that changes in RVR were a function of changes in blood viscosity as a result of cell separation (Pappenheimer and Kinter 1956; Winton 1959) has been abandoned.

The question remains as to how the tone of the renal arterioles changes as a function of changes in BP. According to the so-called "myogenic hypothesis" (which is related to the original Bayliss observation) the tone of the vessel wall reacts directly to distension by an increase in contractile tone. This view is supported by the observation that infusion of papaverine, procaine and CN, in doses capable of paralysing muscle contraction, also results in a disappearance of autoregulation. According to the so-called "juxtaglomerular hypothesis" (Thurau 1966) changes in arteriolar tone in the kidney are associated with changes in the local production of renin and angiotensin-II. (A-II) According to this theory, a transient increase in GFR, results in an increased delivery of Na to the macula densa (at the start of the distal segment of the nephron). Macula densa cells are sensitive to changes in Na concentration in the tubular lumen and this results in an increased production of renin from the juxtamedullary cells and an increased local formation of A-II, which increases the arteriolar tone and decreases GFR and the input of Na to the macula densa. The original state is thus restored. Some reports suggest, however, that autoregulation is not related to changes in the production of renin (Bailie et al. 1972; Schmid 1972). Micropuncture studies (Robertson et al. 1972) have analyzed the problem of autoregulation of RBF as changes in afferent and efferent vascular resistances and so-called "pressure equilibrium". So far, however, these findings have not found a clinical application.

RBF in different parts of the kidney varies. Of the total flow, 90% flows through the cortex and 10% through the medulla. Medullary BF (vasa recta) plays an important role in the medullary counter-current system.

The degree of the medullary osmotic gradient decreases with increasing BF in the medulla (cf.p. 112). Renal vessels are richly supplied with sympathetic nerve fibres from segments T4-L4. These fibres are considered to be vasoconstrictor. According to Smith (1951) in healthy subjects at rest in a reclining position and at normal room temperature, these fibres have a minimal conducting activity, or even none at all. Vasoconstrictor tone significantly increases during body activity, cold, a change to the vertical position and various psychogenic stimuli. If the stimulus is moderate, there is a decrease in RBF, but GFR does not change because the increase in FF can compensate the decrease in plasma flow. If the stimulus is intense, the decrease in RBF is marked (from 1200 ml/min to 200 ml/min) and GFR is also decreased, despite the fact that FF is high. Filtration fraction (FF) (GFR:RPF) depends on the tone of the renal arterioles and glomerular capillary permeability. An increase in arteriolar resistance is associated with an increase in FF, but one cannot on the basis of FF values estimate changes in efferent arteriolar resistance.

Renal haemodynamics is significantly affected also by humoral factors. Adrenaline and nor-adrenaline constrict renal vessels. Low doses decrease RBF with no change in GFR. Administration of larger doses results in a decrease in GFR.

Vasopressin affects renal haemodynamics only in "pharmacological" doses, decreasing RBF and GFR. Serotonin, in pharmacological doses, also decreases RBF and GFR. Vasopressin in "physiological" doses suppresses the renal production of renin.

Renin and angiotensin (A-II) in moderate doses only decrease RBF with no change in GFR. Administration of larger doses results in a decrease in GFR. A-II also causes vasopressin release.

Some substances can increase RBF. It is an old experimental experience that RBF increases after administration of pyrogens (Smith 1951). This reaction is not a function of increased body temperature, since it occurs even if the temperature increase is limited by administration of antipyrine. Pyrogenic hyperaemia also occurs in the denervated kidney. GFR values do not increase under these conditions, so that FF decreases. PGE_1 administration will also increase RBF.

Control of RBF is the result of the action of a number of regulatory systems. It is probable that renin and A-II play a negative feedback role inside the kidney (local A-II production by stimulation of the macula densa) and in the organism in general as a result of changes in systemic BP and the volume of ECF.

Renin is a proteolytic enzyme which converts alpha-2 globulins to free up a decapeptide, A-I. A "converting enzyme" then forms A-II by cleaving off 2 residues. The A-II octapeptide is:
Asp-Arg-Val-Tyr-Ile-His-Pro-Phe.

A-II has a potent effect on arteriolar tone.

As explained on p. 166, A-II changes further to A-III (by loss of the N-terminal residue) which stimulates the cells of the zona glomerulosa of the adrenals to produce aldosterone. Increased aldosterone production then significantly influences tubular transport of Na and K.

The kidneys, however, also have an instrinsic mechanism to increase RBF.

They contain an enzyme which converts A-II to inactive fragments (angiotensinase) and produce prostaglandins in the renal medulla, some of which (PGE_1) increase RBF.

Some pathological processes in the kidney can affect the juxta-glomerular apparatus and decrease the production of renin and aldosterone (hyporeninaemic hypoaldersteronism, p. 166).

RBF can decrease under pathological conditions, mainly as a result of:
1) an increase in arteriolar resistence (without demonstrable anatomical damage)
2) reduction of the vascular bed as a result of obliteration of renal vessels and substitution by connective tissue. Finally, both of these possibilities can be coexistent. Investigation of renal function can assist in the differential diagnosis of the degree to which each of the above possibilities plays a role in the total reduction of flow.

METHODS OF INVESTIGATION

Principles of clinical measurement of renal plasma flow (RPF) and blood flow (RBF)

Methods based upon the Fick or Stewart-Hamilton principles can be used to measure RBF, in analogy to measurement of blood flow through other organs.

1. On the basis of the *Fick principle*, to measure RPF and RBF, we should know the amount of a marker substance excreted per unit time into the urine, and also know the renal A-V difference of the substance.

A further condition is that the marker substance must not be accumulated in the organ, or metabolized or produced there.

If the kidneys excrete per min U_xV of substance x, its concentration in arterial plasma is P_A and in the renal venous plasma is P_{RV}, then according to the Fick principle:

$$RPF(P_A - P_{RV}) = U_xV \qquad (2)$$

From equation (2) it would appear that:

$$RPF = \frac{U_xV}{P_A - P_{RV}} \qquad (3)$$

RBF is calculated on the basis of RPF and the haematocrit (Hct) value:

$$RBF = \frac{RPF}{(1 - Hct)} \qquad (4)$$

In principle, it is possible to measure RPF with any marker substance which is excreted by the kidneys, the A-V difference for which is sufficiently large.

Equation (3) shows that measurement of RPF would be simplified if it were not necessary to measure P_{RV}, which requires catheterization of a renal vein. This can be accomplished if the excretion of x is so intense that P_{RV} approaches nil. In such a case:

$$RPF = \frac{U_x V}{P_A} \qquad (5)$$

This equation is at the same time the classical clearance one.

Para-aminohippuric acid (PAH) satisfies these conditions under conditions of low plasma concentrations (Smith 1940, 1951).

It is necessary, if such a substance x is to be so effectively excreted, for its excretion to involve both glomerular filtration and tubular secretion. The level of the latter process must be such that the tubules "clean out" the plasma in the post--glomerular flow in the peri-tubular capillaries.

For the post-glomerular blood to be completely cleansed of PAH, the following conditions are necessary:

a) the post-glomerular blood must come into contact with tubular segments which can secrete PAH and

b) the intensity of the tubular transport process must be sufficient that with the given plasma concentration, all PAH in the post-glomerular blood must be transported into the tubular lumen.

It is known from renal anatomy that cortical glomeruli break down into a peritubular capillary network. On the other hand, efferent arterioles of juxta-medullary glomeruli turn into the vasa recta. This means that under so-called physiological conditions, part of the blood flow escapes contact with secreting segments of the tubules. In the case of PAH, secretion occurs in the proximal tubule.

In addition, part of the blood flow escapes "cleansing" if it supplies inactive renal elements, such as the capsule.

For these reasons, even under physiological conditions, the PAH concentration in RV plasma is not nil. According to Smith's suggestion, one would consider the clearance of PAH at low plasma concentrations as the "effective RPF" (ERPF) — i.e. the plasma flow which comes into contact with secreting tubular cells.

C_{PAH} can be equal to ERPF under those conditions in which the transport function of the tubules is so large that all peri-tubular plasma is cleared. A further condition is that substance x, once secreted, is not then reabsorbed. This occurs only when plasma concentrations are low. This condition is a function of the investigational technique. On the other hand, the secretory capacity of the tubules can be deranged by pathology so that secretion rates fall below a critical value.

From the above it would appear that measurement of ERPF without catheterizing the renal vein can only be valid under certain circumstances. If one wishes to have precise measurements in the presence of renal pathology, one should obtain renal venous samples. The relation between P_A and P_{RV} can usually be expressed as extraction (E):

$$E = \frac{P_A - P_{RV}}{P_A} \qquad (6)$$

E_{PAH} under normal conditions varies about 90%. With regard to equation (6), it is possible to re-arrange equation (3) to calculate RPF on the basis of PAH as follows:

$$RPF = \frac{C_{PAH}}{E_{PAH}} \tag{7}$$

If RPF is measured with a marker substance, the extraction of which is not large (e.g. inulin) and the urine flow rate is high, it is necessary to use the Fick principle in a corrected form (Wolf 1941). This correction involves taking into account the difference in plasma volume flowing into the kidney (RPF_A) and out of the kidneys (RPF_V). Between these parameters is the relation:

$$RPF_V = RPF_A - V \tag{8}$$

If there is no accumulation, metabolism or neogenesis of the marker substance, the following will be true:

$$RPF_A P_A = U_x V + (RPF_A - V) P_{RV} \tag{9}$$

After re-arrangement, we can derive:

$$RPF_A = \frac{V(U_x - P_{RV})}{(P_A - P_{RV})} \tag{10}$$

Finally we must stress that the condition of nonaccumulation of x in the kidneys is not valid for PAH in acute oliguric states (Balint 1961; 1963). In the latter case it is impossible to determine RPF on the basis of PAH even if the A-V difference is measured directly.

2. Measurement of RBF on the basis of inert gases.

As an example we can use a method based upon N_2O. After a period of inhalation of a mixture of N_2O and O_2, renal tissue is saturated. This saturation is manifested by a disappearance of the A-V difference accross the kidney for this gas. The value of the A-V difference of N_2O change during inhalation. At first the arterial concentration is higher than in the vein to the moment of saturation. When inhalation is stopped, venous concentrations are higher than arterial (Fig. 23).

The sum of all A-V differences of N_2O from the start of inhalation up to saturation of the kidney parenchyma is given by the integral:

$$\int_0^t (P_A - P_{RV}) \, dt.$$

Theoretically, one can use for this calculation area values during the rising or declining phases of the concentration curves. Preference is given to values determined during the rising phase.

The amount of N_2O accumulated in a unit weight of parenchyma (usually, 100 g) can be determined after achieving saturation on the basis of the concentration of N_2O in the blood (P) and knowledge of the so-called partition coefficient (K) which gives the relation between the concentrations of gas in tissue and blood. The equation for calculating flow/100 g tissue is:

$$\text{RBF (ml/100 g tissue)} = \frac{K \times P \times 100}{\int_0^t (P_A - P_{RV})\, dt} \tag{11}$$

From the above it is clear that to determine RBF (ml/100 g tissue weight) by this method we must catheterize the renal vein and we need repeated samples of arterial blood. On the other hand, no urine collection is necessary.

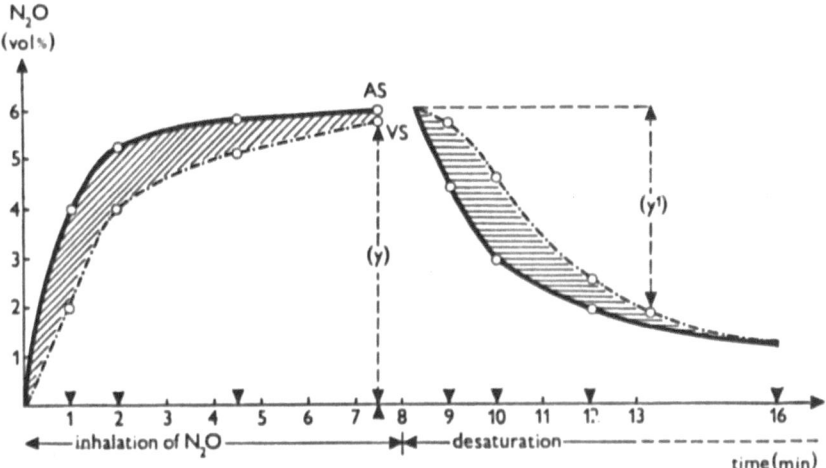

Fig. 23: Time-course of concentration of N_2O in the arterial blood (AS) and renal venous blood (VS) under conditions of inhalation of N_2O (Galnier and Suc 1963).

Renner et al. (1963) carried out a critical analysis of the inert gas methods of determining blood flow and came to the conclusion that they are not precise enough. Large errors occur in calculating the area under the arterial and venous concentration curves. Concentration and achievement of saturation equilibrium are difficult.

3. RBF and RPF in a single kidney on the basis of indicator dilution.

If we inject rapidly into the renal artery a known amount (D) of a marker substance which is neither excreted by the kidney nor is it accumulated or formed by the kidney, and which does not leave the vascular compartment, the same amount of substance must come out of the renal vein.

The concentration of this substance in venous plasma first increases, then decreases. The amount of the substance which in infinitely short time intervals (dt) leaves through the renal vein is given by RPF × Pdt. The integral of those values delimited by the appearance time in the renal plasma and the disappearance time from the same site is equal to the injected quantity D. Therefore:

$$RBF = \text{const } \frac{D}{\int_0^t Pdt} \qquad (12)$$

The value of the constant is given by the characteristics of the recording system. This principle has been used to measure RBF by Reubi et al. (1962, 1964). Both renal artery and vein must be catheterized. The catheter position must be visualized by X-ray. The indicator used was Indocyanine green. Changes in dye concentration in the venous blood are recorded graphically.

This method is not simple and is not suited for routine clinical testing.

Shaldon et al. (1962) used, instead of the bolus technique, the A-V differences measured during continuous infusion. A number of errors can be met with and this method is also not suited for normal clinical measurements.

Of all of the above methods, the original method of Smith et al. (1943) seems to be the most suitable, based upon C_{PAH}. The procedure is described in detail.

MEASUREMENT OF C_{PAH}

The test is carried out in the AM in a separate, quiet room. The patient is either without breakfast or a small breakfast is allowed (tea and bread). The subject should be informed about the technique and the reasons for using it, to exclude undesired emotional side-effects which can influence the results.

The test is carried out in a balanced state of plasma PAH concentration. The bladder is emptied by spontaneous voiding (we catheterize only in special cases). If the test is carried out with a reasonably high urine flow rate with sufficiently long collection periods, spontaneous voiding introduces only an insignificant error. (For details, cf.p. 14).

About 1 hour before the test, the subject drinks about 1 liter of water. ERPF measurement requires low plasma concentration values. These balanced state concentrations should range from 2 to 3 mg%, should not exceed 5 mg% or go below 1 mg%.

First, a bolus load of 8 mg/kg PAH is given i.v. (Smith 1956). Before this bolus a blank blood sample is taken. The last pre-test, pre-load urine is also used as a blank. After the bolus load, an i.v. infusion of PAH is started such that the amount given = the rate of urinary PAH loss. One can only guess from experience at the maintenance dosage. To assist this estimate, we can use C_{cr} values determined in the days before the PAH test. Obviously, C_{cr} and C_{PAH} need not decrease at the same rate in a disease process (as a result of changes in FF) but knowledge of GFR is still useful. If GFR is 50% of normal, C_{PAH} should be in the neighbourhood of 300 ml/min. If P_{PAH} remains at about 2 mg%, each min requires in the infusion: $300 \times 0.02 = 6$ mg PAH.

The required amount of the Na salt of PAH is dissolved in normal saline and we infuse at the calculated rate. The infusion set is the ordinary type or, better, use an infusion pump. The concentration of PAH in the infusion will be determined by the infusion rate. If the infusion rate is, e.g., 2 ml/min, and if we have to give 6 mg PAH/min, then the PAH infusate has to contain a concentration of 300 mg% in concentration.

After 1 hour one can assume that plasma PAH levels are in a balanced state, along with all other subdivisions of its distribution space, and urine collection can start. The time is recorded precisely. The subject is in a reclining position. Since the subject must spontaneously void during the infusion, the infusion tube must be long enough. A flexible i.v. cannula is of advantage. If the subject is correctly instructed, voiding is not difficult.

When spontaneous voiding is used, we usually measure one or two urine collection periods. With a urine flow rate above 3 ml/min, 60-min collection periods suffice.

Blood samples from the contralateral antecubital vein are collected at the start, in the middle and at the end of each urine collection period. Samples of blood are collected in heparinized tubes and immediately centrifuged (because PAH penetrates erythrocytes).

The collection period is ended by spontaneous urine voiding and the time is precisely recorded. There is no harm done if the period is longer, but time must be precisely measured to calculate the urine flow rate.

A sample test is covered by the following protocol:

Healthy male, 40 years of age, wt 78 kg,

$C_{cr} = 110$ ml/min.

We estimate from the GFR that C_{PAH} should be normal.

Loading dose $= 78 \times 8 = 624$ mg.

Maintenance dose $= 600 \times 0.02 = 12$ mg/min.

Urine by spontaneous voiding.

7 : 00 AM, drunk one liter water

8 : 00 AM, voiding. Urine sample (U_0) for blank.

8 : 05 AM, blood sample (B_0), as a blank control.

Immediately give bolus loading dose and the maintenance infusion is connected.

9 : 05 — spontaneous voiding, start urine collection period.

9 : 10 — contralateral antecubital vein used to collect B_1

9 : 30 — contralateral antecubital vein used to collect B_2

10 : 00 — contralateal antecubital vein used to collect B_3

10 : 05 — urine collected, investigation terminated

Volume of urine (V) measured precisely.

Plasma PAH concentrations suggest whether a balanced state existed or not. If separate plasma PAH values do no differ significantly, we calculate a mean concentration. If a balanced state was not achieved, we calculate the area-under-the-curve of the PAH plasma concentrations on the basis of instructions on p. 17.

If a balanced state of plasma PAH concentration was established, clearance values are calculated on the basis of the equation:

$$C_{PAH} = \frac{U_{PAH}V \ (mg/min)}{P_{PAH} \ (mg/ml)} \tag{13}$$

If it was necessary to integrate the curve of plasma PAH concentrations (AUC) we use the equation:

$$C_{PAH} = \frac{U_{PAH}V \ (mg \ per \ collection \ period)}{AUC \ (mg \ min/ml)} \tag{14}$$

The resulting value is then calculated per 1.73 m³ surface area. If the clearance measurement is carried out under the conditions of bladder catheterization, the procedure is the same except that we carry out three urinary collection periods of 10–20 min in duration. Each collection period is terminated by a washout of the bladder with 20 ml of normal saline (warmed to body temperature) and injection of 60 ml air.

Blood samples are taken in the middle of each urine collection period. The time of sampling and of termination of the collection periods are precisely recorded. Determination of the plasma concentration of PAH gives us values to graph on semi-log graph paper vs time, separate points are joined and for each collection period we search out that plasma concentration which precedes by 2 min the midpoint of the urine collection period (cf. p. 18). On the basis of the urinary and plasma concentration values, we calculate the PAH clearance by the classical equation.

Normal C_{PAH} values in healthy controls (adults) under baseline conditions (physical and psychological rest), on a normal diet over the preceding days, and in the AM, give us, according to Smith (1956):

males   654 ± 163 ml/min/1.73 m²
females 592 ± 153 ml/min/1.73 m²

C_{PAH} is affected by a number of factors, detailed on p. 71.

RENAL EXTRACTION OF PAH (E_{PAH}).

Measurement of E_{PAH} requires renal venous catheterization and sampling of arterial blood. We use catheters with a bent end which are introduced into the renal vein through the femoral vein with the aid of a trocar. The catheter position is controlled by X-ray. Sampling of blood through the catheter takes caution. Forced sampling can cause a reflux of blood from the inf. vena cava into the renal vein.

Between blood samplings it is necessary that the catheter be filled with normal saline, so that no coagulation will occur in the lumen. When sampling, the luminal contents of the catheter must be removed to allow for the saline dead space. Arterial blood samples are usually taken from the femoral artery. Both A and V samples must be taken simultaneously.

Measurement of E_{PAH} is carried out under conditions of a balanced state of PAH plasma concentration (between 2 and 3 mg %). On the basis of PAH concentration in arterial plasma (P_A) and in renal venous blood (P_{RV}) we can calculate the value E_{PAH} by equation (6).

Under normal conditions E_{PAH} is 0.925 (0.875–1000) (Bradley et al. 1947). On the basis of this value we can calculate RPF by equation (7).

Average RPF calculated from E_{PAH} in healthy adult males is 720 ml/min. 1.73 m² and in women 660 ml/min/1.73 m². Under pathological conditions, E_{PAH} can be significantly decreased.

CALCULATION OF THE RENAL VASCULAR RESISTANCE

The renal vascular bed has, as with all other vascular beds, a certain degree of flow resistance. The tone of the afferent and efferent arterioles plays an important role in this. Constriction decreases the lumen and resistance increases. According to Poiseuille's law, the rate of flow (Q) is determined as follows:

$$Q = \frac{\pi r^4 \, \Delta P}{8 \eta l} \tag{15}$$

where r = lumen radius, ΔP = pressure drop, η = viscosity and l = length of the flow path.
From equation (15) it would appear that:

$$\frac{\Delta P}{Q} = \frac{8 \eta l}{\pi r^4} \tag{16}$$

The ratio $\Delta P/RBF$ represents the total renal vascular resistance (RVR). Equation (16) shows that the lumen radius (r) is of critical importance. Small changes are raised to the fourth power in effect. This explains why RVR is given mainly by changes in the arteriolar lumina. The flow path (l) does not change, ΔP is based upon levels of renal artery pressure = aortic pressure, but for clinical purposes this can be equated to pressure in the femoral artery.

As an acceptable compromise one can use mean aortic pressure calculated from systolic pressure (P_s) and diastolic pressure (P_d) measured by the normal Korotkoff method. Between these parameters exists the following relation:

$$\overline{AP} = P_d + 1/3(P_s - P_d) \tag{17}$$

Values of renal venous pressure are usually very small compared to $\overline{AP}$, ranging about 10 torr (Smith, 1951). For routine clinical measurement, this value can be ignored, so that a simplified calculation of RVR is as follows:

$$RVR = 1328 \, \frac{\overline{AP}}{RBF} \tag{18}$$

where $\overline{AP}$ is given in torr, RBF in ml/s and, the coefficient 1328 is associated with the transformation of these units into dyn.cm.s.$^{-5}$. If, for example, we find in a subject an arterial BP of 130/80 and RBF = 1200 ml/min = 20 ml/s, the RVR: $1328 \times 97/20 = 6440$ dyn.s.cm^{-5}.

Micropuncture studies enable the measurement separately of the afferent and efferent arteriolar resistances. Such measurements are, of course, not applicable to patients. Indirect calculations of the same are compromised by very risky assumptions (Lamport 1943, Gomez 1951, Schück and Chytil 1955). On the basis of the findings of Goldring et al. (1940) and Bolomey et al. (1949) it would appear that in healthy adult subjects, RVR ranges between 5000 and 7000 dyn.s.cm^{-5}.

FILTRATION FRACTION (FF)

This value gives the ratio between GFR and RPF.

$$FF = \frac{GFR}{RPF} \tag{17}$$

This value is usually given as a percentage. If GFR is measured as C_{in} and RPF = $= C_{PAH}$, then:

$$FF = \frac{C_{in}}{C_{PAH}} \tag{18}$$

FF tells us what fraction of RPF is filtered at the glomerulus. Under normal conditions in healthy adult subjects, FF values are as follows (Smith 1956):
    males 19.2 ± 3.5
    females 19.4 ± 3.9
FF depends upon the effective filtration pressure and the permeability of the glomerular capillaries for water.

With constriction of the renal arterioles, FF increases. Under pathological conditions, when E_{PAH} is decreased and C_{PAH} is not a measure of RPF, the calculated increase in FF is meaningless.

In pathological states, changes in FF can be interpreted as an increase in renal arteriolar resistance or an increase in glomerular capillary permeability.

Interpretation of results

Values of RBF are related to such factors as: sex, age, bodily proportions, body position, ambient temperature, metabolic state, state of hydration and the emotional balance of the subject, etc. These factors will be discussed separately below.

Age

In the first postnatal days (to age 10 days) ERPF values vary about 70 ml/min. This value shows great scatter and depends upon the state of hydration. West et al. (1948) showed that at age about one year, values are attained which, expressed per 1.73 m², correspond to adult values. From age 20 years, C_{PAH} decreases in relation to age. According to Watkin and Schock (1955) this age relation can be expressed as follows:

$$C_{PAH} = 820 - 6.75 \times \text{age (years)} \tag{19}$$

Brod (1973) gives the following values:

age	C_{PAH}(ml/min/1.73 m²)
to 20	638.2 ± 195.2
20–39	592.3 ± 122.7
40–60	493.7 ± 134.8

Diurnal rhythm

According to the findings of Sirota et al. (1950) the diurnal variation in C_{PAH} is minimal; Brod (1973) reports a decrease in C_{PAH} in healthy adults in the night hours.

The diet

In dog experiments it has been shown that the protein content of the diet influences RBF. On a high protein diet RBF in dogs can double (Moustgard 1948). The effect of dietary protein changes in man is far smaller. An increase of 18% has been described after giving a diet containing 220 g protein/day for one week (White and Rolf 1948). A low protein intake (27 g/day) for 10–15 days was associated with a decrease in RBF.

Chasis et al. (1950) did not observe changes in RBF in subjects maintained on the so-called rice diet to which 10 g NaCl was added. However, intake of a rice-diet without NaCl was associated with a tendency to decrease RBF.

Mertz (1976) stresses maintenance of a dietary regime while investigating renal haemodynamics and has reported significant differences related to NaCl intake and state of hydration.

A significant change in RBF occurs in all states related to a decrease in the volume of the ECF.

Physical activity

With physical activity, RBF decreases. It has, for example, been observed that running at full speed for 400 m produces a decrease in RBF of about 61 % (Barclay et al. 1948). Chapman et al. (1948) showed that walking at a rate of 4.8 km/h (at 5°C) for 32 min decreased RBF to 73% of previous values on an average. Walking at a rate of 5.6 km/h (at 10°C) for 32 min decreased RBF to 63% of control values.

Emotional state

An increase in emotional "tone" decreases RBF and increases FF (Smith 1940). This renal vasoconstriction is clearly conditioned by the adrenergic system, since with phenoxybenzamine blockade this reaction disappears (Brod 1973). A similar effect results from a pain stimulus (Wolf 1943).

Ambient temperature

According to Kaufmann et al. (1964) an increase in ambient temperature decreases RPF. A "cold test" has the same effect (Brod 1973).

Pregnancy

RPF at the start of pregnancy increases, reaching maximum values at the end of the first trimester. According to Bucht et al. (1951) RPF values in pregnant women are about 25% higher than the norm.

The increase in RBF is, however, less than the increase in RPF, because the Hct decreases. The increase in ERPF lasts to the mid-point of the 3rd trimester, after which it gradually decreases to normal values by the end of pregnancy (Sims and Krantz 1958).

After delivery, ERPF further decreases to values about 20% lower than in non--pregnant controls. This decrease takes place over several months, and values then return to normal (Sims and Krantz 1958). Neither lactation nor the menstrual cycle per se have an effect on RPF.

MEASUREMENT OF ERPF ON THE BASIS OF RADIONUCLIDES

For estimation of ERPF, [125]I- or ^{131}I-labelled orthoiodohippurate has been shown to closely parallel p-aminohippurate behaviour. Clearance measurements with radio-active indicators can be made either with traditional urine and blood sampling or far more simply with repetitive blood samples only.

The radionuclide frequently used in nephrology contains ^{131}I the nucleus of which contains four neutrons more than nucleus of the stable iodine [127]I does.

Iodine ^{131}I is instable and spontaneously degenerates to a more stable state with simultaneous emission of electrons and gamma photons with a preponderant energy of 364 KeV. There is also a fairly intensive beta radiation, the half-life is eight days. From the aspect of patient exposure and risk Technetium ^{99m}Tc is more suitable for biological purposes. This radionuclide emits only gamma photons with an energy of 140 KeV and its half-life is six hours.

For measurements of the time-course of radioactivity in the kidneys the following counting techniques are used at present.

1. *Scintillation detector technique*

The scintillation counter is sensitive to gamma photons emanating from the kidneys across the lumbar region. The scintillation detectors are shielded by collimators provided with cylindrical hole in the direction of detection. The record is called a renogram or nephrogram. In the past years attempts have been made to distinguish several phases in the nephrogram; the so-called vascular, secretory and excretory phases. A more detailed analysis of this problem has shown, however, that this approach is not correct.

The scintillation detectors must be localized exactly over the renal regions. Many findings may be interpreted falsely as indicating an asymmetry of renal function affection solely due to an incorrect localization of the detectors. Several procedures exist for achieving the best localization of the detectors over the kidneys. For example the kidney region can be localized by using four small detectors and a preliminary injection of a small dose of ^{125}I-Hippuran.

Another factor significantly influencing the nephrogram curve is the radioactivity emanating from pararenal tissues. This factor can be significantly reduced by simultaneous measurement of the activity of ^{131}I-radioiodinated human serum albumin (RIHSA) which must be injected intravenously before the administration of ^{131}I-Hippuran.

A third detector (the first two placed over the kidneys) is placed over a non--specific region, such as the chest. Counts attributable to RIHSA are recorded from body wall tissues by all 3 detectors. This record enables us to correct the ^{131}I-Hippuran curve, which combines body wall transients and the more prolonged phase of renal parenchymal processing. The former can be cancelled out- the renal component remaining in sharper outline.

2. *Gamma camera techniques*

Gamma camera permits the continuous detection, quantitation and spatial localization of gamma photons. The gamma camera converts gamma photons emanating from the patient into a series of electronic pulses representing the X and Y coordinates where the scintillation occurred in the detector. The image represents the distribution of the radioactivity in the field of view of the camera.

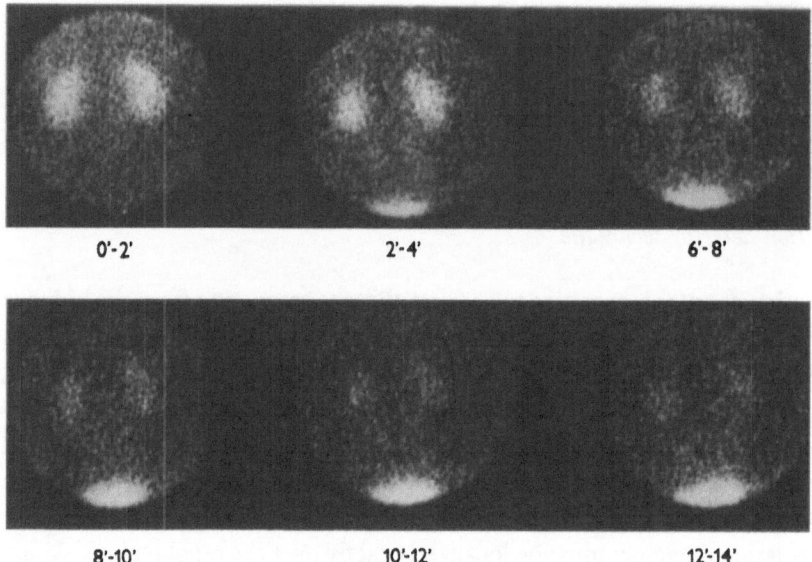

Fig. 24: Scintiphotos of a normal gamma camera dynamic study using ^{131}I-Hippuran. There is symmetrical transit of tracer through both kidneys and its gradual accumulation in the bladder.

This counting technique has the advantage of showing the changes in distribution of activity with time as well as the changes in count rate, but is less sensitive than the scintillation detector. Examples of images of kidneys after ^{131}I-Hippuran administration are shown in Fig. 24.

SLOPE CLEARANCE OF ^{131}I-HIPPURAN

^{131}I-Hippuran after a single bolus injection disappears exponentially so that a semi-log plot of concentration versus time gives us a straight line. The first more rapid phase lasts about 20 min, then a slower phase sets in.

74

The following modifications of slope clearance of ^{131}I-Hippuran are used.

The patient is hydrated by drinking about 0.5 liter of water before the examination. A bolus of ^{131}I-Hippuran is given intravenously and blood is sampled from the contralateral antecubital vein. The time of injection is precisely recorded.

The sampling time depends upon whether we wish to catch the first or only the later exponential phase. If we wish the first phase, we should sample at times 5, 10 and 15 min. The second phase is covered by sampling 20, 30, 50 and 70 min.

Measurement of ^{131}I-Hippuran can be made from plasma or on serum. The values on semi-log graph give a straight line (Fig. 25). Extrapolation of this line down to the ordinate gives the theoretical plasma concentration of ^{131}I-Hippuran at $t = 0$. (P_0)

The graph gives the biological half-life value $(t\ 1/2)$ — time of decrease to 50% of initial value.

On the basis of $t\ 1/2$ we can calculate the elimination constant (K_{elim}) according to the formula:

$$K_{elim} = \frac{0.693}{t\ 1/2} \tag{20}$$

$(0.693 = \ln 2)$

Further, the total plasma clearance of ^{131}I-Hippuran (C_{Hipp}) is calculated as follows:

$$C_{Hipp} = \frac{D}{P_0}\ K_{elim}\ \text{or} \tag{21}$$

$$C_{Hipp} = \frac{D}{P_0} \cdot \frac{0.693}{t\ 1/2} \tag{22}$$

where D is the total injected activity.

If we take into account the first rapid phase, we can proceed in several ways. According to Sapirstein et al. (1955), deviations from the subsequent line in the

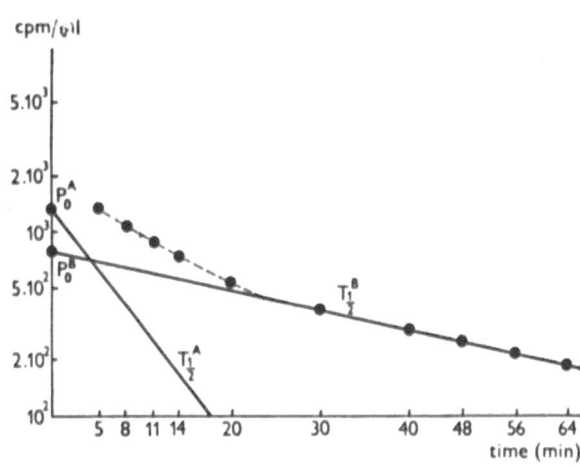

Fig. 25: Graphic evaluation of the clearance of ^{131}I-Hippuran. Analysis of the disappearance curve into two exponentials.

first portion are subtracted from the second line (characterizing a balanced second phase). We measure and construct the second curve and measure t 1/2, and the virtual plasma concentration at t = 0 is derived (Fig. 25).

If the curve of the second phase of balanced disappearance is labelled B, and the first rapid phase A then P_0^A, P_0^B, t $1/2^A$ and t $1/2^B$ are related as follows:

$$C_{Hipp} = \frac{0.693\,D}{P_0^A \times t\,1/2^A + P_0^B \times t\,1/2^B} \tag{23}$$

The second procedure which can be used if the decrease in plasma concentrations is irregular, (so that the two exponentials cannot be distinguished) is to use equation:

$$C_{Hipp} = \frac{D}{AUC} \quad \text{where} \tag{24}$$

AUC = area under the curve of plasma concentrations calculated according to the instructions on p. 17.

Normal values of t 1/2 and C of ^{131}I-Hippuran

On the basis of two probes drawn after 7 and 17 min Rössler (1972) gives the following values:

   t 1/2   men: 10.9 ± 3.5 min
               women: 11.1 ± 2.0 min
   C_{Hipp} men: 684 ml/min/1.73 m^2
               women: 617 ml/min/1.73 m^2

Lerson et al. (1972) on the basis of the points which correspond to 20 and 30 min obtained the following results: t 1/2 19 ± 3.5 min
                         C_{Hipp} 694 ± 108 ml/min

These results correspond to the simplified Hippuran clearance described by Blaufox (1966).

For precise analytical procedure it should be respected that radiolysis of [131]I--Hippuran liberates radioactive iodide which interferes with its application to measurement of renal functions. Lerson et al. (1972) described a purification technique for blood samples that eliminates this at least as a measurement artefact.

Instead of repeated taking off blood samples it is possible to record the activity decrease by means of an external radiation detector placed over the chest. Only one blood sample need be taken at an appropriate time, for example at 13 minutes, and used to calibrate the recorded tissue and blood clearance curve (Britton 1979).

Oberhausen et al. (1972) have recommended for C_{Hipp} measurements with a simple clinical whole-body counter. Using this method no special assumption about a compartment model is necessary. The total body activity is registered at intervals of 30 s. Since the activity already excreted by the kidneys does not belong to this total activity, a lead shield is installed between the kidney-bladder region and the crystal to prevent their detection. From the measured retention curve the differential quotient is numerically calculated at the times when blood samples are taken. In less than half an hour two determinations of clearance rate are performed.

The clearance value is calculated according to the formula:

$$C = \frac{-(dm/dt)}{P_{Hipp}} \qquad (25)$$

where $-(dm/dt)$ = the elimination rate of the marker substance by the kidneys and P_{Hipp} = plasma concentration of Hippuran.

Errors of the slope clearance method

One of the important sources of error in the slope clearance method occurs in obtaining the best straight line from which to estimate P_0 and t 1/2. This error is greater if oedema is present and if renal function is markedly reduced. Another source of the error of the slope method is the fact that under conditions of decreasing plasma concentrations there are significant differences between arterial and peripheral venous plasma concentrations.

The formation of this arterio-venous concentration difference can be explained as follows (Brun et al. 1949, Schück and Buda 1952):
The inferior vena cava takes blood towards the opening of the renal vein. Caval PAH concentration distal to the renal veins is labelled P_V. Under proper low load conditions, the renal vein contains blood with little or no PAH. Mixing of these two flows gives a resulting PAH concentration lower than in the cava distal to the renal veins. The mixed flows get through the heart into the arterial system, where we measure P_A. If cardiac output (CO) mixes these flows, then:

$$(CO - RPF) \times P_V = CO \times P_A \qquad (26)$$

From this equation it would appear that:

$$P_A/P_V = 1 - (RPF/CO) \qquad (27)$$

On the basis of this equation it would appear that the peripheral A-V PAH difference, or the ratio of the A and V concentrations, depends upon the renal fraction of CO.

In general, with various substances (which are not excreted only by the kidneys and the clearance of which does not correspond to RPF) the peripheral A-V difference will be the greater, the more its total clearance approaches CO. Clearly, with substances excreted not just through the kidneys, all known excretion and metabolic mechanisms will have an effect on the peripheral A-V difference.

The existence of a peripheral A-V difference does not play a role in the interpretation of t 1/2, or the elimination constant, because the straight lines of decay of arterial and venous concentrations are parallel.

Radioisotope washout methods

These methods are based upon introduction of a radioactive marker as a bolus in the renal artery, and upon recording the radioactivity by scintillation detector placed over the kidney region. The most widely used isotope is ^{133}Xe. The rate of disappearance depends upon RBF, but also on the volume and density of the kidney and the partition coefficient of the marker substance.

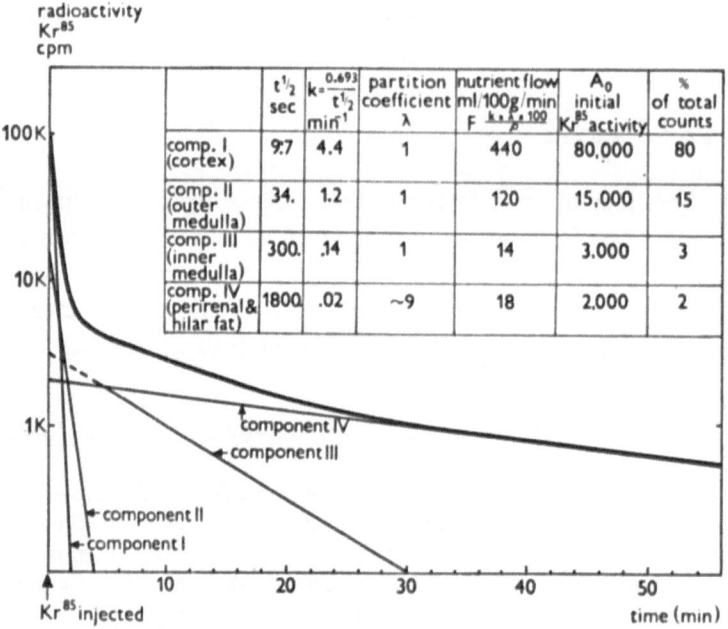

	$t_{1/2}$ sec	$k = \frac{0.693}{t_{1/2}}$ min^{-1}	partition coefficient λ	nutrient flow ml/100g/min $F \frac{k \cdot \lambda \cdot p}{100}$	A_0 initial Kr^{85} activity	% of total counts
comp. I (cortex)	9.7	4.4	1	440	80,000	80
comp. II (outer medulla)	34.	1.2	1	120	15,000	15
comp. III (inner medulla)	300.	.14	1	14	3.000	3
comp. IV (perirenal & hilar fat)	1800	.02	~9	18	2.000	2

Fig. 26: Typical ^{85}Kr disappearance curve (heavy black line) and its analysis into four exponentials. The accompainying table presents derived values from such a curve (Thoburn et al. 1963).

Such washout methods, with either ^{133}Xe or ^{85}Kr, have been used to measure the intrarenal distribution of blood flow (Barger 1966, Thoburn et al. 1963, Ladefoged 1966, Hollenberg et al. 1968, Blaufox et al. 1970). The principle of this method is that the resulting disappearance curve is the sum of several (usually 4) exponentials. Component I (with the fastest disappearance time) = cortical flow, II and III = medullary flow and IV (slowest) = flow in the perihilus fat (Figs. 26 and 27).

Results determined by this method are striking, but the technique must be considered as experimental at present, and not suitable for normal clinical practice.

Fig. 27: ^{133}Xenon disappearance from the kidney of a normal subject. The disappearance curve has been analyzed as the sum of four exponentials (Hollenberg et al. 1970).

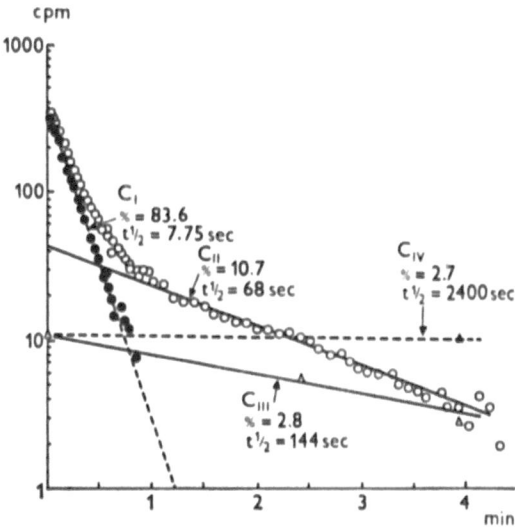

The evaluation of separate ERPF

The empirical interpretation of the renogram by visual inspection can often yield useful information. The relative contribution of each kidney to total renal blood flow can be estimated using the scintillation camera and the initial transit of the tracer through the kidney. The first passage of tracer through the kidney reflects a combination of regional blood flow, blood volume, and extraction of the tracer from the blood into the kidney.

The following method (Brown and Britton 1972, Britton 1979) can be recommended for the estimation of the relative contribution of each kidney to the total function.

The quantity of ^{131}I-Hippuran taken up by a kidney (Q) in a short interval of unit time t, after an intravenous injection, is directly proportional to the supply rate of the substance to the kidney and its extraction (E).

The supply is the product of the mean plasma concentration $\bar{P}$ during time and RPF:

$$Q = \bar{P} \times RPF \times E \qquad (28)$$

As mentioned above, the product $RPF \times E$ represents the effective renal plasma flow (ERPF) and the equation (28) can be simplified as follows:

$$Q = \bar{P} \times ERPF \qquad (29)$$

If Q is measured before any Hippuran has left in the urine, then for the left kidney (L): $Q_L = ERPF_L \times \bar{P}$ and for the right kidney (R): $Q_R = ERPF_R \times \bar{P}$

Since over any small interval of time the mean plasma concentration $\bar{P}$ is the

79

same entering each kidney, then

$$\frac{Q_L}{Q_L + Q_R} = \frac{ERPF_L}{ERPF_L + ERPF_R} = \frac{ERPF_L}{\text{total REPF}} \qquad (30)$$

Measurement of Q_L and Q_R is made after the 90 seconds and before 150 seconds, at which time Hippuran normally starts to leave the kidney. Q_L and Q_R are usually measured at 2 minutes after the injection. The values Q_L and Q_R are measured using a simple scintillation detector or using a gamma camera.

Indications for investigation

Measurements of RBF and RPF are not to be considered as routine clinical tests. Such tests may be of importance in evaluating patients with unilateral renal artery stenosis, in whom the two kidneys must be investigated separately. This investigation usually follows isotopic nephrography.

Measurement of RPF and RBF is usually part of more detailed haemodynamic studies, particularly in patients with arterial hypertension.

Essential hypertension

Hypertensive patients show decreases in RBF and RPF. In the early stages the decrease is related to an increased arterial resistance due to constriction of afferent and efferent arterioles. GFR can be normal at this stage. A characteristic finding is an increased FF.

In more advanced stages, involving the development of vascular nephrosclerosis, anatomical changes in the renal vasculature further contribute to the decrease in ERPF. In such cases, GFR is also decreased.

If the essential hypertension goes into a "malignant" phase, there is a sharp decrease in RBF and GFR, FF is high.

Interpretation of such findings in patients with a depressed GFR should include evaluation of whether E_{PAH} remains normal or not. More precise studies require measurements of RPF on the basis of E_{PAH}.

Nephrogenic arterial hypertension

In patients with chronic renal disease there is a decrease in ERPF as a result of a reduction in the renal vasculature related to the pathology. This situation per se increases renal vascular resistance even if the patient shows no signs of systemic arterial hypertension.

If chronic renal disease is associated with systemic arterial hypertension, both organic and functional changes related to increased renal arteriolar tone summate. In such cases, FF is increased.

Renovascular hypertension

In such cases there may be an asymmetric decrease in ERPF as a result of unilateral renal artery stenosis. On the stenosed side, RVR is determined not only by the tone of the renal arterioles, but also by the antecedent resistance in the renal artery.

There is no simple relation between the decrease in renal artery lumen and the decrease in ERPF, since arteriolar tone also plays a role.

In patients with arterial hypertension of uncertain origin it is of advantage to carry out isotopic nephrography which can reveal renal vascular asymmetry. Detailed isotopic nephrography can give us an estimate of blood flow in each kidney separately.

Evaluation of the asymmetry of pathology of the right and left kidney

Some nephropathies are characterized by a different degree of pathology in the two kidneys. A finding of asymmetric involment of the kidneys may play an important role in the differential diagnosis. Asymmetry in the affection of both kidneys is most frequently caused by chronic pyelonephritis, obstructive uropathies, polycystic kidneys, renal artery stenosis, renal tumors and congenital anomalies. On the other hand, various forms of glomerulonephritis and glomerulopathies affect both kidneys practically to the same degree.

Furthermore, with an established diagnosis of an asymmetric renal affection it is often important to assess the degree of functional impairment of the affected kidney, as well as the functional capacity of the contralateral kidney which may exhibit functional and anatomical compensatory changes. An assessment of these circumstances is important in deciding on possible surgical intervention which would require a reduction of renal parenchyma.

Perfusion of the transplanted kidney

Renal perfusion is evaluated by recording rapid serial images every two or three seconds during the first circulation using ^{99m}Tc-DTPA (diethylenetriaminepentaacetic acid) when the distribution of this radiopharmaceutical is predominantly blood flow dependent.

^{99m}Tc-DTPA is excreted predominantly by glomerular filtration. In moderate and severe rejection there is progressively less renal perfusion. In very severe rejection perfusion is absent and no radiopharmaceutical reaches the bladder. In the differential diagnosis between rejection and acute tubular necrosis comparison of activity curves of ^{99m}Tc-DTPA and ^{131}I-Hippuran is helpful.

Laboratory methods

The easiest method of determining plasma and urine concentrations of PAH continues to be that introduced by Smith et al. (1945).

REFERENCES

Bailie, M. D., Loutzenhiser, R., Moyer, S.: Relation of renal hemodynamics to angiotensin II. in renal hilar lymph of the dog. Am. J. Physiol. *222:* 1075, 1972

Bálint, P.: Le flux sanguin rénal au course de l'hypotensions experimentales. C. R. du I. Congr. Intern. de Nephrologie. Basel Karger, 1961, 207.

Bálint, P.: The reliability of PAH clearance as a measure of renal plasma flow. Proc. Sec. intern. congr. Nephrol. Amsterdam, Excerpta Med. 1963, 84.

Barday, J. A., Cooke, W. T., Kenney, R. A., Marjorie E. Nutt: Effects of water diuresis and exercise on volume compensation of urine. Am. J. Physiol. *148:* 327, 1948

Barger, A. C.: Renal haemodynamics factors in congestive heart failure. Arch. N. Y. Acad. Sci. *139:* 276, 1966

Blaufox, M. D.: Simplified hippuran clearance. Measurement of renal function in man with simplified hippuran clearance. Nephron *3:* 274, 1966

Blaufox, M. D., Fromowitz, A., Gruskin, A., Meng, C. H., Elkin, M.: Validation of the use of Xenon 133 to measure intrarenal distribution of blood flow. Am. J. Physiol. *219:* 440, 1970

Blaufox, M. D., Potchen, E. J., Merill, J. P.: Measurement of effective renal plasma flow in man by external counting methods. J. nucl. Med. *8:* 77, 1967

Bolomey, A. A., Michic, A. J., Michic, C., Breed, E. S., Schreiner, G. E., Lauson, H. D.: Simultaneous measurement of effective renal blood flow and cardiac output in resting normal subjects and patients with essential hypertension. J. clin. Invest. *28:* 10, 1949

Bradley, S. E., Curry, J. J., Bradley, G. P.: Renal extraction of p-aminohippurate in normal subjects and in essential hypertension and chronic diffuse glomerulonephritis. Fed. Proc. *6:* 79, 1947

Britton, K. E.: Radionuclides in the investigation of renal disease. In: Renal disease (Eds. D. Black and N. F. Jones). 4. ed. Oxford, Blackwell Scientific Publ. 1979 pp. 270–304,

Brod, J. The kidney. London, Batterworth, 1973

Brown, N. J. G., Button, K. E.: The theory of renography and analysis of results. In: Radionuclides in nephrology (Eds. M. D. Blaufox and J. L. Funck–Brentano, New York Grune and Stratton, 1972, pp. 315–324).

Goldring, W., Chasis, H., Ranges, A., Smith, H. W.: Relations of effective renal blood flow and glomerular filtration to tubular excretory mass in normal man. J. clin. Invest. *19:* 739, 1940

Gomez, D. M.: Evaluation of renal resistances, with special reference to changes in essential hypertension. J. clin. Invest. *30:* 1143, 1951

Brun, C., Hilden, T., Raaschou, F.: The significance of the difference in systemic arterial and venous plasma concentrations in renal clearance methods. J. clin. Invest. *28:* 144, 1949

Bucht, H.: Studies on renal function in man with special reference to glomerular filtration and renal plasma flow in pregnancy. J. clin. lab. Invest. Suppl. 3 1951

Chapman, C. B., Henschel, A., Mincler, J., Forsgren, A., Keys, A.: The effect of exercise on renal plasma flow in normal male subjects. J. clin. Invest. *27:* 643, 1948

Chasis, H., Goldring, W., Breed, E. S., Schreiner, G. Bolomey, A.: Salt and protein restriction, effects on blood pressure and renal hemodynamics in hypertensive patients. J. am. med. Assoc. *142*: 711, 1950

Forster, R. P., Maes, J. P.: Effects of experimental hypertension on renal blood flow and glomerular filtration rate in intact denervated kidneys of unanesthetized rabbits with adrenal glands demedullated. Am. J. Physiol. *150*: 534, 1947

Hollenberg, N. K., Epstein, M., Rosen, S. M., Basch, R. I., Oken, D. E., Merill, J. P.: Acute oliguric renal failure in man: Evidence for preferential renal cortical ischemia. Medicine *47*: 455, 1968

Kaufmann, W., Nieth, A., Schlitter, J. G.: Nierenhämodynamik bei exogener Wärmebelastung. Klin. Wschr. *42*: 39, 1964

Ladefoged, J., Pederson, F., Dontheil, U., Deetjen, P., Selkurt, E. E.: Renal blood flow measured with xenon-133 wash-out technique with an electromagnetic flowmeter. Pflüger's Arch. ges. Physiol. *284*: 195, 1965

Lamport, H.: Improvements in circulation of renal resistance to blood flow. Charts for osmotic pressure and viscosity of blood. J. clin. Invest. *22*: 461, 1943

Lassen, N. A., Munck, O.: The cerebral blood flow in man determined by use of radioactive krypton. Acta physiol. Scand. *33*: 30, 1955

Lerson, G., Delwaide, P. A., Lejeune, G., Rorive, G., Merchie, G.; The value of two simplified methods for the measurement of renal plasma flow by ^{131}I-Hippuran. In: Radionuclides in nephrology (Eds. M. D. Blaufox and J. L. Funck-Brentano) New York Grune and Stratton, London 1972 241–247

Mertz, D. P.: Quantitative Nierenfunktionsproben. In: Nierenkrankheiten, H. Sarre, 115–139, Thieme, Stuttgart 1976, pp.

Moustgaard, J.: Om proteinstoffernes inflydelse paa nyrenfunktionen hos hund. Kobenhaven Ejvind Christensen, 1948

Oberhausen, E., Kirsch, W., Emrani, I.: Measurement of unilateral renal plasma flow by combination of clearance determination and renograms. In: Radionuclides in nephrology (Eds. M. D. Blaufox and J. L. Funck-Brentano) New York Grune and Stratton, 1972, pp. 233–239

Pappenheimer, J. R., Kinter, W. B.: Hematocrit ratio of blood within mammalian kidney and its significance for renal hemodynamics. Am. J. Physiol. *185*: 377, 1956

Renner, E., Edel, H. H., Buchborn, E.: Critical appraisal of the measurement of renal blood flow using inert gas mixtures. Proc. Sec. intern. Congr. Nephrol. Amsterdam Excerpta Med. 1963, p. 91

Reubi, F. C., Gossweiler, N., Jürtter, R., Huber, A.: Methods of measuring renal circulation in man. Proc. Sec. intern. Congr. Nephrol., Prague and Amsterdam Excerpta Med. 1964, p. 78

Reubi, F. C., Gürtler, G., Gossweiler, N.: A dye dilution method of measuring renal blood flow in man, with special reference to anuric subjects. Proc. soc. exp. Biol. N. Y. *111*: 760, 1962

Robertson, C. R., Deen, W. M., Troy, J. L., Brenner, B. M.: Dynamics of glomerular ultrafiltration in the rat III. Hemodynamics and antiregulation. Am. J. Physiol. *223*: 1191, 1972

Rössler, H.: A semiquantitative evaluation of renograms based on a simultaneously performed simplified slope clearance. In: Radionuclides in nephrology (Eds. M. D. Blaufox and J. L. Funck-Brentano) Grune and Stratton, New York 1972, pp. 221–231

Sapirstein, L. A., Vidt, D. G., Mandel, M. J., Hanusek, G.: Volume of distribution and clearances of intravenously injected creatinine in the dog. Am. J. Physiol. *181*: 330, 1955

Schmid, H. E.: Renal autoregulation and renin release during changes in renal perfusion pressure. Am. J. Physiol. *222*: 1132, 1972

Schück, O., Buda, J.: Arteriovenosní diference kys. paraaminohippurové (PAH). Čas. Lék. čes. *91*: 726, 1952

Schück, O., Chytil, M.: Propočet změn afferentní a efferentní resistence se zvláštním zřetelem ke změnám po fysické práci u zdravých a hypertoniků. Čs. Fysiol. *4*: 472, 1955

Selkurt, E. E., Hall, P. W., Spencer, M. P.: Influence of graded arterial pressure decrement on renal clearance of creatinine, p-aminohippurate and sodium. Am. J. Physiol. *159*: 369, 1949

Shaldon, S., Higgs, B., Chiandussi, L., Walker, G., Garsenstein, M., Ryder, J.: Measurement of renal blood in man with the use of indocyanine green infused into the renal artery. J. Lab. clin. Med. *60*: 954, 1962

Shipley, R. E., Study, R. S.: Changes in renal blood flow, excretion of inulin, glomerular filtration rate, tissue pressure and urine flow with acute alterations in renal artery blood pressure. Am. J. Physiol. *167*: 676, 1951

Sims, E. A. H., Krantz, K. E.: Serial studies of renal function during pregnancy and the puerperium in normal woman. J. clin. Invest. *37*: 1764, 1958

Sirota, J. H., Baldwin, D. S., Villareal, H.: Diurnal variations of renal function in man. J. clin. Invest. *29*: 187, 1950

Smith, H. W.: The physiology of renal circulation. Harvey Lect. *35*: 166, 1940

Smith, H. W.: Principles of renal physiology. New York, Oxford Univ. Press, 1956

Smith, H. W.: The kidney; structure and function in health and disease. New York, Oxford Univ. Press, 1951

Smith, H. W., Finkelstein, N., Aliminosa, L., Crawford, B., Grabar, M.: The renal clearances of substituted hippuric acid derivates and other aromatic acids in dog and man. J. clin. Invest. *24*: 388, 1945

Thoburn, G. D., Kopald, H. H., Herd, I. A., Hollenberg, M., O'Morchoe, C. C. C., Barger, A. C.: Intrarenal distribution of nutrient blood flow determined with krypton[85] in the unanesthetized dog. Clin. Res. *13*, 290, 1963

Thuran, K.: Renal hemodynamics. Am. J. Med. *36*: 698, 1964

Thuran, K.: Influence of sodium concentration at macula densa cells on tubular sodium load. Ann. N. Y. Acad. Sci. *139*: 388, 1966

Watkin, D. M., Shock, N. W.: Agewise standard value for C_{in}, C_{PAH} and Tm_{PAH} in adult males. J. clin. Invest. *34*: 969, 1955

West, J. R., Smith, H. W., Chasis, H.: Glomerular filtration rate, effective renal plasma flow, and maximal tubular excretory capacity in infancy. J. Pediat. *32*: 10, 1948

White, H. L., Rolf, D.: Effects of exercise and some other influences on the renal circulation in man. Am. J. Physiol. *152*: 505, 1948

Winton, F. R.: Present concepts of the renal circulation. Arch. intern. Med. *103*: 495, 1959

Wolf, A. V.: Total renal blood flow at any urine flow or extraction fraction. Am. J. Physiol. *133*: 496, 1941

Wolf, A. V.: The efect of pain on renal function. Res. Publ. assoc. Nerv. and Ment. Dis. *23*: 358, 1943.

PROTEINURIA

The relation between foam formation on the surface of urine and kidney disease was known by Hippocrates (cf. Cameron 1970). An actual demonstration of the presence of protein in the urine, however, had to wait until the dawn of scientific methods. Frederick Dekkers in 1673 started to use a heat coagulation test to demonstrate protein in the urine (cf. Free and Free 1975). The first physician to show clearly that patients with demonstrable anatomical pathology of the kidneys excreted an albuminous protein into the urine was Richard Bright (1836). Twelve years later Watson (cf. Snapper and Kahn 1971) and Bence-Jones (1848) described a quite different protein from that described by Bright in the urine. In 1878, Leube described proteinuria in soldiers after severe exercise, and in the same year Moxon described a postural stimulus to proteinuria (cf. Pesce and First 1979).

In the present century there have been detailed studies of forces which act on the motion of fluid, solutes and macromolecules across the glomerular capillary wall. Recognition of renal tubular proteinuria (Butler and Flynn 1952) turned attention to the tubular reabsorption of proteins. The role of the kidneys in the metabolic homeostasis of plasma low-Dalton proteins and polypeptides was described (Maack et al. 1979, Carone et al. 1979). Attention has been given to the excretion of tissue proteins and antigens (Antoine 1968, Rosemann and Boss 1979). The use of high resolution analytical techniques in the analysis of urine proteins allows us to map total body proteins and polypeptides in health and disease (Anderson and Anderson et al. 1979).

PHYSIOLOGY AND PATHOPHYSIOLOGY (M. ENGLIŠ)

The first step in urine formation is glomerular ultrafiltration. Small non-protein molecules pass through the glomerulus due to hydrostatic and oncotic gradients acting on the capillary wall. The latter acts as a molecular sieve with respect to passage of proteins.

Two theories have been proposed to explain the sieve function of the glomerulus for proteins: the pore theory proposes the existence of protein-permeable pores in a water-permeable, protein-impermeable membrane (Pappenheimer 1953). In contrast, the diffusion theory considers the glomerular capillary wall to be a hydrated gel structure, permeable to proteins as well as water (Chinard 1952). Both theories equally well explain the progressive restriction of substances with increasing Dalton number to membrane passage. In many respects, the two theories agree and complement one another. Present knowledge of the physico-chemical properties of the basal membrane (Misra and Berman 1979) support rather the diffusion theory, but cannot exclude the existence of pores (Bulger 1979).

The permeability of the glomerular wall is of crucial importance to the homeo-stasis of plasma proteins and affects both the amount and the composition of excreted proteins. In animal experiments and clinical research various methods have been used for the study of glomerular permeability, but none of them are suitable for routine clinical use. Analysis of proteinuria therefore gives us indirect but valuable information on the mechanisms involved in the renal handling of proteins and gives us clinically important data on the function of the diseased kidney.

Glomerular capillary structure

Three layers make up the glomerular capillary wall. The internal one is a thin cytoplasmic layer of endothelial cells with frequent oval openings of diameter 60–70 nm (lamina fenestrata); the surface is covered with a hydrated gel with a high content of polyanionic glycoproteins.

The basal membrane of the glomerulus is about 240–430 nm thick. The density of the fibrillar network there in varies from the sub-endothelial (lamina rara interna), to the sub-epithelial (lamina rara externa) and middle (lamina densa) layers. This fibrillar network forms a grid system with holes and the latter are filled with hydrated gel on the fibrillar surface.

The external surface of the basement membrane oriented towards Bowman's capsule is covered by epithelial cells (podocytes, visceral epithelium of Bowman's space). There are plasmatic extrusions foot processes from the podocytes which interdigitate with one another, and together these form a system of slits which are 300–500 nm high and 25–30 nm wide.

The entire wall is therefore a complex ultrafilter with different layers to modu-late transglomerular passage of molecules with greater and greater effective radii (Stokes numbers). Transglomerular motion of neutral molecules decreases sharply if the effective radii increase above 2 nm and is minimal at values greater than 3.4 nm (Wallenius 1954).

The glomerularcapillary wall does not determine molecular motion only according to size. Molecules with the same effective radii (e.g. albumin and dextran) pass the membrane at different speeds. This difference can be explained if we take into account not only size but also net charge. The polyanionic glyco-proteins in the gel are an electrostatic barrier which, under normal conditions, repulse anions, do not influence passage of neutral molecules and interact with cations. Both the lamina rara interna and externa have a much higher charge density than the lamina densa. Of all the structures in the glomerular capillary wall, the epithelial slits and the slit membrane have the highest charge density (Pesce and First 1979).

The physicochemical characterization of the glomerular basement membrane led to a concept that this membrane is a helical glycoprotein gel (Misra and Berman 1979). The configuration of the coiled polyanionic macromolecules form a charge network which — in all probability — forms the basis of both the steric and electrostatic hindrances to transglomerular protein motion. A decrease in this electronegativity alters albumin motion and that of other charged proteins from plasma into the ultrafiltrate. The effect of the electrostatic barrier is manifest more against the motion of albumin and larger proteins than against low-Dalton proteins with less charge/mass. Thanks to this difference the layer of plasma over the lamina fenestrata is more or less albumin — free.

Trans-glomerular passage of any given molecule is also determined by convective and diffusive forces acting on the capillary wall. Renal haemodynamics also affect these forces.

A decrease in RPF is associated with a local increase in protein concentration along the capillary wall, and if FF is raised, trans-glomerular protein motion is also increased. Proteinuria after administration of A-II and nor-epinephrine would appear to result from the ability of these compounds to reduce renal blood flow (Carrie et al. 1980, Montoliu et al. 1979). Renal haemodynamic changes during passive standing, muscular exercise and cold all cause proteinuria, probably in the same manner (Schultze and Heremans 1966).

Tubular reabsorption of proteins

The molecular sieve action of the glomerular capillary wall is very effective and under normal conditions in man very little protein is filtered. Recent micropuncture studies in rats have shown a mean albumin concentration of less than 10 mg/liter in proximal luminal fluid (Oken 1976). If we extrapolate this value to man, about 1.5 g albumin should be filtered/day. If daily excretion is 10–40 mg albumin, it is clear that tubular reabsorption is greater than 95%. Excreted albumin in patients with severe tubular damage and only slight glomerular damage, and during experimental inhibition of protein reabsorption in man (Solling et al. 1979), tends to confirm this hypothesis.

Data on albumin concentration in more distal nephron segments, known so far only in animals, are very varied and no immediate conclusions can be drawn (Carone et al., cited by Oken, 1976). Some observations suggest that albumin concentration does not change along the proximal tubule, i.e. albumin and water are reabsorbed at the same rate (Oken et al. 1972). The maximal tubular reabsorptive capacity for albumin is not precisely known. Most investigators assume that Tm_{alb} is in the region of the plasma threshold of albumin, and a 3-4-fold increase of the filtered load results in saturation of the reabsorptive capacity (Maack et al. 1979).

The tubular reabsorption of albumin and other proteins involves binding of the luminal protein to the brush border of proximal tubular cells. Apical vacuoles form and fuse with primary lysosomes to form secondary phagolysosomes, where hydrolysis occurs (Maack et al. 1979, Carone et al. 1979). It is probable that vacuole formation involves binding the luminal protein to the vacuolar wall and concentrating it. (Maack et al. 1979).

Low-Dalton proteins and polypeptides pass the glomerular capillary wall with ease and their concentration in the glomerular filtrate attains levels in excess of 50% of those in plasma. Plasma microproteins are filtered in this manner (alpha$_2$-microglobulins, beta$_2$-microglobulin, postgamma globulin, monomeric and dimeric polyclonal light chains and IgG fragments) along with biologically active polypeptides (growth hormone, insulin, pro-insulin, glucagon, small vasoactive peptides) and enzymes (amylase). Since these latter substances are present in relatively high concentrations in the glomerular filtrate, it would appear that filtration is the main mechanism of removing small proteins from the vascular compartment.

Urinary excretion of low-Dalton proteins is very small under normal conditions; the degree of their estimated reabsorption appears to be higher than for albumin and can reach 100% (e.g. beta$_2$-microglobulin and light chains) (Solling et al. 1979). Exceptions to this are lysozyme — only 75% is reabsorbed even if plasma concentrations are high (Maack and Shermann 1974) — and amylase, with 45% reabsorption (Selling et al. 1979). The Tm of low-Dalton proteins seems to exceed the plasma threshold considerably as compared to Tm_{alb}. It would also appear that tubular reabsorption of these proteins is effective since even with water or osmotic diuresis their excretion rate does not increase (Wibell and Karlsson 1976).

There is no doubt that reabsorption of low-Dalton proteins relates to a different process in the tubules than reabsorption of albumin and larger proteins. Convincing evidence for selective reabsorption of separate micro-proteins is lacking, however, and the existence of specific membrane receptors for individual proteins is very questionable (Maack et al. 1979). On the other hand, there are clear differences in the excretion of individual proteins in various tubular lesions and particularly in the transplanted kidney (Boesken 1975).

During the process of reabsorption the content of the apical vacuoles is subject to the hydrolytic action of tubular lysozymes. It can be assumed that the rate of intracellular hydrolysis depends on the chemical resistance of the individual molecules. Proteins difficult to hydrolyze can accumulate in tubular cells and damage or destroy them.

Higher Dalton proteins penetrate into the glomerular filtrate with greater difficulty than albumin. Practically nothing is known of their concentration in the filtrate or in the tubular fluid along the nephron. It is assumed that their reabsorption is non-selective (as with albumin) and that tubular function does not affect the ratio in which albumin and larger molecules are filtered (Stolte et al. 1979).

Small linear polypeptides are handled by mechanisms different from those that process proteins. Hydrolysis starts with binding to the brush border, which is rich in hydrolytic enzymes, and hydrolytic fragments are reabsorbed rather than the original peptide (Carone et al. 1979).

Contraluminal secretion of plasma proteins is improbable; if it exists at all, the rate is negligible. This process can be important, however, with some polypeptides and is very probable with insulin (Pesce and First 1979).

Urinary proteins of renal origin

Tamm—Horsfall's uromucoid (mucoprotein, mucoglycoprotein) is produced by the epithelial cells of the collecting ducts and in the loops of Henle. The daily excretion is considerable — up to 40 mg (Pesce and First 1979). An increase in electrolyte content and a decrease in pH support aggregation and gel formation of Tamm—Horsfall uromucoid (Wieslander et al. 1977). This process is the basis for the matrix formation of urinary casts. Co-precipitation of Tamm — Horstfall uromucoid with some low-Dalton proteins, e.g. (myoglobin, Bence — Jones protein) results in an increase in renal toxicity and this can contibute to acute renal failure (Clyne et al. 1979).

IgA is produced in tubular cells and in the mucous membranes of the urogenital tract. The daily excretion is about 1.1 mg, of which more than 90% is secretory IgA (Bienenstock and Tomasi 1968).

Renal tissue antigens (brush border antigens, ligandin, basement membrane antigen, tubular antigens) represent quantitatively a very small component of excreted proteins. Under normal conditions their urinary presence is a manifestation of metabolic turnover of corresponding tissues (Rosemann and Boss 1979).

Excretion of proteins by the healthy kidney

The urine of healthy subjects contains daily about 400 mg of non-dialyzable solids (King and Boyce 1963). If only the polypeptide moieties of excreted urocolloids are taken into account, daily excretion is about 30–150 mg protein. Data vary widely according to the method used. Mean values of daily excretion from 30 to 150 mg, with extreme individual variation from 10 to 300 mg, are seen. The excretion of 150 mg protein/day can be taken as an approximate upper level of normal (Robinson 1979). Daily protein excretion is not very age-dependent, is somewhat higher in males than in females, and clearly higher during the day than during the night (Robinson 1964). The following haemodynamically related changes may increase daily protein excretion over and above the upper limit of normal: blood pressure and volume changes, blood volume redistribution with a change in body position, muscular exercise, cold and increased body temperature.

About 40% of total urinary protein is represented by albumin, which is identical in its properties to plasma albumin. Some concentrating procedures and freezing at $-20°C$ can cause partial polymerisation of albumin (Boesken et al. 1977). About further 20% of urinay protcins is represented by IgG monomers and dimers of light chains kappa and lambda, fragments of IgG, monomeric IgA and secretory IgA. The following are present as traces only: pro-albumin, $alpha_1$-lipoprotein, $alpha_1$-antitrypsin, orosomucoid, Gc globulin, haptoglobins, $alpha_2 HS$-glycoprotein, $alpha_2 zn$-glycoprotein, transferrin, haemopexin, the C 4 component of complement, etc. Immunological methods have been used to demonstrate occasionally in the urine of healthy subjects: $alpha_2$-macroglobulin, fibrinogen and IgM; it cannot be excluded that the measurements detected only antigenically compatible fragments of these proteins (Berggard 1970, Schultze and Heremans 1966, Hemmingsen and Skaarup 1975, Pesce and First 1979). A common property of all proteins in this group is a Dalton number lower than 200,000.

The remaining 40% of urinary protein represents a heterogenous group both in terms of origin and properties. In this group are low-Dalton plasma proteins (e.g. $beta_2$-microprotein, $alpha_2$-microproteins, $alpha_1$-microprotein, post-gamma globulin lysozyme), biologically active peptides (erythropoietin, stances, insulin, etc.), enzymes (plasmin, pepsin, amylase) and a large group of thus far uncharacterized tissue proteins, antigens, polypeptides and peptides. Many of the last group are rich in protein-bound carbohydrate and it can be assumed that for the most part we are dealing with degradation products of structural macromolecules of various, mainly connective, tissues (Schultze and Heremans 1966).

CLASSIFICATION OF PROTEINURIA

1. *Classification with respect to the localization of protein transport*

Most cases of pathological proteinuria can be subdivided into three basic groups:

a) Glomerular proteinuria results from an increase in permeability. As long as the wall of the glomerular capillaries retains the ability to differentiate between proteins according to the size, charge and shape of the molecules, albumin and similar proteins (alpha$_1$-antitrypsin, orosomucoid and transferrin) will be excreted into the urine. More extensive glomerular changes, with disturbance of the structure of the basal membrane, are associated with a low selectivity of protein filtration and excretion of immunoglobulins or even plasma macroproteins into the urine. The glomerular differential capacity for filtration is not operative in haemorrhagic nephropathy with coarse ruptures of glomerular capillaries and penetration of red blood cells into the filtrate.

b) Tubular proteinuria is a reflection of a decrease or disappearance of tubular reabsorptive capacity for proteins. This is characteristic for chronic intoxication with Cd and phenacetine, Balkan nephropathy and in some congenital diseases (Wilson's disease, galactosaemia, Fanconi syndrome). Proteinuria associated with K depletion, the advanced stages of interstitial nephropathy, polycystic kidneys, and acute renal failure are also tubular in origin. Tubular proteinuria is less frequent than glomerular and is often associated with glomeruler damage. The amount of urinary protein excretion in tubular proteinuria is usually less than 1 g/day; greater losses usually mean that both glomeruli and tubules have been damaged.

c) Overflow (pre-renal) proteinuria. This type occurs without damage to the glomeruli or tubules when the plasma concentration of low-Dalton proteins is raised (alpha$_1$-antitrypsin, orosomucoid) or when similar proteins appear in the plasma (Bence-Jones protein, haemoglobin, myoglobin, tissue degradation products).

2. *Classification with respect to the selectivity of glomerular protein excretion*

The general relationship between molecular mass of a protein and its clearance has given rise to a concept of selectivity (Hardwicke and Squires 1955). If we compare log mass of several differently-sized proteins, e.g. alpha$_1$-antitrypsin, orosomucoid, transferrin, albumin, IgG, alpha$_2$-macroglobulin, etc. with log of their clearance, a straight line results on the log-log graph; (Blainey 1960, Hardwicke and Soothill 1961, Joachim et al. 1964). A similar and simpler approach is to compare the clearances of two proteins of different mass, e.g. albumin and IgG, transferrin and IgG, transferrin and alpha$_2$-macroglobulin (Cameron and Blandford 1966, McLean and Robson 1966, Poreh and Berlyne 1974). According to the slope of the regression line, or the index, high, intermediary, poor and non-selectivity have been identified (Manuel and Revillard 1970). The theoretical basis of this concept of selectivity is far from complete. Glomerular filtration of proteins and their tubular reabsorption do not depend to the same degree on molecular mass. If proteinuria is less than 3 g/day one can assume that Tm_{prot} has not been attained and reabsorption influences clearance of proteins. In such a case, a measure of "selectivity" is not reliable (Renner et al. 1975). For the same reasons, selectivity in tubular dysfunction cannot be reliably determined, nor can it be applied to protein excretion in healthy subjects.

Immunochemical methods of determining protein, which are usually used for tests of selectivity, do not respect mass differences in the same antigen. Such differences between plasma and urine proteins can develop and affect the results of the measurement.

Construction of a regression line is often difficult because of scatter (Bienenstock and Poortmans 1970, Pesce and First 1979). On the other hand, comparison of results of measurements of plasma protein clearances with other methods of demonstrating selectivity, mainly polyacrylamide electrophoresis, show a clear validity for some areas of investigation.

The relation between the degree of selectivity and morphological changes in the kidneys can be really accepted only in patients with minimal change nephrotic syndrome, who as a group tend to have highly selective proteinuria.

Other forms of glomerular disease, renal amyloidosis, diabetic nephropathy and even orthostatic and exercise proteinuria, are usually non-selective. Determination of selectivity offers no help in distinguishing between these and other pathological entities. Selectivity and non-selectivity patterns may be encountered in the same morphological entity. Progression of chronic disease and a decrease in GFR is associated with an irreversible decrease of selectivity.

3. *Classification with respect to routine clinical investigation*

A. Intermittent proteinuria

A transient proteinuria can be caused by functional changes in the kidney and need not be due to a pathological process affecting the kidney. This type of proteinuria is called **functional proteinuria.** Very likely the increased urinary protein excretion here is caused by haemodynamic changes. A decrease in renal blood flow very likely facilitates the diffusion of protein molecules across the capillary wall.

The following conditions can cause the intermittent functional proteinuria.
a) postural proteinuria. Posture can affect protein excretion in healthy

subjects, but the excretion rate of protein remains within normal limits. In some cases, however, upright posture can produce manifest proteinuria without any signs of disease. When these subjects are recumbent, the protein excretion is within normal limits.

The majority of subjects with postural proteinuria are growing youngsters, thin, with marked lordosis of the lumbar spine and underdeveloped musculature. In quality the proteinuria appears to be mainly glomerular and quite unselective.

The prognosis of subjects with postural proteinuria appears to be excellent, but according to some authors (King 1959, Thompson et al. 1970) in some of these subjects persistent proteinuria developes. Extended observations in such patients are required to define more precisely the long-term consequences (Kassirer and Gennari 1979). The daily loss of protein in these subjects does not usually exceed 1.0–1.5 g/day.

Position-dependent proteinuria is very common in kidney pathology. For example, in chronic glomerulonephritis the protein excretion in the day time is often 2–4 times greater than at night. These position-dependent changes of protein excretion cannot, of course, be labeled as postural proteinuria.

b) exercise proteinuria. Proteinuria after muscular exercise occurs in 10–30% of exercising subjects. Literary data vary, obviously because the exercise stimulus is so variable. If the exercise lasts some time, the protein excretion is increased from 0.04 mg/min at rest to about 0.7 mg/min, i.e. by a factor of 10–15 times. After ceasing the exercise, excretion of protein can continue to increase up to 4.0 mg/min (Poortmans and Van Kerchove 1972, Poortmans 1972).

This type of proteinuria originates both at glomeruli and in the tubules (Poortmans and Vancalck 1978). With extreme exercise, red blood cells also appear in the urine, as do roughly granulated casts.

In clinically latent cases of renal impairment, we can utilize short periods of exercise to provoke proteinuria, e.g. in diabetes mellitus without manifest proteinuria (Fabre et al. 1975, Mogensen et al. 1979, Meyer et al. 1980, de Seigneux et al. 1980). A significant increase of protein excretion which need not exceed the upper limit of normal and a clear qualitative change in excreted protein composition are the first signs of diabetic renal damage.

c) protein excretion can be increased also by emotional stress.

Is summary, these types of intermittent proteinuria can be caused by changes in renal function. Nevertheless, if there is an underlying pathological process, it is possible that protein excretion can manifest itself after adequate stimuli. For these reasons the diagnosis of functional intermittent proteinuria is difficult, and long-term follow-up of these subjects is indicated.

B. Persistent proteinuria

This type of proteinuria is characterized by an increase in protein excretion above normal in all samples on repeated testing.

This pattern of proteinuria is a sign of renal disease. In these cases further investigation of quantity and quality of excreted protein is valuable. Regardless of the cause of proteinuria, pathological degrees may be influenced by the same haemodynamic effects which may change protein excretion in healthy controls.

METHODS OF INVESTIGATION

1. BEDSIDE AND LABORATORY SCREENING METHODS FOR PROTEINURIA

Commercially available "dip-sticks" allow a ready and acceptable demonstration of proteinuria.

False positive results can occur with analysis of strongly alkaline urines, excessively long exposure of the papers to the urine, the presence of too high a concentration of quarternary ammonium bases and urea, and a sticking of vaginal secretion to the indicator zone of the insert (Thysell 1969). Most of these methods show proteinuria if the urinary concentration of albumin is higher than 100 mg/l. Dip-sticks underestimate proteinuria containing non-albuminous proteins to a significant degree: (e.g. non-selective and tubular proteinuria and Bence Jones proteinuria).

The sulfosalicylic acid method is one of the best and simplest demonstrations of proteinuria available. False positive results can be conditioned by the excretion of injected contrast substances containing organically bound iodides, a high concentration of some drugs such as sulfonamides and antibiotics in pyuria and a high concentration of uric acid. The sulfosalicylic acid method does not detect glyco-peptides and glyco-proteins which are often excreted in inflammatory processes. The sensitivity of this method is 100 to 200 mg/l, and the non-albumin urinary proteins react for better than with dipsticks. For this reason, this method is more suitable for laboratory screening.

The subjective error in both methods can be considerable. A less experienced technician usually overestimates the results rather than the reverse (Gyure 1977). Stress should be laid on the fact that fluid intake, tubular water reabsorption and hemodynamic changes which influence renal excretion independent of any disease can all affect the results of these tests. Marginal results can therefore not be used. In such cases one should take into account urine specific gravity and then repeat the tests.

2. THE 24-HOUR PROTEIN EXCRETION

As already mentioned above, the upper normal limit of normal protein excretion in healthy subjects is 150 mg/day.

Investigation of 24-hour protein excretion helps in the diagnosis of the renal disease. It is generally accepted that persistent proteinuria greater than 4 g/day is always a result of glomerular disease. Heavy proteinuria (greater than 4 g/day) usually leads to the development of nephrotic syndrome. Persistent proteinuria less than 4 g/day is seen in both interstitial and glomerular diseases. If such a proteinuria is not associated with clinical signs of the disease, it is called **asymptomatic proteinuria.** Because there may occur fluctuations of day-to-day protein excretion, quantification of proteinuria should be based on repeated measurement of 24-hour protein loss. The daily protein loss should be expressed in relation to body surface area (g/day/1.73 m²) especially in children.

Investigation of 24-hour protein excretion is important with respect to the evaluation of the effect of the therapy and the progress of the disease.

When interpreting 24-hour protein excretions it should be taken into account that the total urinary excretion is the sum of protein excretion of individual nephrons. With some simplification the ratio $U_{Pr}V/C_{cr}$ indicates the protein excretion rate per nephron. In healthy subjects the ratio $(U_{Pr}V/C_{cr})$. 100 does not exceed 0.1 mg/min/100 C_{cr}.

From the practical point of view it is important that for calculation of this ratio the quantitative urine collection is not necessary, since:

$$\frac{U_{Pr}V \,(mg/min)}{C_{cr} \,(ml/min)} \, 100 = \frac{U_{Pr}\,(mg\%)}{\dfrac{U_{cr}}{P_{cr}}}$$

If the excretion of protein molecules is caused predominantly by their penetration across glomerular capillary wall and their tubular reabsorption can be neglected, the ratio $U_{Pr}V/C_{cr}$ indicates the theoretical minimal value of the protein concentration in the glomerular fluid.

In patients with heavy proteinuria the ratio $(U_{Pr}V/C_{cr}) \times 100$ can reach values about 100 or more.

Investigation of subjects with postural proteinuria

The patient collects the urine during recumbent and upright positions separately. In the evening, immediately before the patient goes to the bed, he empties his bladder and collects the urine until the morning of the next day — which is usually accomplished by a single voiding at the time of arising. The reclining urine sample is collected for 6 to 8 hr. The next day the patient collects the urine during the day-time for 16 to 18 hr.

The amount of excreted protein in both the samples is extrapolated to 24 hr.

The subject with postural proteinuria has increased protein excretion when in the upright position, but normal protein excretion in the recumbent position. This means that the latter extrapolated value does not exceed 150 mg/day.

Provocation of proteinuria by physical exercise

Physical exercise has been introduced as a provocation test for early renal abnormalities in diabetes mellitus as well as in hypertension. Vittinghus and Mogensen (1982) used the following work loads:
300, 450, 600, 750, 900 and 1200 kpm/min on a bicycle ergometer for 20 min each.

Healthy subjects showed an exercise induced albumin excretion at 1200 kpm/ /min, while beta-2-microglobulin excretion was undisturbed. (Three of ten healthy subjects developed increase in albumin excretion at 900 kpm/min).

The values of albumin excretion before and during graduated exercise found by Vittinghus and Mogensen (1982) are given in the following table.

Table 1

	Before exercise	300	450	600	750 kpm/min	900	1200
albumin excretion (µg/min)	7.0 (± 4.4)	6.4 (± 4.0)	6.8 (± 3.5)	6.7 (± 3.2)	6.4 (± 2.6)	15.8 (± 18.3)	147.6 (± 156.6)

The results indicate that healthy persons have to exercise at very hard levels in these short-term experiments before an increase of albumin excretion appears.

CLEARANCES OF INDIVIDUAL PROTEINS AND INVESTIGATION OF THE SELECTIVITY OF PROTEINURIA

A timed urine collection and one blood sample are necessary. The clearance values are calculated in the usual manner (see p. 262).

The measurement of clearances of individual proteins enables us to evaluate the selectivity of proteinuria. Furthermore, this investigation helps in the differentiation of glomerular and tubular proteinuria.

In clinical practice the clearances of the following proteins are usually investigated: albumin, IgG and beta-2-microglobulin. Normal clearance values of these proteins are as follows (Viberti et al. 1982):

protein	clearance (ml/min/1.73 m^2)
albumin	$1.4 \pm 0.1 \times 10^{-4}$
IgG	$0.69 \pm 0.3 \times 10^{-4}$
beta-2 microglobulin	$5.1 \pm 0.6 \times 10^{-2}$

The clearance of albumin (Stokes radius of 36 Å) and IgG (Stokes radius of 50 Å) gives some idea of the transglomerular flux of large protein molecules. Beta-2-microglobulin (Stokes radius 16 Å) penetrates the glomerular capillary wall and is reabsorbed by the tubules. The clearance of beta-2-microglobulin measures the tubular function with respect to reabsorption of microproteins. Healthy subjects excrete daily about 100 μg of beta-2-microglobulin (Evrin et al. 1971).

In clinical practice the selectivity of proteinuria can be evaluated on the basis of the measurements of the clearance ratio of IgG/albumin or IgG/transferrin (Cameron and Blandford 1966). Patients with a clearance ratio of IgG/albumin or IgG/transferrin of less than 0.10 are considered to have highly selective proteinuria. If this clearance ratio is 0.5 or more, the proteinuria is considered to be poorly selective.

Investigation of protein selectivity on the basis of the slope of the relationship between the clearance ratio of various proteins to albumin and the molecular size of a number of plasma protein is not suitable for clinical practice.

Interpretation of changes in clearance values of individual proteins with respect to the sieving properties of the glomerular membrane is not simple. Inferences about glomerular sieving from clearances of large molecular weight proteins are possible in conditions of clinical proteinuria on the assumption that (since albumin loss is substantially through glomerular filtration), the tubular reabsorptive mechanism becomes saturated. Thus nearly all filtered proteins are excreted in the urine. As mentioned above, if proteinuria is less than 3 g/day one can assume that the Tm of proteins has not been attained. Blainey et al. (1979) assume that any patient in whom the clearance of albumin exceeds 0.02 per cent of GFR (about 2 g/day in an adult) must have an increase in glomerular permeability.

In the interpretation of glomerular proteinuria it is necessary to take into account that the glomerular membrane, under normal conditions, is also an electrostatic barrier because the sialic acid containing glycoprotein restricts penetration of anionic proteins like albumin. Enhanced transglomerular transport of the highly anionic albumin molecule can be caused by a loss of electrostatic retardation due to a decrease in sialoprotein content in the basement membrane and the epithelial podocytes (Carrie et al. 1981, Bohrer et al. 1977, Bennett et al. 1976).

An increase of beta-2-microglobulin clearance as a symptom of tubular dysfunction must be interpreted with caution. In patients with reduced GFR and plasma levels of beta-2-microglobulin greater than 50 mg/l, the tubular reabsorptive mechanism for this protein can be saturated and increased urinary excretion of beta-2-microglobulin can be caused by its increased glomerular filtration in residual nephron (Karlsson et al. 1980).

POLYMER CLEARANCES

Inert polymeric macromolecules such as dextran and polyvinylpyrollidone have been used for the investigation of permeability of the glomerular membrane. These molecules are neither reabsorbed nor secreted by the renal tubules and they are available in a wide range of molecular size (Hulme and Hardwicke 1968). The clearance of dextrans (C_D) is usually expressed in relation to GFR. This ratio is called the fractional dextran clearance or the sieving coefficient (Θ):

$$\Theta = \frac{C_D}{C_{in}} = \frac{U_D/P_D}{U_{in}/P_{in}} \tag{1}$$

It has been shown that Θ decreases with increasing of the molecular size. Investigation of polymer clearance involves a slow intravenous administration of polydisperse preparations and collection of urine and serum. The polymers are separated on the basis of molecular size, and the clearance of each fraction is determined. Dextran-40 (Rheomacrodex) can be used for the measurement of fractional dextran clearances.

In patients with chronic renal disease an increase in fractional clearance of polymers has usually beeen found. At present the measurement of polymer clearances is reserved for research.

Indication for investigation

Measurement of urinary protein excretion is one of the basic tests in the diagnosis and management of patients with renal disease. The following indications are to be stressed here:

Screening of renal disease

Semiquantitative tests for proteinuria can detect previously unrecognized renal impairment. As mentioned above, the semiquantitative tests done on random urine samples may be positive when total daily protein excretion is still within normal limits. On the other hand, it can be negative in patients with increased protein excretion.

For these reasons investigation of proteinuria must be based on the measurement of a 24-hour urine sample. The measurement of 24-hour protein loss is also necessary for detection of microproteinuria which can be the sign of an early glomerular lesion.

Differential diagnosis of postural proteinuria and proteinuria caused by renal disease

A diagnosis of postural proteinuria can be made only if the protein excretion in the recumbent position does not exceed the normal level.

If the result of the investigation indicates postural proteinuria, further investigation should establish whether in the given case it only expresses functional changes, or is a sign of renal disease.

Postural proteinuria can be a sign of a minimal glomerular lesion and may occur in the healing phase of various glomerular diseases.

Differential diagnosis of renal diseases and the quantification of proteinuria

There is no relationship between the severity of renal impairment and the amount of urinary protein loss. Patients with heavy proteinuria (for example 20 g/day) may have a normal GFR. On the other hand, in some patients with chronic renal failure only microproteinuria is present and can be overlooked by routine urine examination.

Nevertheless, quantification of proteinuria can assist in the differential diagnosis of chronic renal diseases.

Heavy proteinuria (urinary protein loss greater than 4 g/day) is an indication of glomerular disease and is often associated with the nephrotic syndrome. In the latter patients urinary protein loss can reach 10–20 g/day, and in some cases even greater values.

Patients with various forms of interstitial nephritis (chronic pyelonephritis, analgesic nephropathy, urate nephropathy) or renal impairment caused by metabolic changes like potassium depletion or hypercalcaemia, and patients with polycystic kidneys or obstructive nephropathy usually have a protein excretion less than 4 g/day. Proteinuria of this magnitude can be observed in patients with various forms of glomerulopathies.

Nephrotic syndrome and the investigation of selectivity of proteinuria

Patients with nephrotic syndrome due to minimal change disease have highly selective proteinuria (Blainey et al. 1979). On the other hand, patients with nephrotic syndrome due to other pathological processes usually have non-selective proteinuria.

The investigation of selectivity of the proteinuria can help in the differential diagnosis of nephrotic syndrome but the precise diagnosis of the glomerular disease cannot be made without renal biopsy.

Arterial hypertension

Urinary excretion of protein in patients with essential hypertension is low; it usually does not exceed 2–3 g/day. In patients with renovascular hypertension the urinary protein loss is also low. In cases with accelerated hypertension the protein excretion rapidly increases and heavy proteinuria is one of the characteristic signs of patients with malignant hypertension.

Renal impairment in primary non-renal diseases

The course of many non-renal diseases can be associated with secondary renal impairment. Examples of this include diabetes mellitus, gout and various haematologic diseases. Screening of the renal impairment in these conditions includes investigation of urinary protein excretion.

As mentioned above the physical exercise provocation test can assist in the recognition of an early glomerular lesion.

Tubular syndromes

There is an association between light chain proteinuria and tubular nephropathies (Engle and Wallis 1957, Maldonado et al. 1975, Smithline et al. 1976). In patients with light chain proteinuria due to overproduction the following tubular syndromes have been described:

Fanconi syndrome, distal tubular acidosis, nephrogenic diabetes insipidus and their combination.

Detailed investigation of urinary protein excretion is indicated in such patients.

Laboratory methods (M. Engliš)

For routine measurement of the 24-hour protein excretion, the most frequently used method is the biuret reaction. The biuret reaction is sufficiently specific but is not accurate with low protein concentrations. Measurements of low concentrations therefore require us to concentrate the urine, or to precipitate out the urinary proteins. Both these procedures detract from the specificity of the analysis.

Turbidimetric methods using sulphosalicylic acid, trichloracetic acid or phosphotungstate precipitates do not give accurate results, because not all the proteins form the same type of precipitate with reference to volume.

100

For routine practice, there are very suitable methods recently introduced by Yatzidis (1977) and Iwata and Nishikaze (1979).

The reference standards are two in number: determination of protein N by a modified Kjeldahl method, and double-gel filtration according to Doetsch and Gadsden (1975).

Electrophoresis of urinary proteins

The high resolution of present-day electrophoretic techniques can be used to advantage for qualitative analysis of urinary proteins.

Electrophoresis in agarose or acrylamide gels, which are the most suitable for this purpose, require in most cases previous concentration of the urine to at least 10–15 g/l. Ultrafiltration through a semi-permeable membrane is the best method of concentration. Commercially available materials for this include Visking tubing (Union Carbide) or collodion sacks (Sartorius). The Minicon apparatus (Amicon), membrane type B-15, normally used to concentrate urine, cannot be recommended because beta$_2$-microglobulin passes through the membrane. Petersson et al. (1969) have found a recovery of albumin of 93%, beta$_2$-microglobulin 82% and total proteins in the urine 98% when using Visking tubing for concentration. Recovery figures are far poorer if the initial volume is small (0.1–0.2 ml) (Sehti et al. 1977).

Agarose electrophoresis (Johansson 1972) allows analysis and comparison of a number of urine and plasma samples at once under identical conditions (Figs. 28–30).

Glomerular and tubular types of proteinuria can be clearly recognized by electrophoresis, along with mixed forms and excretion of Bence-Jones protein. Electro-

Fig. 28: Agarose gel electrophoresis of urinary proteins: S-normal human serum, ALb-albumin, Atα-$_1$anti-trypsin, Tf-transferrin, C-3 component of complement, Ig-immunoglobulins. 1-selective glomerular proteinuria (minimal change nephrotic syndrome (dominated by albumin, α-$_1$antitrypsin and transferrin). 2-nonselective glomerular proteinuria (diabetic nepropathy). Note the presence of the intense immunoglobulin zone.

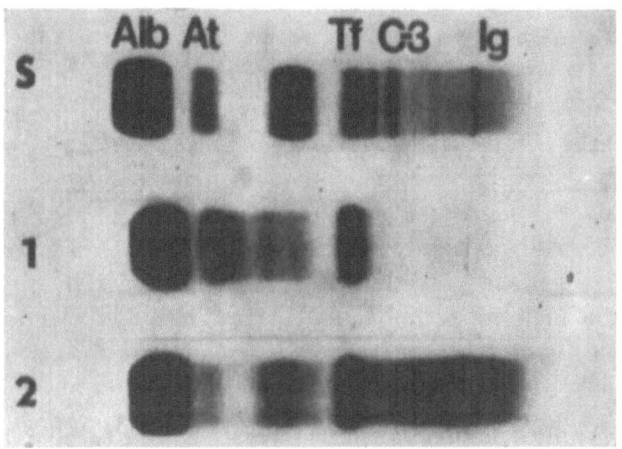

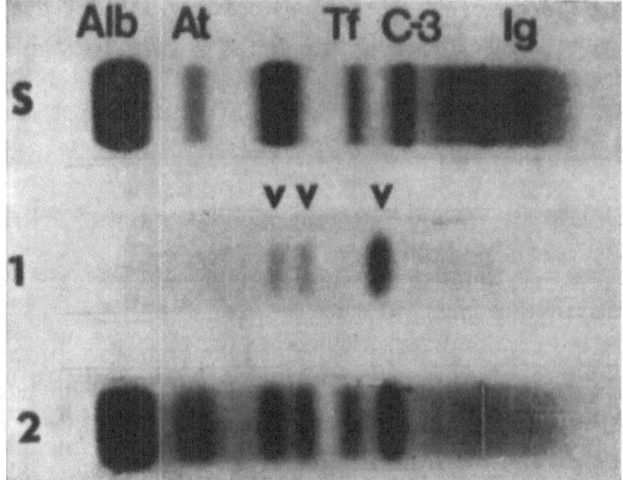

Fig. 29: Agarose gel electrophoresis of urinary proteins:
S-normal human serum, for
explantation see Fig. 28.
1-tubular proteinuria with
arrows indicating two faint
bands of α-2microglobulins
and a single intense band of
$\beta_2$microglobulin.
2-mixed glomerulo-tubular
proteinuria

phoresis in glomerular proteinuria (Fig. 28) in many ways resembles electrophoresis of serum: the dominant zone is albumin, the electrophoretic mobilities of the other zones, in particular alpha$_1$-beta and gamma, are practically the same as the corresponding zones in plasma. The electrophoretic pattern of urine in tubular proteinuria (Fig. 29) is very different from that seen in glomerular proteinuria. In cases of pure tubular proteinuria, where the degree of glomerular damage is very small, the electrophoretic pattern is striking; there is a characteristic zone of beta$_2$-microglobulin which can be easily recognized by its mobility between the transferrin and beta$_{1C}$ globulin zones. Similarly characteristic findings are usually two zones for alpha$_2$ — microglobulin. Cases of pure tubular proteinuria are rare, but mixed glomerular-tubular proteinuria is not, particularly in such "tubular" lesions as chronic Cd intoxication, K depletion, and chronic renal failure.

Electrophoresis of urinary proteins is particularly suitable to identify Bence Jones protein (Fig. 30). With no renal functional damage, the latter protein is practically completely excreted. The electrophoresis shows 1, 2 or more atypical zones which correspond to the monomeric or polymeric forms. The presence of zones of beta$_2$-microglobulin and alpha$_2$-microglobulins are manifestations of simultaneous overloading and relative insufficiency of tubular reabsorption.

In recent years there is more frequent use of acrylamide-gel electrophoresis in the analysis of proteinuria (Alt et al. 1979, Balant and Fabre 1979, Fabre et al. 1975, Sehti et al. 1977, Stolte et al. 1979, Boesken 1975, Manuel et al. 1975, Leskovar and Kratzer 1979). The small pores in this gel allow separation not only according to charge but also according to molecular mass. In homogenous gels (usually we use 5–20% gel) separation of proteins according to size is not propor-

Fig. 30: Agarose gel electrophoresis of urinary proteins: S-normal human serum, for explantation see Fig. 23.

1a-overflow proteinuria (IgG myeloma) dominated by a single intense band of Bence Jones protein. The corresponding band of monoclonal light chains in serum (1b) is missing due to the very efficient renal extraction of the pathological low-Dalton protein.

2a-albuminuria with traces of 7 S IgG immunoglobulin (IgGmyeloma) due to the high concentration of monoclonal IgG in serum (2b).

3a-fixed orthostatic proteinuria of low selectivity. The band of the macromolecular C-3 component of complement is indicated by arrow.

3b-electrophoretic pattern of a morning urine sample from the same patient.

4-hematuria; the intense broad zone of free hemoglobin covers completely the transferrin band, the faint band indicated by arrow corresponds to red cell stroma protein.

5-electrophoretic pattern of urinary proteins in uremia: a mixed glomerulo-tubular proteinuria, often with three faint bands (indicated with arrows) in the fast gama region.

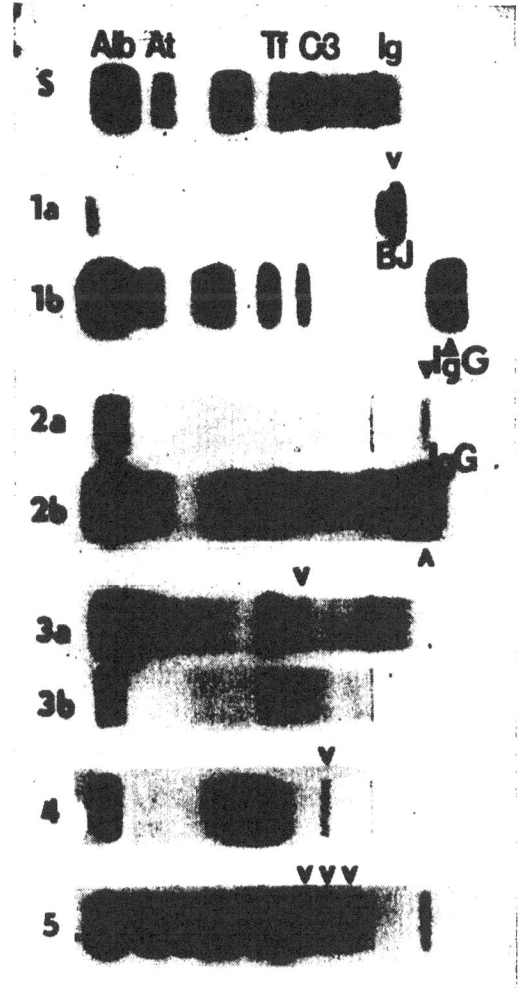

tional. In gradient gels, in which gel concentration and thus pore size gradually change, proportionality can be achieved as a function of molecular mass.

Densitometric quantitation of individual electrophoretic bands is not of great importance with polyacrylamide electrophoresis. Identification of the separate bands can be dificult, but also of importance for, e.g. albumin dimers, haemoglobin, recognition of individual low-Dalton proteins, etc. The great advatage of polyacrylamide gels is realiable separation of urinary proteins, according to their mass, into three groups: albumin and proteins with a lower and a higher Dalton number than albumin. Densitometric quantitation of groups is simple and the ratio of low-Dalton to high-Dalton proteins gives us useful information on the origin and the selectivity of the proteinuria (Boesken 1979, Sehti et al. 1977, Stolte et al. 1979). In this manner we can determine the ratio only of two proteins of different mass, identification of which is not difficult, e.g. transferrin and IgG (Boesken et al. 1975). Some micro-modifications of electrophoresis with acrylamide gel are highly sensitive and allow us to analyze unconcentrated urine samples. It has been shown that this technique can be used to demonstrate the first, but significant, qualitative changes in protein excretion in patients without manifest proteinuria (Balant and Fabre 1979, Fabre et al. 1975).

REFERENCES

Anderson, N. G., Anderson, N. L., Tollaksen, S. L.: Proteins in human urine: I. Concentration and analysis by two-dimensional electrophoresis. Clin. Chem. *25:* 1199, 1979

Alt, J. M., Jänig, H., Schurek, H. J., Stolte, H.: Study of renal protein excretion in chronic pyelonephritis. Contr. Nephrol. 16: 37–43, 1979

Antoine, B., Neven, Th.: Pathological urinary excretion of tissue macromolecules (histuria). J. lab. clin. Med. *71:* 101, 1968

Balant, L., Fabre, J.: Clinical relevance of different electrophoretic methods for the analysis of urinary proteins. In: Current Problems in Clinical Biochemistry, vol. 9. U. C. Dubach, W. Schmidt (eds.), H. Bern, Huber, 1979

Bence Jones, H.: On a new substance occurring in the urine of a patient with mollities ossium. Phil. Transac. Royal Soc. London, I., 1848

Bennett, C. M., Glassock, R. J., Chang, R. L. S., Deen, W. M., Robertson, C. R., Brenner, B. M.: Permselectivity of the glomerular capillary wall: Studies of experimental glomerulonephritis in the rat using dextran sulfate. J. clin. Invest. *57:* 1287, 1976.

Bergaard, I.: Studies on proteins, glycoproteins and mucopolysaccharides in normal human urine. Acta Soc. Med. Upps. *66:* 230, 1961

Bergaard, I.: Plasma protein in normal human urine. In: Proteins in normal and pathological urine. Y. Manuel, J. P. Rewillard (eds.) Basel Karger, 1970

Bienenstock, G. M., Tomasi, T. B. Jr.: Sectory IgA in normal urine. J. clin. Invest. *47:* 1162, 1968

Bienenstock, J., Poortmans, J.: Renal clearance of 15 plasma proteins in renal disease. J. lab. clin. Med. *75:* 297, 1970

Blainey, J. D., Brewer, D. B., Hardwicke, J.: Proteinuria and the nephrotic syndrome. In: Renal disease (Eds. D. Black and N. F. Jones). 4 ed. Oxford, Blackwell, 1979, pp. 383–399.

Blainey, J. D., Brewer, D. B., Hardwicke, J., Soothill, J. F.: The nephrotic syndrome. Diagnosis by renal biopsy and biochemical and immunological analyses related to the response to steroid therapy. Quart. J. Med. *29:* 23, 1960

Boesken, W.H.: Disclelectrophoretic molecular weight analysis of urinary proteins. Contr. Nephrol. *1:* 143, 1975

Boesken, W. H., Schindera, F., Billingham, M., et al.: Polymeric albumin in the urine of patients with nephrotic syndrome. Clin. Nephrol. *8:* 395, 1977

Boesken, W. M.: Diagnostic significance of SDC-PAA electrophoresis of urinary proteins. In: Current Problems in Clin. Bioch., vol. 9. U. C. Dubach, W. Schmidt (eds.). Bern, H. Huber, 1979

Bohrer, M. P., Baylis, C., Robertson, C. R., Brenner, B. M.: Mechanism of the puromycin-induced defects in the transglomerular passage of water and macromolecules. J. clin. Invest. *69:* 152, 1977

Boileau, M., Fuchs, E., Barry, J. M., Hodges, C. V.: Stress haematuria: Athletic pseudonephritis in marathoners. Urology, *15:* 471, 1980

Bright, R.: Cases and observations, illustrative of renal disease accompanied with the secretion of albuminous urine. Guy's Hospital Reports, *I:* 338, 1836

Bulger, R. E.: Kidney morphology. In: Diseases of the kidney. L. E. Earley, C. W. Gottschalk, (eds.) Boston, Little, Brown 1979

Butler, E. A., Flynn, F. V.: The proteinuria of renal tubular disorders. Lancet *II:* 978, 1958

Cameron, J. S., Blandford, G.: The simple assessment of selectivity in heavy proteinuria. Lancet *II:* 242, 1966

Cameron, J. S.: The history of proteinuria. In: Proteins in normal and pathological urine. Manuel, J., Revillard, J. P., Betuel, H. (Eds.). Baltimore, Univ. Park Press, 1970

Carone, F. A., Bansk, D. B., Post, R. S.: Micropuncture study of albumin excretion in the normal rat. 66th Meeting of the Amer. Assoc. of Pathologists and Bacteriologists, San Francisco 1969 Amer. J. Pathol. *55:* 19a, 1969

Carone, F., Peterson, D. R., Oparil, S., Pullman, T. N.: Renal tubular transport and catabolism of proteins and peptides. Kidney int. *16:* 271, 1979

Carrie, B. J., Hilberman, M., Schroeder, J. S., Myers, B. D.: Albuminuria and the permselective properties of the glomerulus in cardiac failure. Kidney int. *17:* 507, 1980

Carrie, B. J., Salyer, W. R., Myers, B. D.: Minimal change nephropathy: An electrochemical disorder of the glomerular membrane. Am. J. Med. *70:* 262, 1981.

Chinard, F. P.: Derivation of an expression for the rate of formation of glomerular fluid (GFR). Applicability of certain physical and physicochemical concepts. Am. J. Physiol. *171:* 578, 1952

Clyne, D. H., Kant, K. S., Peace, A. J., Pollak, V. E.: Nephrotoxicity of low molecular weight serum proteins: Physicochemical interaction between myoglobin, hemoglobin, Bence-Jones proteins and Tamm-Horsfall mucoprotein. In: Current Problems in clin. Biochem. vol. 9. U. C. Dubach, W. Schmidt (Eds.), H. Huber. Bern 1979

Doetsch, K., Gadsden, R. H.: Determination of urinary total protein by use of gel filtration and a modified biuret method. Clin. Chem. *21:* 778, 1975

Engle, R. L., Wallis, L. A.: Multiple myeloma and the adult Fanconi syndrome. Am. J. Med. *22:* 5, 1957.

Evrin, P. E., Wibel, L.: The serum levels and urinary excretion of Beta$_2$-microglobulin in apparently healthy subjects. Scand. J. clin. lab. Invest. *29:* 69, 1972

Fabre, J., Balant, L. Ducrey, J., Giromini, M.: Proteinuria in diabetes. Abstr. No. 579 of the VIth Int. Congress Nephrol., Florencia, Italy 1975

Free, A., Free, H.: Urinalysis in clinical laboratory practice. West Palm Beach, CRC Press 1975

Gyure, W. L.: Comparison of several methods for semiquantitative determination of urinary protein. Clin. Chem. *23:* 876, 1977

Hardwicke, J., Squire, J. R.: The relationship between plasma albumin concentration and protein excretion in patients with proteinuria. Clin. Sci. *14:* 509, 1955

Hardwicke, J., Soothil, J. F.: Glomerular damage in terms of „pore size". In: Ciba Foundation Symposium on Renal Biopsy G. E. W. Wolstenholme, M. P. Cameron, (eds.) Churchill, London 1961

Hemmingsen, L., Skaarup, P.: The 24-hour excretion of plasma proteins in the urine of apparently healthy subjects. Scand. J. clin. lab. Invest. *35:* 347, 1975

Hulme, B., Hardwicke, J.: Human glomerular permeability to macromolecules in health and disease. Clin. Sci. *34:* 515, 1968.

Iwata, J., Nishikaze, O.: New micro-turbidimetric method for determination of protein in cerebrospinal fluid and urine. Clin. Chem. *25:* 1317, 1979

Joachim, G. R., Cameron, J. S., Schwartz, M., Becker, E. L.: Selectivity of protein excretion in patients with the nephrotic syndrome. J. clin. Invest. *43:* 2332, 1964

Johansson, B. G. Agarose gel electrophoresis. Scand. J. clin. lab. Invest. *29:* Suppl. 124: 7–19, 1972

Karlsson, F. A., Wibell, L., Ervin, P. E.: Beta-2-microglobulin in clinical medicine. Scand. J. clin. lab. Invest *40* (suppl. 154): 27, 1980

Kassirer, J. P., Gennari: Laboratory evaluation of renal function. In Strauss and Welt's Diseases of the kidney. Third ed. (Eds. L. E. Early and. C. W. Gottschalk). pp 41–91. Boston, Little, Brown, 1979.

King, J. S., Jr., Boyce, W. H., Little, J. M., Artom, C.: Total nondialyzable solids (TNDS) in human urine. I. The amount and composition of TNDS from normal subjects. J. clin. Invest. *37*: 315, 1958

Leskovar, P., Kratzer, M.: Electrophoretische Erfassung der einzelnen Harnproteinfraktionen. Med. Welt, *30*: 47, 1777, 1979

Maack, T. M., Sherman, R. L.: Proteinuria. Am. J. Med. *56*: 71, 1974

Maack, T., Johnson, V. Kau, S. T. et al.: Renal filtration, transport and metabolism of low molecular-weight proteins. A review. Kidney. int. *16*: 251, 1979

MacLean, P. R., Robson, J. S.: A simple method for determining selectivity of proteinuria. Lancet *I*: 539, 1967

Maldonado, J. E., Velosa, J. A., Kyle, R. A., Wagoner, R. D., Holley, K. E., Salasa, R. M.: Fanconi syndrome in adults: A manifestation of a latent form of myeloma. Am. J. Med. *58*: 354, 1975.

Mannuel, Y., Revillard, J. P.: Study of urinary proteins by zone electrophoresis. In: Proteins in normal and pathological urine. Mannuel Y., Revillard, J. P., Betiel, H. (eds.) S. Karger, Basel 1970, pp. 153–171

Mannuel, Y., Colle, A., Leclercq, M., Tonnelle, C.: Low molecular weight proteinuria. Contr. Nephrol. *1*: 156, 1975

Misra, R. P., Berman, L. B.: The molecular basis of proteinuria. JAMA *242*: 757, 1979

Mogensen, C. E., Vittinghus, E., Solling, K.: Abnormal albumin excretion after two provocative renal tests in diabetics: physical exercise and lysine injection. Kidney int., *16*: 385, 1979

Montolu, J., Botey, A., Torras, A. et al.: Renin-induced massive proteinuria in man. Clin. Nephrol. *11*: 267, 1979

Myer, R., Marshall, W., Jones, R. H. et al.: Characterization of diabetic proteinuria. La Ricerca Clin. Lab. *10*: 143, 1980

Ohen, D. E., Flamenbaum, W.: Micropuncture studies of proximal tubular albumin concentrations in normal and nephrotic rats. J. clin. Invest. *50*: 1498, 1970

Oken, D. E., Cotes, S. C., Mende, C. W.: Micropuncture study of tubular transport of albumin in rats with aminonucleoside nephrosis. Kidney int. *1*: 3, 1972

Oken, D. E.: Proteinuria and aminoaciduria. In: Pathophysiology of the kidneys. Ed.: N. A. Kurtzman, SpringfieldThomas, 1976

Pappenheimer, J. R.: Passage of molecules through capillary walls. Physiol. Rev. *33*: 387, 1953

Pesce, A. J., First, M. R.: Proteinuria. M. Dekker, Inc., New York 1979

Peterson, P. A., Ervin, P. E., Bergaard, I.: Differentiation of glomerular, tubular and normal proteinuria: determination of urinary excretion of Alpha2-macroglobulin, albumin and total protein. J. clin. Invest. *48*: 1189, 1969

Peterson, P. A., Evrin, P. E., Bergaard, I.: Determination of urinary excretion of Alpha2-microglobulin, albumin and total protein. J. clin. Invest. *48*: 1189, 1969

Poortmans, J. R., van Kerchove, E.: La proteinurie d'effort. Clin. Chim. Acta 7: 229, 1962

Poortmans, J. R.: Effect of exercise on the renal clearance of amylase and lysozyme in humans. Clin. Sci. *43*: 115, 1972

Poortmans, J. R., Vancalck, B.: Renal glomerular and tubular impairment during strenous exercise in young women. Europ. J. clin. Invest. *8*: 175, 1978

Poreh, S., Berlyne, G. M.: Renal protein clearances and selectivity of proteinuria in renal amyloid complicating familial mediterranean fever. Nephron, *13*: 221, 1974

106

Renner, E., Heinecke, G., Lange, H.: Clinical value of the renal protein clearance determination. Contr. Nephrol. *1*: 134, S. Karger, Basel 1975

Robinson, R. R., Glenn, W. G.: Fixed and reproducible orthostatic proteinuria. J. lab. clin. Med. *64*: 717, 1964

Robinson, R. R.: Isolated proteinuria in asymptomatic patients. Kidney int. *18*: 395, 1980

Rosenmann, F., Boss, J. H.: Tissue antigens in normal and pathologic urine samples: A review. Kidney int. *16*: 337, 1979

Schultze, H. E., Heremans, J. F.: Molecular biology of human proteins. Amsterdam, Elsevier, 1966

Sehti, K., First, M. R., Pesce, A. J. et al.: Proteinuria following renal transplantation. Nephron *18*: 49, 1977

de Seigneux, R., Schwarz, R., Balant, L., Fabre, J.: Aspects initiaux des alterations de la proteinurie ches les diabetiques. Schweiz. med. Wschr. *110*: 295, 1980

Smithline, N., Kassirer, J. P., Cohen, J. J.: Light-chain nephropathy: Renal tubular dysfunction associated with light-chain proteinuria. N. Engl. J. Med. *29*: 71, 1976.

Solling, K., Mogensen, C. E., Vittinghus, E., Brock, A.: The renal handling of amylase in normal man. Nephron *23*: 282, 1979

Snapper, I., Kahn, A.: Myelomatosis. Basel, S. Karger, 1971

Stolte, H., Alt, J., Schurek, H. J.: Experimentelle und klinische Untersuchungen zur Differentialdiagnostik der Proteinurie. Klin. Wschr. *57*: 1069, 1979

Thompson, A. L., Durrett, R. R., Robinson, R. R.: Fixed and reproducible orthostatic proteinuria: VI. Results of a 10-year follow up evaluation. Ann. intern. Med. *73*: 235, 1970.

Thysell, H.: A comparison between Albustix, Hema-Combistix, Labstix, the sulphosalicylic-acid test, Heller's nitric acid test and a biuret method. Acta med. Scand. *185*: 401, 1969

Viberti, G. C., MacIntosh, D., Bilous, R. W. et al.: Proteinuria in diabetes mellitus: role of spontaneous and experimental variation of glycemia. Kidney int. *21*: 714, 1982

Vittinghus, E., Mogensen, C. K.: Graded exercise and protein excretion in diabetic man and the effect of insulin treatment. Kidney int. *21*: 725, 1982

Wallenius, G.: Renal clearance of dextran as measure of glomerular permeability. Acta Soc. Med. Upp. *59*: 1, 1954

Wibell, L., Karlsson, A.: Urinary excretion of Alpha$_2$ microglobulin after the induction of diuresis. Nephron *17*: 343, 1976

Wieslander, J., Byrgen, P., Heinegard, D.: Determination of the Tamm-Horsfall glycoprotein in human urine. Clin. Chim. Acta *78*: 391, 1977

Yatzidis, H.: New colorimetric method for quantitative determination of protein in urine. Clin. Chem. *23*: 811, 1977

CONCENTRATING ABILITY

Historical remarks

In 1879 Koranyi observed — as far as is known for the first time — that the diseased kidney produces urine of lower osmotic concentration than a healthy organ does. Although at that time nothing was known about the mechanism of concentrating urine, Koranyi's finding stimulated clinical interest in functional investigation of the kidneys. Unfortunately, at the beginning of the twentieth century measurement of the osmotic concentration of biological fluids by freezing point depression was not an easy method suitable for routine use.

Thanks to Volhard (1910) measurement of urine osmolality was substituted by a simple estimation of specific gravity. Because of this, measurement of renal concentrating capacity became part of routine clinical investigation.

Following publication of Volhard's paper, measurement of renal concentrating ability remained for many years one of the most important criteria of adequacy of kidney function despite the fact that concentrating capacity does not show a clear relation to the quantity of functional renal parenchyma.

Measurements of concentrating capacity in clinical practice which involve water intake restriction (unpleasant for the patient) lost their importance with the discovery that the quantity of functional renal parenchyma can be estimated on the basis of endogenous creatinine clearance or, more approximately, by plasma creatinine concentration.

Physiological and pathophysiological laboratories remained interested in investigating renal concentrating capacity for a number of reasons. Homer Smith (1951, 1956) showed the possibility of applying clearance methods to investigate concentrating ability and also calculate other functional parameters.

Measurement of osmolar clearance (C_{osm}), tubular reabsorption of solute free water ($T^c_{H_2O}$) and solute free water clearance (C_{H_2O}) were used more for research on physiological, pathophysiological and pharmacological problems (e.g. localization of the site of drug action in the nehron) rather than for clinical practice.

In 1951, Wirz, Hargitay and Kuhn showed that the countercurrent system in the medulla plays an important role in the formation of concentrated urine. This discovery stimulated intensive research (based predominantly on micropuncture studies) and helped interpret many physiological and pathophysiological problems of urine concentration. Of great physiological significance was Verney's discovery (1947) of the regulation of secretion of antidiuretic hormone and its influence on tubular reabsorption of water. Cellular mechanisms of antidiuretic hormone (vasopressin) action have been elucidated only in recent years.

Clinical interest in investigation of concentrating ability was revived by studies on interstitial nephritis, in particular chronic pyelonephritis. It has been suggested that these pathological processes can affect the concentrating ability prior to a decrease in the glomerular filtration rate (GFR). Unfortunately, this clinical problem has not yet been unequivocally solved.

Discrepancies in various published findings on the concentrating ability of the kidneys under various pathological conditions may be due to the different criteria used for assessing "normality". For instance, the following values of concentrating ability (sp. grav.) have been taken as sufficient or "normal": Volhard et al. (1910) 1025–1030, Alving and Van Slyke (1934) 1026, Addis and Shevky (1922) 1032, Reubi (1970) 1028, Mertz (1963) 1026, Brod (1973) 1028, Sarre (1976) 1028–1030, Papper (1979) has argued that a "specific gravity greater than 1020 can be accepted as demonstrated ability to concentrate urine and the matter need not be pursued with more detailed tests".

When measurements of urine osmolality have been used, a value of 900 mOsm/l has been taken as an index of normal concentrating ability: Epstein et al. (1957), Isaacson (1960), Lindeman et al. (1960), Hulet and Smith (1961) and Mertz (1963). Although it is well known that concentrating ability declines with age (Bock and Krecke 1957, Nádvorníková 1968), this factor is rarely taken into account in clinical practice.

In the authors' view, when comparing the results of various investigators in this field it is necessary to distinguish between results reflecting the maximum concentrating ability and those indicating merely that concentrating ability is "sufficient", or is not severely affected.

Measurement of urine osmolality is generally accepted as an important investigation in the differential diagnosis of acute renal failure. It also helps in the differential diagnosis of polyuric states.

Although at present the value of measurement of concentrating ability for the differential diagnosis of glomerular and tubular diseases remains questionable, it can be accepted that in some cases of chronic renal disease the decrease in GFR can be preceded by impairment of maximum concentrating ability.

For precise clinical diagnosis it is not sufficient to state that renal function is normal only on the basis of measurement of endogenous creatinine clearance (or plasma creatinine concentration). Such a conclusion should also be based on measurement of concentrating ability which depends on many partial functions of the nephron.

PHYSIOLOGY AND PATHOPHYSIOLOGY

The countercurrent mechanism and formation of concentrated urine

Concentrated urine is formed in the collecting ducts from isosmotic tubular fluid because of diffusion of water into the surrounding hyperosmotic interstitium.

The hyperosmolarity of the medullary interstitium increases from the corticomedullary border towards the tip of the papilla. The difference in osmotic concentration between these parts of the medulla is called the medullary osmotic gradient.

The medullary osmotic gradient is created by the action of the countercurrent system. The processes causing the tubular fluid osmotic difference between the descending and ascending limbs of the loops of Henle are fundamental for estalishment of this gradient. A further basic condition is continuous countercurrent flow of the tubular fluid between both the limbs.

According to present knowledge (Kokko 1977, Rector 1977) the osmotic difference between the descending and ascending limbs of the loop of Henle is developed by a mechanism briefly described as follows (and schematically presented in Fig. 31):

Active transport of NaCl not accompanied by water takes place in the thick portion of the loop of Henle. This transport of NaCl increases the osmotic concentration of the outer part of the medullary interstitium. This increase induces water diffusion from the proximal portion of the collecting duct into the medullary interstitium. Since the permeability of the proximal part of the collecting duct for urea is low, the concentration of the latter substance in tubular fluid increases. Since the distal part of the collecting duct is permeable for urea, the latter diffuses

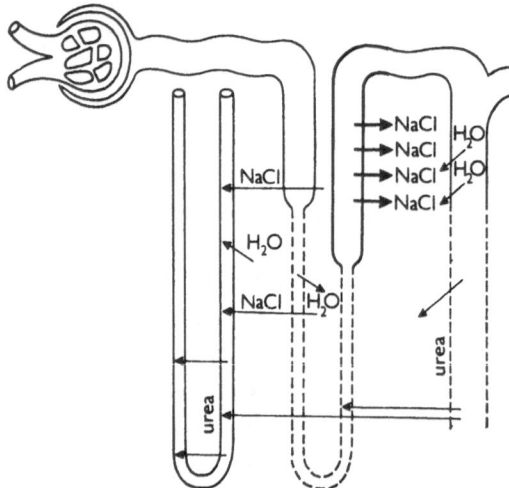

Fig. 31: Schematic presentation of the tubular transport of water, NaCl and urea in the nephron with respect to the action of the countercurrent system. Heavy lines indicate active transport (Deetjen et al. 1976).

110

at this point into the surrounding medullary interstitium. Due to this urea diffusion the osmotic concentration in the medulla increases and induces water diffusion from the tubular fluid of the descending limb of the loop of Henle into the interstitium (this limb of the loop of Henle is permeable for water but relatively impermeable for NaCl). The tubular fluid in the descending limb of the loop of Henle becomes hyperosmotic in relation to that in the ascending limb (which is not permeable for water but allows some diffusion of NaCl). In this manner there develops the osmotic concentration difference between tubular fluid in the descending and ascending limbs. Thanks to continuous countercurrent flow of fluid in both limbs, the medullary osmotic gradient is created. The loop of Henle operates as a countercurrent multiplier.

Urea diffuses from the medullary interstitium also into the tubular fluid in the loop of Henle. Since the urea concentration in the tubular fluid coming into the descending limb is lower than in the medullary interstitium, a concentration difference develops between the urea concentration in the tubular fluid in the descending and ascending limbs of the loop of Henle.

Progressive rise in the concentration of NaCl and urea in the medullary interstitium is created in the loop of Henle and collecting tubule. Since the capillaries are permeable to NaCl and urea, these solutes enter the descending vasa recta and leave from the ascending vasa recta. Conversely, water leaves the descending vasa recta, causing plasma protein concentration to increase. In the ascending vasa recta the sum of osmotic pressure and oncotic pressure results in capillary fluid uptake.

The function of the medullary countercurrent system can be altered by various pathological processes. These may be classified as follows:

1. Anatomical deformation of the medulla

Pathological processes such as hydronephrosis can deform the morphological substrate of the countercurrent system. Consequently, formation of the medullary osmotic gradient can be diminished by prolonged ureteral obstruction and deformation of the pyramids. It can be assumed that pathological changes in the medullary interstitium (cellular infiltration, scarring, etc.) can affect the movement of osmotically active substances between the limbs of the loop of Henle and the vasa recta, and consequently can affect the formation of the medullary osmotic gradient.

Deformation of the renal pyramids can be visualized by intravenous urography. This investigation provides useful information on the morphology of the apices and, indirectly, of the pyramids. A characteristic X-ray picture accompanies obstructive uropathy, chronic pyelonephritis, polycystic kidneys and papillary necrosis.

2. Decrease of tubular transport of osmotically active substances with subsequent decrease of tubular reabsorption of water

A decrease in fractional reabsorption of solutes and water is accompanied by an increase in the flow rate of tubular fluid. It has been shown (Malvin and Wilde 1959) that under conditions of an experimentally induced osmotic diuresis the medullary osmotic gradient is diminished (there is a "washout" of the medullary osmotic contents).

Under pathological conditions osmotic diuresis occurs in residual nephrons. This is due to a decrease in fractional reabsorption by the tubules of NaCl, and by an increase in the plasma concentration of urea. The decrease in fractional NaCl reabsorption in residual nephrons is, in most cases, due to a functional adaptation of residual renal parenchyma (Platt 1950, 1952, Bricker et al. 1965, Gottschalk 1971). The increase in plasma urea concentration is caused predominantly by a decrease in GFR.

The decrease in fractional tubular reabsorption of osmotically active substances is clinically demonstrable by measurement of fractional excretion of osmotically active substances (FE_{osm}) and water (FE_{H_2O}). For details see p. 160.

In healthy subjects on a normal diet and fluid intake FE_{osm} does not go above 4% and FE_{H_2O} above 2.0%. Under pathological conditions, FE_{osm} and FE_{H_2O} can reach 30% or more. Under these conditions, maximum urinary osmolarity is decreased.

For interpretation of the decreased concentrating ability in an individual case it is worthwhile measuring FE_{osm} and FE_{H_2O}.

In the initial stages of chronic renal disease values of FE_{osm} and FE_{H_2O} need

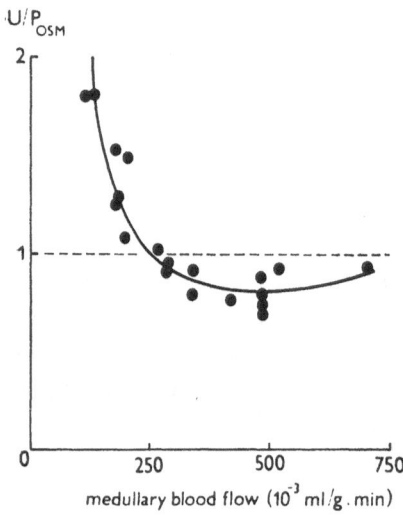

Fig. 32: Relationship between medullary blood flow and the osmotic concentration index $(U/P)_{osm}$ (Thurau 1964).

not be increased, but in cases with a significantly decreased GFR such is usually the case.

3. Concentrating ability can be affected by changes in the *distribution of intrarenal blood flow*. Experimentally it has been shown (Thurau 1964) that an increase in medullary blood flow is accompanied by a decrease in urine osmolarity (Fig. 32). Clinical investigation of the distribution of intrarenal blood flow is not a simple procedure, and at present not applicable for routine clinical examination. For clinical investigation of intrarenal blood flow distribution, the use of isotopic methods is necessary (see p. 78).

Clinically, the possibility of an alteration in concentrating ability due to changes in intrarenal blood flow distribution should be borne in mind in cases of alterations in the systemic circulation, e.g. acute hypotension, shock and acute renal failure.

4. The function of the medullary countercurrent system depends on an adequate blood level of the *antidiuretic hormone* (ADH, vasopressin, VP). Decreased production of VP, or nephron resistance to it, is accompanied by a decrease in maximum concentrating ability.

In cases of very low blood levels of VP the osmotic concentration of the urine is below that of the plasma. For precise clinical diagnosis of inadequate VP production or resistance of the distal nephron to this hormone, special methods have been evaluated (see p. 151).

Cases with permanent production of hypoosmotic urine are often analyzed in cooperation with an endocrinologist. Estimation of blood levels of VP can be made with RIA and changes in blood levels after various stimuli can be followed.

METHODS OF INVESTIGATION

MAXIMUM CONCENTRATING ABILITY

Maximum urinary osmolarity in healthy subjects is about 1200 mOsm/l, or about a four-fold increase over plasma osmolar concentration (McCance 1945, Raisz and Scheer 1959). Such measurements are unpleasant for the patients because they involve restriction of water intake for some time and require the patient's cooperation.

How long is it necessary to restrict water intake to reach maximum urinary osmolarity?

As can be seen in Fig. 33, urinary osmolarity increases in healthy subjects under conditions of restriction of water intake, to maximum values in 28 to 32 hours. Max. U_{osm} stabilizes at about 1000 mOsm/l, but can reach higher values in some

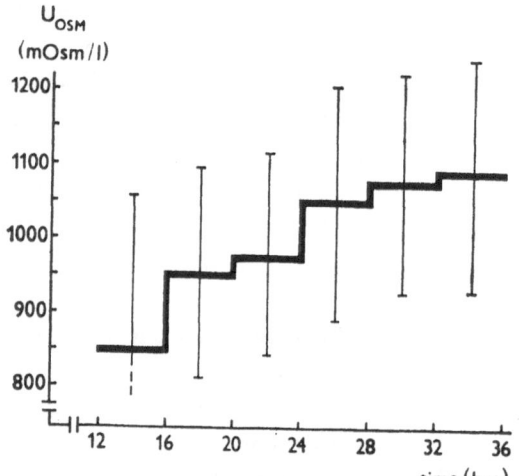

U_{OSM}
$(mOsm/l)$

Fig. 33: Time-course of urinary osmolarity (U_{osm}) during 36hr water intake restriction.

cases. The standard deviation is about 100 mOsm/l. In Fig. 33 it can be seen that the U_{osm} value reached after 24 hr of restriction of water intake does not, in most cases, represent a maximum value. In some subjects, urine osmolarity can slightly decrease after reaching a maximum value (Stříbrná et al. 1965). This latter U_{osm} decrease can be related to a decrease in urinary Na concentration and increased Na fractional tubular reabsorption, caused by restriction of extracellular fluid volume.

In some subjects the time necessary to reach maximum U_{osm} is significantly shorter. Formation of hyperosmotic urine is influenced by the level of fluid intake in the days preceding the investigation (de Wardener and Herxheimer 1957).

With increased water intake before the investigation (e.g. in patients with psychogenic polydipsia or in those drinking large quantities of beer or wine) max. U_{osm} is lower than in healthy subjects with a normal fluid intake. On the other hand, some subjects maintain themselves on a lower volume of voluntary fluid intake and elaborate practically permanently a more concentrated urine. In the latter subjects, max. U_{osm} is achieved after a shorter period of fluid intake restriction than in healthy subjects with a normal fluid intake. This finding (volume of fluid intake) can be important to the therapy of patients with urolithiasis.

Urine collection

The examination begins in the evening. At 6:00 or 7:00 P.M. fluid intake is cut off. The next morning, after 12 hr of fluid intake restriction, the subject voids and the first collection period begins. Urine is collected by spontaneous voiding in 4 hr intervals. If possible, urine osmolality is measured immediately after voiding. If the required U_{osm} value (with respect to age) is achieved, the investigation can

114

be terminated. To investigate the max. concentrating ability, six urine collection periods are required.

Diet

During the investigation, intake of fluids and foods rich in water content (fruits and vegetables) must be excluded.

Since the concentrating ability of the kidneys depends on the solute excretion rate, it is necessary to take into account the protein and salt content of the diet. It has been shown that under conditions of high protein intake the osmotic concentration index U_{osm}/P_{osm} is 10–15% higher than with a low protein intake (McCance 1945, Epstein et al. 1957, Meroney et al. 1958). It has furthermore been shown that the addition of urea to the diet of subjects on a low protein diet is accompanied by an increase in urine osmolarity (Levinsky and Berliner 1958). This effect of urea addition to the diet does not result in increases in U_{osm} in subjects on a normal protein intake (Raisz et al. 1959).

Since such an investigation is contraindicated in subjects with advanced renal disease and elevated plasma urea concentration, proper protein intake (about 1.0–1.5 g/kg/day) should be given.

From a quantitative point of view it should be remembered that about 5.5 mmol urea are produced by metabolism of 1 g protein. The decrease in NaCl content in the diet does not seem to affect max. urine osmolality significantly (Levitt et al. 1959, Schück et al. 1970).

Under these conditions, lower concentrations of Na and Cl in the urine are compensated by an increased urea concentration. A very high intake of NaCl can affect the formation of maximally concentrated urine because of the increased solute excretion.

Age

Maximum concentrating ability depends on the age of the subject. With ageing, max. U_{osm} achieved during 36 hr water intake restriction declines. This relationship can be seen in Fig. 34 (Nádvorníková 1968).

As explained below, ageing also affects the U_{osm} value reached after 24 and 16 hr water intake restriction, as well as after dDAVP administration. Therefore, the results of measurement of concentrating ability should be interpreted with respect to the age of the subject.

Relationship between urine osmolarity and specific gravity

The value of osmotic concentration of a solution depends on the number of particles per unit volume. The specific gravity of a solution, in addition to the

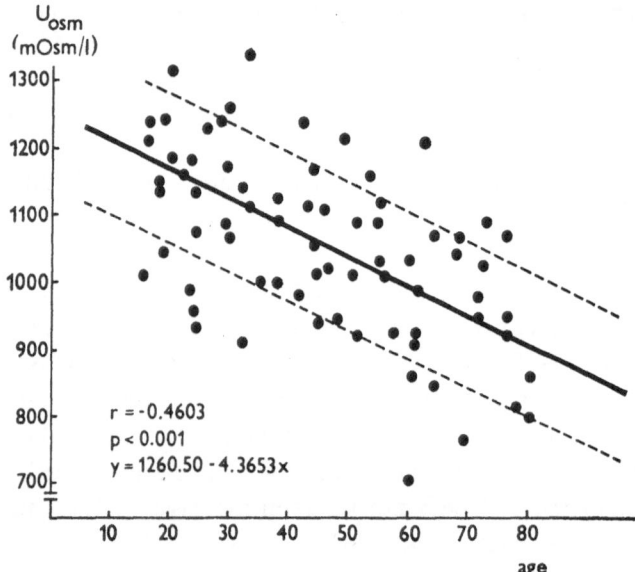

Fig. 34: Correlation graph in healthy individuals of maximal urine osmolarity (U_{osm}) after 36hr dehydratation vs age of subjects in years.

number of dissolved particles, also depends on the molecular weight of the substance.

Osmotic concentration is usually expressed as mOsm/l of solution (osmolarity) or mOsm/kg of water (osmolality).

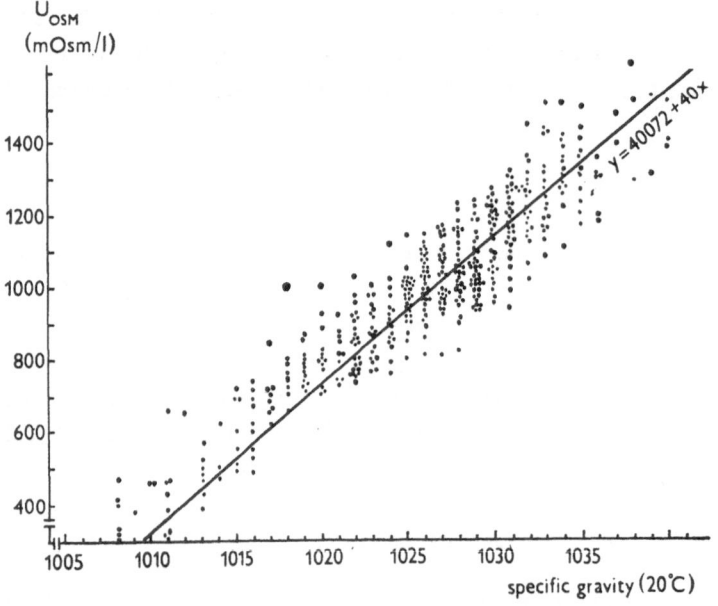

Fig. 35: Relationship between urine specific gravity and osmolarity.

There is a simple linear relationship between osmolarity and specific gravity if only one substance is dissolved in water. Urine is a complex solution of many substances, and therefore the relation between urinary osmolarity and specific gravity (Fig. 35) can be taken only as a useful approximation of urine osmolarity, but this substitution is not acceptable for an exact investigation. Specific gravity depends significantly on urine temperature at the time of measurement. Urine temperature should be adjusted to the temperature for which the urinometer has been calibrated. If this condition is not fulfilled, the following corrections have to be made: for each 3°C above or below this temperature 0.001 should be added to or subtracted from the value observed. If proteinuria is present, 0.003 should be subtracted from the observed reading for each 10 g of protein/l. In diabetic patients with glucosuria, a correction factor of 0.003 to 0.004 for each 10 g glucose/l is sometimes employed.

Glassware should be clean and free of detergent which may alter the surface tension and apparent specific gravity. Each new urinometer should be calibrated in distilled water. Urinary excretion of iodinated compounds can significantly increase specific gravity and therefore investigation of concentrating ability should not be carried out several days after intravenous urography.

Urinary osmolarity after 36 hr restriction of water intake

The values of urine osmolarity achieved in healthy subjects of various age after 36 hr water intake restriction are given in table 1. In each group, 9–13 healthy subjects were investigated.

Table 1

Age group (years)	Mean $U_{osm} \pm$ SD	Mean $U_{osm} - 1$ SD
15–20	1182 ± 83	1099
21–30	1160 ± 82	1078
31–40	1090 ± 129	961
41–50	1073 ± 105	968
51–60	998 ± 126	872
61–70	980 ± 135	846
71–80	936 ± 96	840

For practical use, values in table 1 can be approximated as follows:
Healthy subjects 15–30 years old should produce urine under these conditions with osmolarity 1000 mOsm/l (specific gravity 1030), subjects 31–50 years old: osmolarity 900 mOsm/l (sp. grav. 1028), subjects 51–80 years old: osmolarity 800 mOsm/l (sp. grav. 1026).

As explained above, urinary osmolarity need not reach a max. value after 24 hr restriction of water intake. Nevertheless, in healthy subjects U_{osm} values after 24 hr restriction of water intake are high, and therefore, on the basis of this investigation, a severe impairment of concentration ability can either be diagnozed or excluded.

Values of urine osmolarity achieved in healthy subjects of various ages after 24 hr restriction of water intake are given in table 2:

Table 2

Age group (years)	Mean $U_{osm} \pm$ SD	Mean U_{osm} − 1 SD
15–20	1019 ± 97	922
21–30	1021 ± 86	935
31–40	914 ± 136	862
41–50	977 ± 136	841
51–60	870 ± 150	720
61–70	876 ± 120	756
71–80	856 ± 102	754

According to the data in table 2, healthy subjects 15–30 years old should achieve under these conditions a urine osmolarity of 900 mOsm/l (spec. gravity 1028), 31–50 years old: 800 mOsm/l (sp. grav. 1026), 51–80 years old: 700 mOsm/l (sp. grav. 1023).

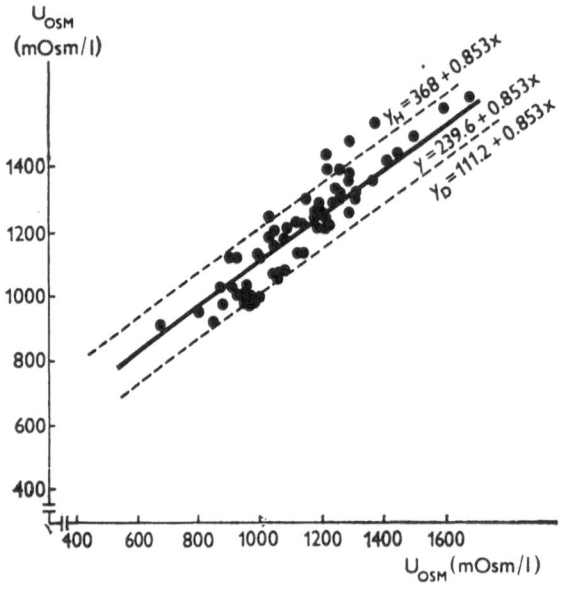

Fig. 36: Correlation graph of maximal urine osmolarity (U_{osm}) after 36hr dehydratation (abscissa) vs U_{osm} after 24 hr dehydratation 24hr dehydratation (ordinate).

The U_{osm} values reached after 24 hr of restriction of water intake are in linear relation to those reached after 36 hr restriction of water intake, as shown in Fig. 36.

The degree of scatter is not negligible, and therefore max. U_{osm} cannot be predicted with certainty on the basis of urinary osmolarity achieved after 24 hr restriction of water intake.

Urinary osmolarity after 16 hr restriction of water intake

It is an established clinical experience that the morning urine specimen is relatively concentrated because of the diurnal rhythm involving water intake restriction during the night. For these reasons, to know the value of morning urine osmolarity is of interest for evaluation of concentrating ability. From this point of view urine osmolarity was analyzed in subjects of various ages after 12 to 16 hours of restriction of water intake. These values are given in table 3:

Table 3

Age group (years)	Mean $U_{osm} \pm$ SD	Mean $U_{osm} - 1$ SD
15–20	980 $\pm$ 107	873
21–30	988 $\pm$ 94	894
31–40	857 $\pm$ 210	647
41–50	860 $\pm$ 262	598
51–60	814 $\pm$ 200	614
61–70	703 $\pm$ 196	507
71–80	689 $\pm$ 150	539

From table 3 it is clear that under these conditions urine osmolarity is also related to age and relatively high values are observed in young subjects. For practical use, the values given in Table 3 can be approximated as follows:

Under these conditions in the age group 15–30 years the urinary osmolarity should reach 850 mOsm/1 (sp. grav. 1026), 31–60 years 600 mOsm/1 (sp. grav 1020), 61–80 years: 500 mOsm/1 (sp. grav. 1018).

Urine osmolarity and specific gravity values reached after 16 hr restriction of water intake do not represent max. U_{osm}, but are useful for recognizing severe impairment.

Scatter of U_{osm} and specific gravity values over 24 hr under conditions of free fluid intake

In healthy subjects on a normal diet with fluid intake 1.0 to 1.5 1/day the urine remains hypertonic throughout the day. An increased intake of fluids is accompanied by a decrease in U_{osm} and of spec. gravity. With high fluid intake,

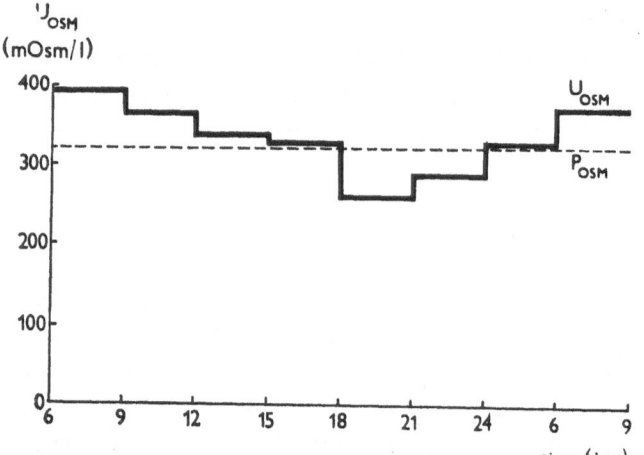

Fig. 37: Time-course of urine osmolarity (U_{osm}) during 24hr in a patient with chronic renal failure. U_{osm} oscillates about the level of plasma osmolarity (P_{osm}).

hypoosmotic urine can be transiently produced. As stated above, the highest U_{osm} and spec. gravity values are observed in the morning urine.

The diurnal rhythm of U_{osm} can be altered in patients with nocturia on the basis of cardiac or renal disease. This rhythm is also usually altered in patients with diabetes mellitus (U_{osm} depends on the rate of glucose excretion) and in patients treated with diuretics.

If urine is collected at intervals of 3–4 hr and U_{osm} and sp. grav. are measured, it is possible to recognize or exclude isosthenuria, i.e. a severe defect of concentrating ability manifest by permanent production of urine with U_{osm} about 300 mOsm/l. An example of such an investigation is shown in Fig. 37.

In some patients with chronic renal insufficiency urine osmolarity can remain below plasma levels over 24 hours. Such a case is seen in Fig. 38. Permanently

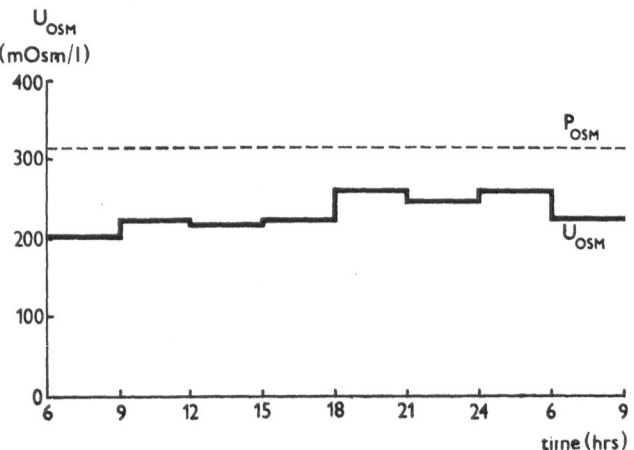

Fig. 38: Time-course of urine osmolarity (U_{osm}) during 24hr in a patient with chronic renal failure. U_{osm} is permanently below the level of plasma osmolarity (P_{osm}).

120

hypoosmotic urine can be theoretically caused by increased thirst in these patients or can be due to resistance of the residual nephrons to the action of VP (cf. p. 140).

Urine osmolarity in the newly born and children

Urine osmolarity in the first days of life usually varies between 200 and 400 mOsm/ /l, and specific gravity varies about 1012. Breast feeding is accompanied by a de- crease in urine osmolarity to values about 100 mOsm/l and in sp. grav. to 1002–1006 (Poláček 1975). At the end of the first month, values about 1000 mOsm/l occur but individual differences are large. Further increases in U_{osm} are relatively slow in appearing.

In healthy children, after reaching the age of two years, urine osmolarity after 12 hr restriction of water intake reaches 870 mOsm/l or greater (Edelman et al. 1967, Poláček 1975).

Lehotská et al. (1981) examined the morning urine specimen in newly born and children, and found the following values:

Table 4

Age (months)	$U_{osm}(\pm 1\ SD)$
–1	227 ($\pm$92)
–2	247 ($\pm$97)
–3	239 ($\pm$95)
–4	386 ($\pm$165)
–5	513 ($\pm$316)
–6	788 ($\pm$440)
–7	847 ($\pm$227)
–8	865 ($\pm$279)
–9	781 ($\pm$152)
–10	759 ($\pm$301)
–11	1003 ($\pm$110)
–12	1074 ($\pm$267)
12–24	884 ($\pm$307)

URINE OSMOLARITY AFTER VP OR dDAVP ADMINISTRATION

To avoid unpleasant restriction of water intake, concentrating ability has been investigated after administration of VP. Administration of 5 IU VP-tannate in oil and measurement of U_{osm} and urinary spec. gravity over the next 24 hr has been recommended. Under these conditions urinary spec. grav. should reach 1020-

'(de Wardener 1956). For investigation of concentrating ability aqueous VP solution has also been recommended (Wrong 1962).

Values of urine spec. grav. after VP administration are significantly lower than those obtained after restriction of water intake. This difference is greater in healthy subjects than in patients with impairment of kidney function.

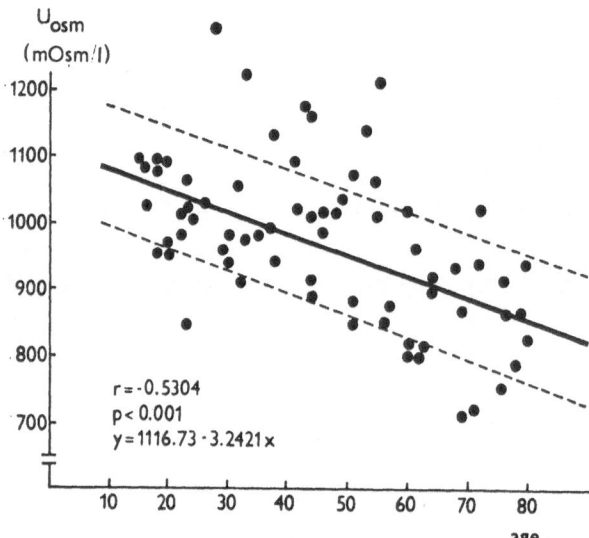

Fig. 39: Correlation graph in healthy individuals of maximal urine osmolarity (U_{osm}) after 12hr dehydratation + dDAVP administration vs age of the subject in years.

The test with vasopressin-tannate in oil should not be carried out in very young children because of the possibility of water intoxication. Administration of VP is contraindicated in patients with ischaemic heart disease.

In recent years, an antidiuretically potent analog of VP, desmopressin (1--desamino-/8-D-Arg/-VP, dDAVP), has been used for the investigation of concentrating ability (Aronson and Svenningson 1974, Monson and Richards 1974, Pacovský and Holeček 1976, Némethová et al. 1977, Delin et al. 1978, Radó 1978, Curtis and Donovan 1979, Nádvorníková at al. 1978, 1980). The following modification of the dDAVP test provides useful information on concentrating ability (Nádvorníková et al. 1980):

1. *After 12 hr restriction of water intake,* 10 µg dDAVP is given intranasally into both nostrils with the head in a supine position. The urine is then collected in four one-hour collection periods.

Urine osmolarity after dDAVP administration depends significantly on age. Fig. 39 shows the inverse relation between max. U_{osm} reached after dDAVP administration and age. For these reasons, values which should be reached after dDAVP should be interpreted with allowance made for this variable. Table 5 gives values of U_{osm} in healthy subjects in various age groups.

Table 5

Age group (years)	Mean $U_{osm} \pm$ SD	Mean $U_{osm} - 1$ SD
15–20	1037 $\pm$ 63	974
21–30	1020 $\pm$ 120	900
31–40	1029 $\pm$ 103	926
41–50	1026 $\pm$ 87	939
51–60	971 $\pm$ 140	831
61–70	857 $\pm$ 72	785
71–80	858 $\pm$ 79	779

From this table it is evident that after dDAVP administration high values of U_{osm} are obtained. In healthy subjects 15–30 years old, mean U_{osm} reached significantly lower values after dDAVP than after 36 hr restriction of water intake. In subjects 31–80 years old, mean U_{osm} after dDAVP was slightly lower than after 36 hr restriction of water intake, but these differences were either insignificant or only reached borderline significance (Fig. 40).

For practical use, values given in table 5 can be approximated as follows: Healthy subjects aged 15–50 years produced, following dDAVP, a urine osmolarity of at least 900 mOsm/l. In subjects aged 51–80 years, U_{osm} under the above conditions should reach at least 750 mOsm/l.

In patients with chronic renal disease a good correlation was observed between U_{osm} after dDAVP and U_{osm} after 36 hr restriction of water intake (Fig. 41).

2. *The dDTVP test without previous water intake restriction.* In 15 healthy subjects we have compared the maximum urinary osmolarity after 12 hr restriction of water intake and the intranasal administration of 10 μg dDAVP (A) with values

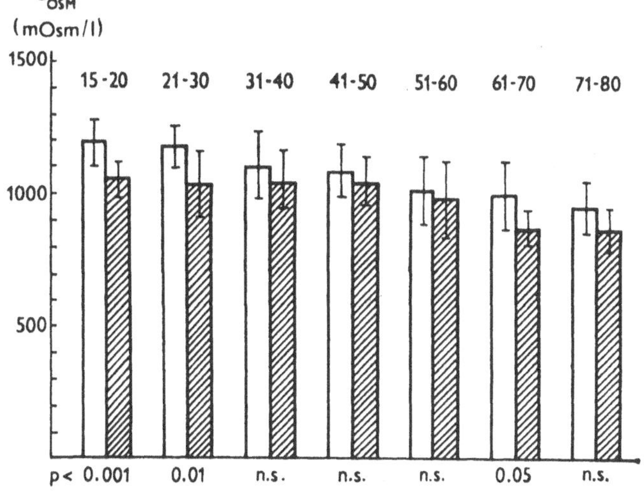

Fig. 40: Comparison of the maximal values of urine osmolarity (U_{osm}) after 36hr dehydratation (white columns) and U_{osm} after 12hr dehydratation + dDA.P administration (hatched columns) in various age groups of healthy subjects.

123

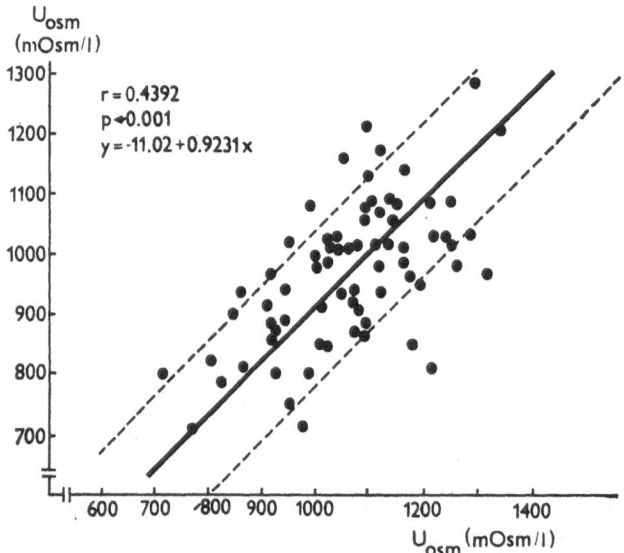

Fig. 41: Correlation graph in patients with chronic renal diseases of maximal value of urine osmolarity (U_{osm}) after 36hr dehydratation (abscissa) vs U_{osm} after 12hr dehydratation + dDAVP administration.

of U_{osm} achieved under conditions of free water intake, and the intranasal ad-ministration of the same amount of dDAVP (B).

The urine was collected in four one hour intervals. The time interval between these investigations was one week.

The following table indicates the maximum values of U_{osm} achieved under these conditions.

	A	B
$U_{osm} \pm SD$	1043	987
(mOsm/l)	($\pm$ 122)	($\pm$ 152)

There was no significant difference between the average values of U_{osm} achieved under these conditions. These results suggest that the dDAVP test can be used in the general practice in the following simplified modification:

In the morning (without any previous water intake restriction) 10 µg dDAVP is given intranasally. Urine is collected 2–3 and 3–4 hours after dDAVP administration.

The dDAVP test provides useful information on the concentrating capacity. On the basis of this investigation, impairment of concentrating ability can be recognized, particularly in subjects older than 30 years.

124

In newborns, Svenningsen et al. (1974) found after dDAVP administration an average U_{osm} of 385 mOsm/l in children 1–3 weeks old, and 565 mOsm/l in children 4–6 weeks old.

Lehotská et al. (1981) found the following values after dDAVP intranasally:

Table 6

Age (months)	$U_{osm}(\pm 1\ SD)$ (mOsm/kg)
–1	671 ($\pm$160)
–2	742 ($\pm$167)
–3	899 ($\pm$118)
–4	896 ($\pm$213)
–5	979 ($\pm$164)
–6	990 ($\pm$223)
6–12	934 ($\pm$178)

TUBULAR REABSORPTION OF SOLUTE-FREE WATER

As stated above, hyperosmotic urine is formed from isosmotic tubular fluid in the collecting ducts due to diffusion of water. The virtual volume of solute-free water ($T^c_{H_2O}$) reabsorbed in the collecting ducts in healthy subjects under normal conditions amounts to 1.0–1.5 ml/min. $T^c_{H_2O}$ is calculated according to the formula:

$$T^c_{H_2O} = C_{osm} - V$$

where C_{osm} = osmolar clearance and V = rate of urine flow.

Under conditions of restriction of water intake, the diference $C_{osm} - V$ does not significantly increase. A characteristic time course of $T^c_{H_2O}$ over 36 hr of restriction of fluid intake is shown in Fig. 42.

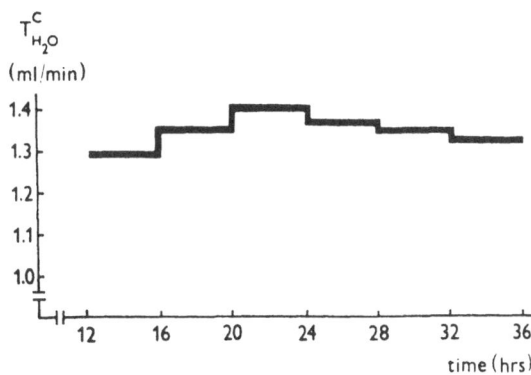

Fig. 42: Time-course of tubular re-absorption of solute-free water ($T^c_{H_2O}$) in healthy subject during 36hr dehydratation.

125

The value of $T^c_{H_2O}$ (ml/min/100 ml GFR) achieved in various age groups are given in the following table:

Table 7

Age group (years)	$T^c_{H_2O}$(ml/min/100 ml GFR)	
	36 hr water intake restriction	dDAVP test
15–20	1.26 ($\pm$0.34)	1.26 ($\pm$0.34)
21–30	1.36 ($\pm$0.41)	1.33 ($\pm$0.59)
31–40	1.39 ($\pm$0.41)	1.39 ($\pm$0.29)
41–50	1.41 ($\pm$0.26)	1.39 ($\pm$0.47)
51–60	1.46 ($\pm$0.39)	1.25 ($\pm$0.52)
61–70	1.50 ($\pm$0.44)	1.46 ($\pm$0.57)
71–80	1.51 ($\pm$0.31)	1.40 ($\pm$0.36)

The value of $T^c_{H_2O}$ increases significantly under conditions of osmotic diuresis and can reach values of 5.7 ± 2.0 ml/min (Zak et al. 1954). Baldwin and al. (1955) reported mean value of maximal value of $T^c_{H_2O}$ $5.1 + 1.5$ ml/min per 100 ml C_{In}.

In healthy subjects such a value of $T^c_{H_2O}$ can be achieved, for example, after infusion of hypertonic mannitol.

Usually, 500 ml 10% mannitol (W/v) is administered i.v. over 1.5–2.0 hr. Rapid infusion of hypertonic mannitol is associated with an acute expansion of extracellular fluid volume, which is contraindicated in patients with cardiovascular disease. The osmotic diuresis which results from hypertonic mannitol infusion causes increased urinary electrolyte excretion and changes in the composition of the ECF.

Measurement of $T^c_{H_2O}$ is not carried out at present as a clinical diagnostic procedure. This investigation has rather been used for physiological and pharmaco-

Table 8

Age group (years)	$\dfrac{U_{cr}}{P_{cr}}$	
	36 hr water intake restriction	dDAVP test
15–20	261 ($\pm$75)	191 ($\pm$56)
21–30	226 ($\pm$66)	213 ($\pm$90)
31–40	221 ($\pm$52)	191 ($\pm$49)
41–50	201 ($\pm$61)	195 ($\pm$66)
51–60	170 ($\pm$40)	179 ($\pm$65)
61–70	175 ($\pm$33)	159 ($\pm$40)
71–80	160 ($\pm$45)	154 ($\pm$51)

logical research on, e.g. localization of the site of action of diuretics in the nephron (if the assumption is allowed that $T^c_{H_2O}$ reflectes NaCl transport in the loop of Henle).

In patients with chronic renal disease the value of $T^c_{H_2O}$ calculated per 100 ml GFR was found to be normal (Baldwin et al. 1955). In terminal stages, $T^c_{H_2O}$ decreases and in cases with isosthenuria this value can reach zero. In patients in the polyuric phase of chronic renal disease $T^c_{H_2O}$ can be negative.

Values of U_{cr}/P_{cr} indicating the fractional water reabsorption in various age groups are seen in the following Table 8 (36 hr water deprivation vs. dDAVP):

Values of U_{cr}/P_{cr} after 36 hr water intake restriction were significantly lower ($P < 0.01$) in the age group 51–80 than in subjects 15–40 years old.

Indications for measurement of renal concentrating ability

1. Recognition of the initial stages of renal impairment in chronic renal disease

As mentioned above, measurement of concentrating ability does not provide information on the quantity of functional renal parenchyma (as opposed to endogenous creatinine clearances). On the other hand, this measurement can in some cases detect renal impairment prior to a decrease in C_{Cr}. Some investigators have stressed that early impairment of the concentrating ability is a characteristic feature of interstitial nephritis, particularly chronic pyelonephritis (Brod 1955, Kleeman et al. 1960). This assumption has not gone without challenge (Mertz 1976).

Fig. 43 shows values of max. U_{osm} in patients in the initial stages of various

Fig. 43: Maximal urine osmolarity (U_{osm}) in initial stages of various chronic renal diseases (endogenous creatinine clearance was within normal limits). The empty marks denote patients with normal maximal U_{osm} (with respect to age). The full marks denote patients with decreased maximal U_{osm}).

○ ● patients with chronic pyelonephritis

□ ■ patients with chronic glomerulonephritis

△ ▲ patients with essential hypertension

▽ ▼ patients with other chronic renal diseases (mostly with urolithiasis and polycystic kidneys)

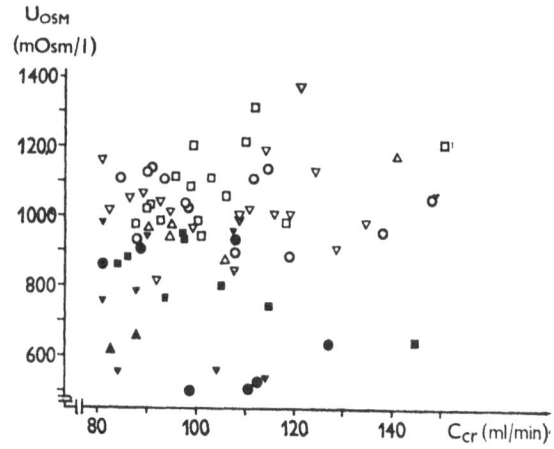

chronic renal diseases. It is clear that in about 1/3 rd of patients, maximum concentration ability was impaired despite normal C_{Cr} values.

The practical use of such measurement can be summarized as follows:

a) In some young subjects genetically destined to develop polycystic kidneys, the clinical picture in the initial stages of the disease need not be clear, and the questions of parents as to whether their child suffers from this hereditary disease cannot be answered with certainty. Investigation of maximum concentrating ability can detect initial impairment of the kidneys (Prát 1961, Defronzo and Thier 1971, Martinez-Moldonaldo 1972). Early impairment of concentrating ability is characteristic also for medullary cystic disease (Gardner 1971, Defronzo and Thier 1976) and medullary sponge kidney (Gardner et al. 1971).

b) In patients with chronic urinary tract infection (diagnosis based on repeated bacteriological studies) and analgesic abuse there often occurs a question of whether the kidneys are involved.

Intravenous urography can give the most critical information. However, at times X-rays need not be conclusive in the initial stages. In such cases, investigation of the max. concentrating ability can be of use. Impairment of this function will implicate renal involvement.

c) Investigation of renal concentrating ability can assist the diagnosis of initial impairment of tubular function in patients with general metabolic disorders such as chronic potassium depletion with kaliopenic nephropathy (Schwartz and Relman 1953), or hypercalcaemia, (Epstein et al. 1958).

d) In patients with various forms of glomerulonephritis or other glomerulopathies, investigation of the renal concentrating ability does not assist the diagnosis which should be made on the basis of the histology of renal biopsy material.

2. Differential diagnosis of acute renal failure

This is based on many investigations, among them being measurements of urinary osmolarity and Na concentration.

If acute renal failure is caused by severe dehydration and renal function prior to this was normal, the kidney elaborates a small volume of urine of high osmolarity and spec. gravity. On the other hand, if the acute oliguric state is caused by tubular impairment, urinary osmolality is at the plasma level and isosthenuria develops.

In patients with acute renal failure caused by an acute reduction of ECF volume and water depletion, urine osmolality does not decrease below 500 mOsm/l, and in some cases can attain values of 1000 mOsm (Heinze 1976). In such cases, urine sp. grav. does not drop below 1020. On the other hand, in patients with acute renal failure caused by severe tubular impairment, urine osmolality is about 300 mOsm/l (does not exceed 350 mOsm/l), and urine sp. gravity is about 1010.

Additional useful information is provided by measurement of Na and urea creatinine concentrations.

In patients with acute renal failure due to dehydration, urinary Na concentration is below 20 mmol/l and fractional Na excretion is less than 1 %.

In patients with acute renal failure due to acute tubular damage, urinary Na concentration is above 40 mmol/l, and the fractional Na excretion is greater than 2 %.

All the above laboratory data must be interpreted in the context of other investigations and the clinical status, but in any case of high urinary osmolality severe tubular impairment can be excluded. Pre-existing renal diseases can significantly modify the reaction of the kidneys to dehydration, and the above criteria may fail. The past history of the patient is clearly important.

Contraindications for measuring maximum concentrating ability

Restriction of water intake is contraindicated in patients with advanced stages of chronic renal disease, and in patients with chronic renal insufficiency. Usually, the investigation is not performed in patients with C_{cr} less than 50 ml/min or endogenous plasma creatinine above 2 mg %. In these patients the measurement results are of little value for diagnosis and the investigation can be of no harm to the patient. In dehydrated subjects restriction of water intake is contraindicated. In such cases urine osmolality and sp. grav. should provide the required information. Furthermore, the investigation should not be carried out in oedematous patients. In the latter, ECF volume is increased and restriction of water intake does not provide an adequate increase in plasma osmolality. Hence, stimulation of "osmoreceptors" to increase VP production is subnormal. In some oedematous patients, VP production is increased and urine of high osmolality is produced spontaneously. Restriction of water intake should be forbidden in patients with active urinary tract infection and in patients with urolithiasis.

Finally, it should be stressed that investigation of maximum renal concentrating ability requires the collaboration of the patient, so that full disclosure to the latter is necessary.

Laboratory methods

For osmotic concentration of the urine and plasma, various types of instruments are used. These are based on measurement by thermistor of depression of the freezing point or of increase in vapour pressure. The reproducibility of most instruments is adequate above 100 mOsm/kg, with an error of 2-3 %. Required fluid volumes for measurement are 0.2 ml or less. Specific gravity of urine is measured with a urinometer, and several conditions must be respected to obtain accurate values, such as fluid temperature, presence of protein and glucose, etc. (see p. 117). Each instrument should be periodically calibrated in distilled water and measurements should always be made at the calibration temperature (usually 15 or 20°C).

REFERENCES

Addis, T., Shevky, M. C.: A test for the capacity of the kidney to produce a urine of high specific gravity. Arch. intern. Med. *30*: 559, 1922

Alving, A. S., VanSlyke, D. D.: The significance of concentration and dilution test in Bright's disease. J. clin. Invest. *13*: 969, 1934

Aronson, A. S., Svenningsen, N. W.: DDAVP test for estimation of renal concentrating capacity in infants and children. Arch. Dis. Childh. *49*: 654, 1975

Baldwin, D. S., Berman, H. J., Heinemann, H. O., Smith, H. W.: The elaboration of osmotically concentrated urine in renal disease. J. clin. Invest. *34*: 800, 1955

Bastl, C. P., Rudnick, M. R., Narins, R. G.: Diagnostic approaches to acute renal failure. In: Acute renal failure (Eds. R. M. Brenner and J. H. Stein), New York, Edinburgh, London, Melbourne, Churgill Livingstone 1980

Bock, K. D., Krecke, H. J.: Der Konzentrationsversuch als klinische Nierenfunktionsprobe. Grundlagen, Methodik und Beurteilung. Dtsch. Arch. klin. Med. *204*: 599, 1957

Bricker, N. S., Klahr, S. Parkerson, M., Schultze, R. G.: Renal function in chronic renal disease. Medicine *44*: 263, 1965

Brod, J.: Chronická pyelonefritis. Praha, Stát. zdrav. nakl. 1955

Brod, J.: The kidney. London, Butterworth 1973

Curtis, J. R., Donovan, B. A.: Assessment of renal concentrating ability. Brit. med. J. *1*: 304, 1979

De Fronzo, R. A., Thier, S. O.: Functional abnormalities in renal cystic diseases. In: Cystic diseases of the kidney (Ed. K. D. Gardner) New York, London, Sydney Toronto, Wiley 1976, pp. 65–81

Delin, K., Aurell, M., Ewald, J.: Urinary concentration test with desmopressin. Brit. med. J. *1*: 757, 1978

DeWardener, H. E.: Vasopressin tannate in oil and the urine concentration test. Lancet, *1*: 1037, 1956

DeWardener, H. E., Herxheimer, A.: The effect of high water intake on the kidney's ability to concentrate the urine in man. J. Physiol. (London) *139*: 42, 1957

Edelman, C. R. Jr., Barnett, N. L. et al.: Standardised test of renal concentrating capacity in children. Am. J. Dis. Child. *114*, 639, 1967

Epstein, F. H., Kleeman, C. R., Hendrikx, A.: The influence of bodily hydratation on the renal concentrating process. J. clin. Invest. *36*: 629, 1957

Epstein, F. H., Kleeman, C. R., Pursel, S., Hendrikx, A.: The effect of feeding protein and urea on renal concentrating process. J. clin. Invest. *36*: 635, 1957

Gardner K. D.: Cystic disease of the kidney. New York, London, Sydney, Toronto, Wiley, 1976 New York 1964. Boston New York, N. Y.

Gottschalk, C. W.: Function of chronically diseased kidney. The adaptive nephron. Circulat. Res. Suppl. II. *28*: pp. II-1-II-3 1971

Heinze, V.: Akutes Nierenversagen. In: Nierenkrankheiten. H. Sarre, pp. 425–469 Stuttgart; Thieme 1976

Hulet, W. H., Smith, H. W.: Postural natriuresis and urine osmotic concentration in hydropenic subjects. Am. J. Med. *30*: 8, 1961

Isaacson, L. C.: Urinary osmolality in thirsting normal subjects. Lancet *1*: 467, 1967

Kleeman, C. R., Hewitt, W. L., Guze, L. B.: Pyelonephritis. Medicine 39: 3, 1960

Kokko, J. P.: The role of renal concentrating mechanisms in the regulation of serum sodium concentration. Am. J. Med. 62: 165, 1977

Korányi, A. V.: Physiologische und klinische Untersuchungen über den osmotischen Druck thierischer Flüssigkeiten. Z. klin. Med. 33: 1, 1897

Lehotská, V., Lichardus, B., Némethová, V., Škultétyová, M.: Antidiuretinový (DDAVP) test na vyšetrenie koncentračnej schopnosti obličiek dojčat. Čs. Pediat. 36: 324, 1982

Levitt, M. F., Levy, M. S., Polimeros, D.: The effect of a fall in filtration rate on solute and water excretion in hydrogenic man. J. clin. Invest. 38: 463, 1959

Lindeman, R. D., Van Buren, H. C., Raisz, L. G.: Osmolar renal concentrating ability in healthy young man and hospitalized patients without renal disease. New Engl. J. Med. 262: 1316, 1960

Malvin, R. L., Wilde, W. S.: Washout of renal countercurrent sodium gradient by osmotic diuresis. Am. J. Physiol. 197: 177, 1959

Martinez-Moldonado, M., Yium, J. J., Eknoyan, G. Suki, W. N.: Adult polycystic kidney disease: studies of the defect in urine concentration. Kidney int. 2: 107, 1972

McCance, R. A.: The excretion of urea, salts, and water during periods of hydropenia in man. J. Physiol. (London) 104: 196, 1945

Meroney, W. H., Rubini, M. E., Blythe, W. B.: The effect of antecedent diet on ruine concentrating ability. Ann. intern. Med. 48: 562, 1958

Mertz, D. P.: Untersuchungen über den Harnkonzentrierungsmechanismus während Hydropenie. I. Beziehung zwischen maximalem spezifischem Harngewicht und Harnosmolarität bei nierengesunden und nierenkranken Personen. Z. klin. Med. 157: 517, 1963

Mertz, D. P.: Semiquantitative Niereninfektionsproben. In: Nierenkrankheiten. H. Sarre, Stutgart, Thieme, 1976, pp. 101–115

Monson, J. P., Richards, P.: Desmopressin urine concentration test. Brit. med. J. 1: 24, 1974

Nádvorníková, H.: Konzentrations- und Dilutionsfähigkeit der Niere bei Erwachsenen und im Alter. Z. ges. inn. Med. 24: 810, 1968

Nádvorníková, H., Schück, O., Cort, J. H.: Možnosti vyšetřování koncentrační schopnosti ledvin na podkladě DDAVP (1-deamino-(8-D-arginin)-vasopressin) testu. Vnitř. Lék. 24: 1026, 1978

Nádvorníková, H., Schück, O., Cort, J. H.: A standardized desmopressin test of renal concentrating ability. Clin. Nephrol. 14: 142, 1980

Némethová, V., Lichardus, B., Lehotská, V.: Erfahrungen mit einem DDAVP Schnelltest zur Bestimmung der Konzentrationsfähigkeit. Mschr. Kinderheil. 125: 165, 1977

Pacovský, V., Holeček, V.: Dlouhodobé zkušenosti s léčením diabetu insipidu syntetickými analogy neurohypofysárních hormonů. Sbor. lék. 78: 149, 1976

Papper, S.: Clinical nephrology. 2. ed. Boston, Little and Brown, 1978

Pascal, R. P.: Medullary cystic disease of the kidney. Am. J. clin. Path. 59: 659, 1973

Platt, R.: Sodium and potassium excretion in chronic renal failure. Clin. Sci. 9: 367, 1950

Platt, R.: Structural and functional adaptation in renal failure. Brit. med. J. 1: 1372, 1952

Poláček, E.: Nephrologie dětského věku. Praha, Avicenum, 1975

Prát, V.: Klinický obraz polycystických ledvin u dospělých. Praha, Stát. zdrav. nakl., 1961

Raisz, L. G., Scheer, R. L.: Studies on the renal concentrating mechanism II. Effect of small acute changes in solute excretion. J. clin. Invest. 38: 1725, 1959

Radó, J. P.: 1—Desamino—8—D—arginine vasopressin (DDAVP) concentration test. Am. J. med. Sci. 275: 43, 1978

Rector, F. C.: Renal concentrating mechanisms. In: Disturbances in Body Fluid Osmolality. Eds. T. E. Andreoli, Grantham, J. J., Rector, F. C. Jr. Bethesda, Am. Physiol. Soc. 1977, pp. 179–196

Reubi, R.: Nierenkrankheiten. Bern, Stuttgart, Wien, Huber, 1970

Rjabov, C. I., Natočin, J. V., Bondarenko, B. B.: Diagnostika bolezněj poček. Leningrad, Medicina., 1979

Sarre, H.: Nierenkrankheiten. 2 Aufl. Stuttgart, Thieme, 1959

Schwartz, W. B., Relman, A. S.: Metabolic and renal studies on chronic potassium depletion resulting from overuse of laxatives. J. clin. Invest. *32,* 258, 1953

Schück, O., Stříbrná, J., Kuhn, E., Brodan, V.: Vliv sníženého příjmu Na v potravě na tvorbu hypertonické moči. Čas. Lék. čes. *109:* 285, 1970

Smith, H. W.: The kidney; structure and function in health and disease. New York, Oxford Univ. Press, 1951

Smith, H. W.: Principles of renal physiology. New York, Oxford Univ. Press, 1956

Stříbrná, J., Šmahelová, R., Schück, O.: Příspěvek k hodnocení tzv. koncentrační schopnosti ledvin. Vnitř. Lék. *11:* 1170, 1965

Svenningsen, N. W., Aronson, A. S.: Postnatal development of renal concentration capacity as estimated by DDAVP-test in normal pashyxiated neonates. Biol. Neonat. *25:* 230, 1974

Thurau, K.: Fundamentals of renal circulation. Proc. II. int. Congr. Nephrol. Prague 1963. New York, Excerpta Med. Found. Anest., 1964, p. 51

Verney, F. B.: The antidiuretic hormone and the factors which determine its release. Proc. roy. Soc. B *135:* 25, 1947

Volhard, F.: Über die functionelle Unterscheidung der Schrumpfnieren. Verh. dtsch. Ges. min. Med. *27:* 735, 1910

Wirz, H., Hargilay, B., Kuhn, W.: Lokalisation des Konzentrierungsprozesses in der Niere durch direkte Kryoskopie. Helv. physiol. pharmacol. Acta *9:* 196, 1951

Wrong, O. M.: Tests on renal function. In: Renal disease (Ed. D. Black). Oxford, Blackwell Sci. Publ., 1962

Zak, G. A., Brun, C., Smith, H. W.: The mechanism of osmotically concentrated urine during the antidiuretic state. J. clin. Invest. *33:* 1064, 1954

DILUTION OF THE URINE

Historical remarks

As with renal concentrating capacity, investigation of the ability of the kidney to dilute urine was introduced at the beginning of this century by Volhard (1910). Clinical experience with this investigation demonstrated, however, that inability of the kidneys adequately to decrease osmolality (as measured by urea) and specific gravity occurred, or was measurable, only in the late stages of chronic renal disease. This resulted in some degree of abandonment of this test in chronic renal disease since there was not the advantage to be gained of early diagnosis of functional impairment, nor was there any great value in differential diagnosis (Nonnenbruch 1941). This development is in sharp contrast with the increase in use and importance of the opposite test — concentrating capacity.

However the dilution test did not quite disappear from the repertoire of functional renal tests for a number of reasons:

1. Abnormal excretion of a water load can involve a relatively inadequate response in decreasing the endogenous secretion of VP. Recent studies comparing plasma levels of VP analyzed by RIA with plasma osmolality (Robertson et al. 1977) have shown that the syndrome of inappropriate ADH secretion (SIADH) may have a number of different aetiologies.

2. Various pathological processes can affect renal function and leave the body in a state of constant spontaneous water diuresis. Functional investigation here can differentiate between a renal or a central (VP secretion) mechanism.

3. Thanks to the work of Homer Smith (1951, 1956), clearance methods were adapted to measurement of diluting capacity. Estimates of the clearance of solute-free water (C_{H_2O}) became the basis of localization of the site of action of many substances on tubular transport of osmotically active solutes (Na in particular) in the nephron. Measurement of C_{H_2O} under conditions of maximal water diuresis has been and continues to be useful in studies of the action of drugs on the kidney, and in studying detailed alterations in a number of pathological states.

Measurement of C_{H_2O} under conditions of maximal water diuresis makes it possible to evaluate tubular reabsorption of Na in the distal nephron, and combined

133

with measurement of other parameters such as C_{Na} and C_{Cl} also gives an indirect measure of tubular reabsorption of Na in the proximal nephron (i.e. that segment proximal to the dilution site in the tubule).

The impossibility of using micropuncture techniques in patients is thus at least partially compensated for by using the above techniques to localize changes in tubular Na transport.

Similar to investigation of renal concentrating ability, the availability of sensitive osmometers to clinical laboratories give us more accurate data in dilution testing, particularly since specific gravity measurements are of little assistance at low urine osmolalities. Most osmometers, however, do not behave in a linear manner at levels below 100 mOsm, and detailed standard curves must be repeatedly measured for very accurate results.

PHYSIOLOGY AND PATHOPHYSIOLOGY

The human body is most usually in a state in which it is necessary to conserve water by forming hypertonic urine. Under some conditions (excessive intake) the water excess must be excreted by diluting the urine.

Verney (1946) demonstrated that maintenance of water balance and osmotic homeostasis is part of the function of the neurohypophysis. Further work showed that antidiuretic hormone (VP) is synthesized as part of a large protein in the supra-optic nucleus of the hypothalamus, cleaved enzymatically into nonapeptide cyclic fragments there, the latter then re-associating themselves by low affinity attachment to carrier proteins known as neurophysins provided the pH is in the region 4–6. This hormone-carrier complex is transported along the axonal cytoplasm from the hypothalamus to bulbar nerve endings in the neurohypophysis, where it is stored in a bound form in visible granules. Release of VP from the neurohypophysis involves exocytosis into capillary blood collection and distribution, the blood pH of 7.4 favoring dissociation of the hormone from the carrier. The exocytotic release mechanism is triggered by two known stimuli, in order of quantitative significance: change in ECF osmotic pressure and change in ECF of blood volume. The afferent receptors of the latter signal are thought to be localized in the pulmonary veins and the left atrial wall. The afferent receptors for the former signal are thought to be in the brain stem, perhaps in the hypothalamus, but earlier work on vacuole-containing osmoreceptor cells has not stood the test of time and further observation.

No matter where the osmoreceptor cells are located, we can still speak of a thirst centre in the lateral hypothalamus (Andersson 1957). On the basis of the present knowledge we can summarize the thirst-VP-renal tubule axis as a functioning system thus:

134

In the presence of a negative water balance (excess loss or inadequate intake) there is a rise in plasma osmolality. The rise in P_{osm} causes a) a release of VP, and b) the sensation of thirst. The former increases water reabsorption in the distal nephron — thirst leads one to drink. It is surprising that if renal losses do not play a role in re-establishing osmotic balance, thirst alone can do so with remarkable precision which approaches that of the best osmometers. This is summarized below schematically:

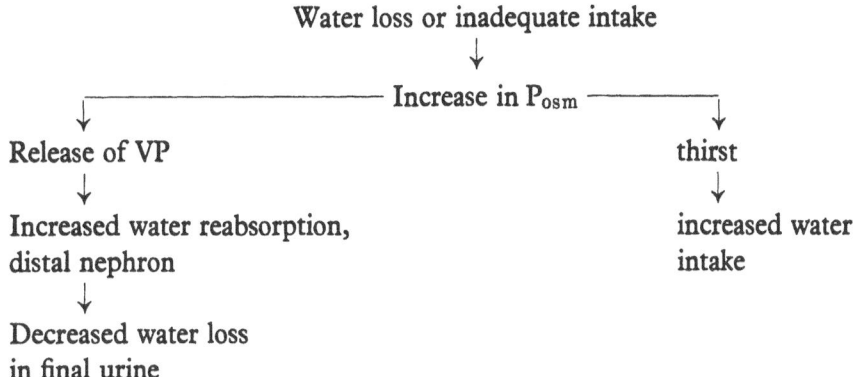

Increased water intake results in a decrease in P_{osm}, decrease in endogenous secretion of VP and resultant decrease in water reabsorption in the distal nephron with accompanying diuresis.

Micropuncture studies in animals have given us more detailed information on the site of action of VP in the nephron. Walker et al. (1941) and later Wirz (1951, 1956) and Gottschalk and Mylle (1959) showed that the tubular fluid in the proximal section is isotonic with plasma. This latter relation remains throughout the course of an induced water diuresis and also during the formation of concentrated urine. The proximal tubular wall is freely permeable for water and VP plays no role in its movement. Formation of a hypotonic urine occurs in the distal nephron. As has already been explained in diagrams of the function of the countercurrent system (see p. 110), NaCl is actively transported by the thick limb of the ascending portion of the loop of Henle, from the lumen into the surrounding interstitium. This dilutes the tonicity of the luminal fluid. With adequate plasma levels of VP in the distal tubule the luminal fluid returns to plasma osmolality and luminal osmolality can increase above plasma levels in the collecting ducts.

With VP secretion inhibited, the walls of the distal tubule and the collecting ducts become relatively impermeable for water. Luminal hypotonicity in the outflow from the thick ascending limb of the loop of Henle is further heightened by distal tubular reabsorption of osmotically active solute unaccompanied by water transport.

Under conditions of water diuresis the medullary osmotic gradient is decreased, but does not completely disappear (Bray 1960, Ullrich and Jarausch 1956). Since water permeability of the collecting ducts is low when plasma levels of VP are low, any existing interstitial medullary osmotic gradient cannot pull water out of the luminal fluid.

The question arises whether, during maximal water diuresis, the wall of the distal nephron is completely impermeable for water. Berliner and Davidson (1957) showed in dog experiments that in conditions of diabetes insipidus, if there is a slowing of flow rate of luminal fluid in the distal nephron (e.g. because of a decrease in GFR), urine osmolality can increase.

Functionally, the dilution segment of the nephron starts at that point in the ascending limb of the loop of Henle at which luminal osmolality decreases from higher-than P_{osm} levels to P_{osm}. Calculation of C_{H_2O} involve the distal nephron, starting from that point at which luminal osmolality decreases to values below P_{osm}.

The mechanism by which VP alters water permeability in the distal nephron can be summarized, according to the present state of the art, as follows (Schwartz et al. 1960, Leaf and Frazier 1961, Orloff and Handler 1967, Schafer et al. 1977, Dousa and Valtin 1974, 1976):

VP binds to receptors on the basal-lateral surface of the tubular cell plasma membrane (it also penetrates tubular cells, but for what purpose, if any, is not known). The receptor-peptide complex, once triggered, activates adenyl cyclase, which catalyzes the formation of 3',5' — cyclic-adenosinmonophosphate (cAMP) from its precursor, ATP. The cAMP increases the synthesis of protein kinase which phosphorylates proteins which act on the apical plasma membrane of tubular cells. This effect of the phosphorylated protein is aided by and dependent upon microtubular and microfilamentous organelles within the cell (Ross et al. 1976); cAMP is broken down to the inactive nucleotide 5' — AMP. This reaction is further accelerated by phosphodiesterase (cf. Fig. 44). The microtubular stage of the sequence alters water permeability.

In recent years work has accumulated showing an interaction between VP and

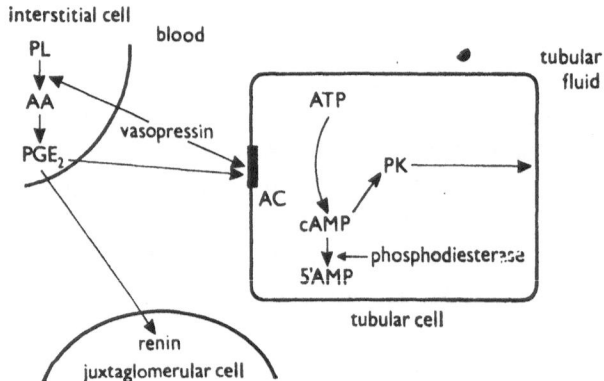

Fig. 44: Schematic presentation of the mechanism of action of vasopressin in the nephron (Pl = = phospholipids, AA = arachidonic acid, AC = adenylcyclase, ATP = adenosine triphosphate, cAMP = cyclic adenosinemonophosphate, PK = protein kinase). (Adapted from Dunn and Hood 1977)

136

renal medullary prostaglandins. It has been shown that VP (but not dDAVP) stimulates the formation of prostaglandins and that the latter antagonize the hydro--osmotic action of VP (Urakabe et al. 1975, Andersson et al. 1975, Zusman et al. 1977, Walker et al. 1977).

VP increases the release of arachidonic acid from phospholipids. The former is important for the formation of PGE_2. The latter prostaglandin possibly plays a role either in VP binding to its receptor or in the action of the receptor-peptide activated complex on adenyl cyclase (Dunn and Hood 1977).

Prostaglandins may have an effect on the renal excretion of salt and water by the further mechanism of increasing cortical blood flow in the kidneys. PGE_2 also increases renin output either by increasing synthesis or release.

The mechanism of action of VP on tubular cells is still not completely clear. Animal experiments have also shown an effect of VP on Na transport and urea excretion. These actions on the excretion of water, Na and urea can be dissociated by combination with other drugs and by synthetic alterations in the VP molecule.

For clinical purposes, the causes of the inability of the kidney sufficiently to dilute urine can be subdivided into two:

1. *Inability to decrease urine osmolality due to the existence of osmotic diuresis*

The higher the rate at which osmotically active solutes are excreted, the higher the minimal osmolality which the kidneys can attain under conditions of maximal water diuresis.

Patients with chronic renal disease can develop a state of osmotic diuresis because of a rise in plasma osmolality (e.g. urea concentration) and because of a decrease in the rate of reabsorption of osmotically active solutes (in particular, a decrease in proximal Na reabsorption). In patients with a large reduction in the number of functional nephrons there is, in all probability, an increase in individual nephron GFR in the residual functional units. This results in a greater delivery of isotonic luminal fluid to the diluting segment of the nephron. This automatically results in a decrease in the attainable minimal osmolality of the luminal fluid in the subsequent portions of the nephron.

Clinically, we can estimate the intensity of the osmotic diuresis by calculating the fractional excretion of osmotically active solutes (FE_{osm}). When total GFR decreases to levels of 20–30 ml/min, FE_{osm} markedly increases in patients with chronic renal disease. In other words, at this stage of chronic renal disease a defect in the ability of the kidney to dilute urine begins to be evident.

Fig. 45 shows the relation between FE_{osm} and the minimal U_{osm} in patients with chronic pyelonephritis. It is clear that U_{osm} values increase in direct relation to levels of FE_{osm}.

The functional importance of this disturbance is clear — if FE_{osm} is decreased

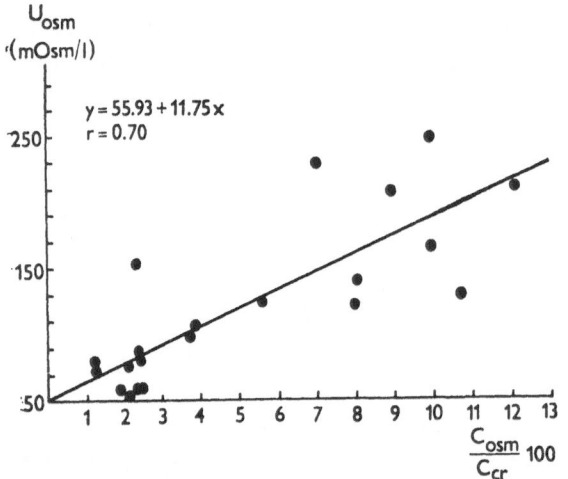

Fig. 45: Relationship between fractional excretion of osmotically active substance. (C_{osm}/C_{cr} 100) and minimal urine osmolarity (U_{osm}) after water load (22 ml/kg) in subjects with chronic renal diseases.

by, for instance, a decrease in Na intake and a consequent decrease in Na excretion, the kidneys are able to form urine of lower osmolality and in some cases dilution capacity can become "normal".

Fig. 46 shows the relation between minimal U_{osm} values under conditions of normal Na intake (150 mmol NaCl/day) and with a low salt intake (30 mmol/day). As can be seen, a decrease in salt intake results in a decrease in minimal U_{osm}.

Since the level of osmotic diuresis in residual nephrons has an adaptive and variable character, the decrease in dilution capacity of the kidneys in patients with advanced chronic renal disease cannot be considered per se as a defect in tubular function. This means that if a decrease in NaCl reabsorption in the residual nephrons is adequate, fluid volume homeostasis can be maintained. Abnormal dilution capacity can be considered a direct tubular malfunction if decreased re-

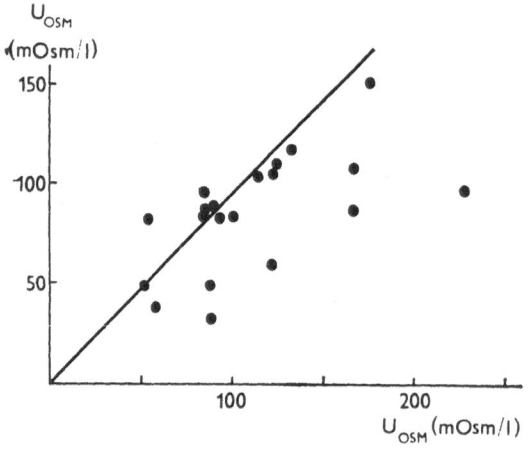

Fig. 46: Relationship between minimal urine osmolarity (U_{osm}) after water load (22 ml/kg) in patients with chronic pyelonephritis under conditions of normal salt intake (abcissa) nad low salt intake (ordinate).

absorption of osmotically active solutes (even with a normal total kidney GFR) is the result of malfunction of transport processes for these solutes.

If an increase in plasma urea levels plays an important role in the development of osmotic diuresis, then both the level of the osmotic diuresis, and the resulting loss of diluting capacity are mainly a function of the decrease in GFR.

The ability of the diluting segment of the nephron to reabsorb osmotically active solute without water, even in patients in an advanced stage of chronic renal disease, is manifest by the fact that despite the inability to achieve sufficiently low U_{osm} values after a water load, the excretion of solute free water related to GFR (C_{H_2O} /GFR) × 100 is normal. This latter value may even be higher than that achieved by healthy subjects, probably because the inflow of isotonic fluid from the proximal tubule into the diluting segment of the nephron is high. Nevertheless, in a few cases, even the excretion of solute-free water is decreased. This latter situation can only be interpreted as evidence of decreased reabsorption of osmotically active solutes in the diluting segment of the nephron.

A decrease in total GFR may modify the renal reaction to a water load by decreasing the % of the load excreted per unit time following ingestion, even in cases in whom U_{osm} decreases to very low values.

2. Failure of renal diluting capacity due to extrarenal causes

A standard water load cannot produce hypotonic urine if the decrease in P_{osm} is not accompanied by a decrease in secretion of VP. This situation may prevail in a number of pathological states, collected together under the heading "inappropriate secretion of ADH" (SIADH). SIADH can result from a number of CNS afflictions, but also from lung disease and tumours variously located. The mechanism of increased VP production is by no means uniform in all cases.

Present findings suggest that one cause may be in the CNS and involve autonomous hyperproduction of VP (e.g. in some tumours) or in an abnormal relation between P_{osm} and VP release (Robertson et al. 1977).

In some cases of pulmonary disease, changes in intrathoracic blood volume can be a source of continual stimulation of baroreceptors leading to VP hypersecretion (Cohen et al. 1977). In some cases of lung tumour (oat cell carcinoma) it would appear that the tumor itself is capable of producing and releasing an "anti-diuretic principle" (Padfield et al. 1977, Coscia et al. 1977).

Increased endogenous VP secretion occurs in women with idiopathic oedema during orthostasis (Thibonnier et. al. 1981). This can be considered a physiological response to changes in the distribution of ECF volume associated with increased capillary permeability and increased transudation of ECF in the lower extremities during orthostasis.

Abnormality of the dilution capacity of the kidneys can be conditioned by a number of endocrine irregularities. It has been shown that ACTH and gluco-corticoids are required for a normal ability to dilute urine (Schrier et al. 1977, Balment et al. 1976).

There is no single mechanism to explain how glucocorticoids affect the dilution capacity of the kidneys (Fichman 1978). These steriods have a direct effect on the permeability of the collecting ducts for water and inhibit hypothalamic production of VP. In addition, they indirectly influence urine dilution by affecting the transport of Cl and Na ions in the thick ascending limb of the loop of Henle.

Abnormality of urine dilution also occurs in hypothyroidism. This has also been associated with increased plasma levels of VP (Seif et al. 1977, Fanestil 1977). Again, there appears to be no single mechanism of action of thyroid hormones on the kidney. In animal experiments thyroxin stimulates VP-induced, cAMP--mediated, water and Na transport.

Tri-iodothyronin is an inhibitor of phosphodiesterase. Indirectly, thyroid hormones also influence Na transport by an action on Na-K dependent ATP-ase. By increasing cardiac output they also have an indirect action on renal haemody-namics and Na excretion.

The relation of the renin-angiotensin system to abnormalities of urine dilution is not clear at this time. Angiotensin-II affects the thirst center and indirectly can alter water excretion by altering renal haemodynamics (Johnson and Malvin 1977).

Robertson et al. (1977) also include in the SIADH category cases in whom abnormal urine dilution could be explained by an increased sensitivity of the distal nephron to VP (perhaps because of a decrease in prostaglandin production).

Pathological states associated with permanent water diuresis

These can be classified as follows:

1. Central diabetes insipidus (DI). This involves inadequate production of VP and, according to Randall et al. (1959), can be subdivided into two forms:

a) Primary: Idiopathic cases with a tendency towards familial incidence. This form can become manifest at any age in either sex (as opposed to hereditary nephrogenic DI which always becomes evident in early childhood).

b) Secondary: This follows on skull trauma, as an aftermath of neurosurgery in the cranium or primary and metastatic tumours in the CNS. Metastasis of lung and breast carcinomata seems to have a predeliction for the hypothalamus. Second-ary DI has also been observed in some granulomatous diseases (sarcoidosis, tuberculosis) and in encephalitis, meningitis, brain aneurysms and so-called "brain death" as a result of brain hypoxia.

2. Nephrogenic DI is characterised by a resistance of the distal nephron to VP. This syndrome is usually congenital, may also be acquired and may possibly involve a lack of or change in the conformational requirements of antidiuretic receptors in the distal nephron.

a) Congenital variant. There is some evidence that this form of nephrogenic DI involves an absolute or relative inability of tubular cells to react to VP by increasing cAMP production (Epstein 1977). There is a further possibility that this disturbance is also associated with an increased production of medullary prostaglandins since in some cases urine flow can be decreased by the administration of indomethacin (Wohltman et al. 1977). Since the lack of a cAMP response to VP. has not been confirmed in all such cases investigated, it is also possible that the disturbance lies in a post-cAMP molecular event.

The congenital form seems to have at least two forms: an absolute lack of response to dDAVP and relative lack-so that the excessive water turnover can be normalized, but with 20–40 x the usual dDAVP dosage.

b) Acquired form. Tubular resistance to VP agonist triggering of antidiuretic receptors can result from a number of pathological processes involving the kidney. Such resistance has been reported in various forms of tubulo-interstitial nephritis such as: kaliopenic nephropathy, urate and phenacetine nephropathies, pyelonephritis, medullary cystic disease, state following relief of an obstruction to urine flow, the diuretic state following acute tubular necrosis and with hypergammaglobulinaemias of various origin (myeloma, sarcoidosis, Sjörgren syndrome and amyloid disease). Furthermore, some drugs such as Li, demeclocydine and methoxyfluorane can also result in a tubular cell resistence to the action of VP. Some of these drugs can also affect appreciation of the thirst afferent signal and VP production in the CNS.

3. Psychogenic polydipsia. In such cases the lack of release of VP is the result of excessive water intake. In most cases this is a psychological disorder and psychiatric investigation is indicated. One simple test is a therapeutic trial with dDAVP — central DI patients welcome the therapy, psychogenic polydipsia patients admit that their water turnover has decreased but do not welcome the therapy at all.

Recently, a number of drugs have been found to affect the "thirst center" in the hypothalamus, or appreciation of a thirst signal (cf. mention of angiotensin II above). Diuretics (saluretics) with the additional action of increasing kaliuria, and laxatives, may also play a similar role. In addition to an effect directly on the distal nephron, Li salts and chlorpropamide also appear to have a central action on the "thirst centre".

Excess water intake, because of stimulation of a "thirst centre", can also be met with in patients in an advanced state of chronic renal failure (particularly in the course of a chronic dialysis programme maintaining the patients).

METHODS OF INVESTIGATION

A maximal water diuresis is produced by oral intake of a water load. The load can be a single "bolus" test, after which a diuretic response reaches its peak for a short time only, or, once reached, the peak urine flow can be maintained by replacing the water losses as they occur. A maximal diuretic state of long duration (as long as the load is maintained) can thus be produced. Water diuresis can also be induced by infusion of hypotonic NaCl or dextrose solutions. VP production can be inhibited by administration of ethanol.

Investigational conditions

Since the dilution capacity of the kidneys depends on the rate of excretion of osmotically active solutes, the diet must be taken into account. In our own experience, the subjects are kept on a standard diet with a normal protein and NaCl content for several days before testing. Water intake during this same preparatory period is ad libitum. If the subject to be tested is dehydrated at the time of testing, the administered water load will be retained and no diuresis will result.

The investigation should take place at a normal room temperature. Cold inhibits VP secretion and excessive heat can result in excessive extrarenal water loss. For these reasons, body wt. should be measured before, and at the end of the investigation. If a decreased diuresis results in fluid retention, an increase in body wt. will be recorded. The subject cannot be allowed to smoke during any test, since nicotine stimulates VP secretion.

The investigation is usually carried out with the subject seated, but in some patients — e.g. with idiopathic oedema — the subject should be reclining and the test should be repeated a few days later with the subject moving about in a vertical position. If during orthostasis there is excess transudation of EFC volume, VP release can thereby be stimulated.

All painful procedures should be avoided (including blood sampling) during the investigational period. Pain can decrease urine flow rate per se, both haemodynamically and by virtue of VP secretion. The psychological state of the subject can also influence the response to a water load. Emotion can also result in an osmotic diuresis. The investigation should therefore be carried out in a quiet isolated treatment room.

Before and during the test no drug administration (other than a purposefully tested substance) can be allowed.

The definition of a maximal water diuresis

Maximal water diuresis represents a minimal U_{osm} which an additional water load or a further decrease in P_{osm} will not further decrease. It is assumed that this state represents the maximal attainable suppression of VP release. RIA estimates of arginine-vasopressin levels in plasma during the peak of water diuresis have given results of 0.16 ± 0.1 pg/ml. AVP plasma levels in dehydrated subjects were $3.2 \pm \pm 2.5$ pg/ml (Thomas and Lee 1976).

Fig. 47 shows the relation between P_{osm} and U_{osm} during maximal water diuresis. in a healthy subject. It can be seen that after attaining a certain level of P_{osm}.

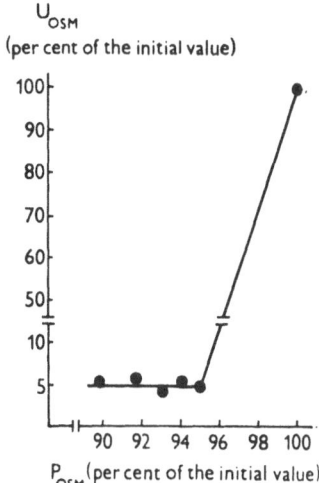

Fig. 47: Relationship between the decrease of plasma osmolarity (P_{osm}) and the decrease of urine osmolarity (U_{osm}) under conditions of maintained maximal water diuresis. (Water intake exceeded urinary excretion of solute-free water).

in a given subject, a further decrease induced by further water intake (exceeding excretion rate) does not result in a further decrease in U_{osm}. From data in 9 healthy volunteers it has been calculated that a water load of 22 ml/kg results in a minimal value of U_{osm}. This is slightly higher than the usually accepted water dosage level of 20 ml/kg.

Under these conditions FE_{H_2O} varies about 15%. This is in good agreement with data from micropuncture studies in rats which show that the volume of tubular urine at the start of the distal tubule and the net reabsorption of Na in the distal segment of the nephron also vary about a figure of 15%. In agreement with Smith's views (1951, 1956) it can be assumed that during maximal water diuresis tubular reabsorption of water in the distal segment of the nephron is negligibly small.

Clinical evaluation of dilution capacity

1. The usual evaluation of the dilution capacity of the kidney involves measurement of U_{osm}. This is certainly more accurate than measurement of urine specific gravity. Physiologically, however, it would be more correct to evaluate U_{osm} in relation to P_{osm}. The (U_{osm}/P_{osm}) ratio is called the *concentration index*. Since P_{osm} can vary only to a very limited degree, the U_{osm} value alone is usually of clinical value.

If we make the assumption that during maximal water diuresis water reabsorption in the distal segment of the nephron is negligible, then the concentration index is a measure of that portion of total osmotically active solute, still present in the lumen at the start of the dilution segment, which actually appears in the final urine.

If, for example, the concentration index at the peak of a water diuresis decreases to 0.2, then 20% of the total osmotic load in the lumen in the thick segment of the loop of Henle finds its way into the final urine. Thus, $(U_{osm}/P_{osm}) \times 100$ under conditions of maximal water diuresis gives us the *distal exretion fraction of osmotically active solutes*. Then $(1 - (U_{osm}/P_{osm}) \times 100 =$ the *distal fractional reabsorption of osmotically active* solutes.

2. The dilution capacity of the kidney can be evaluated from the diuresis which follows the oral water load. This can be accomplished in a number of ways:

a) we can measure the *maximal urine flow rate* in ml/min (V) . V, however, is a function of both the decrease in water reabsorption in the diluting segment and the level of GFR. With a GFR of 120 ml/min the rate of urine flow (with $FE_{H_2O} = 15\%$) can reach 18 ml/min, but with GFR = 30 ml/min (with the same FE for water) the maximal rate of urine flow can only reach 4.5 ml/min.

b) *Cumulative excretion of water.* In this case we measure the total volume of urine excreted after administration of the water load, usually over a 3–4 hr period. Usually, this total value is expressed as a % of the water load volume.

c) The maximal rate of urine flow per min. or s. as related to GFR, i.e. *the maximal value of FE_{H_2O}.* In patients in an advanced state of chronic renal disease the initial value of FE_{H_2O} is already above normal because of the osmotic diuresis in residual nephrons.

3. The degree of water diuresis can be evaluated as the *clearance of solute--free water* (C_{H_2O}). This parameter expresses the rate of urinary excretion of "pure" water, i.e. water not containing osmotically active solutes. The equation for this calculation is:

$$C_{H_2O} = V - C_{osm} \tag{1}$$

C_{H_2O} is usually expressed in relation to GFR as a % value : $(C_{H_2O}/GFR) \times 100$. Evaluation of the dilution capacity of the kidney by the latter expression is of value, particularly in cases where a water diuresis is superimposed on an existing osmotic diuresis. In such cases U_{osm} does not decrease to very low values after a water load, but $(C_{H_2O}/GFR) \times 100$ is found to be within normal limits or even slightly above, apparently because of the increased luminal load of osmotically active solute in the diluting segment of the nephron. Since distal reabsorption of osmotically active solute (T^d_{osm}) is quantitatively due mainly to distal reabsorption of Na (T^d_{Na}) and accompanying anions, we can indirectly estimate distal reabsorption of Na in terms of C_{H_2O}. Since Na^+ reabsorption is mainly accompanied by a univalent anion (mainly Cl^-), the relation between T^d_{osm} and T^d_{Na} can be expressed, in simpli-

144

fied form, as follows:

$$T_{Na}^d = \frac{T_{osm}^d}{2} = \frac{C_{H_2O} \times P_{osm}}{2} \tag{2}$$

Equation (2) suggests a simple linear relation between values of T_{Na}^d and C_{H_2O}. On more detailed analysis of distal reabsorption of Na one should, however, take into account that part of Na transport at this site is in exchange for K^+ and NH_4^- and that the latter process is reflected neither in a change in luminal osmolality nor in the calculated value for C_{H_2O}.

SIMPLE ("BOLUS") WATER LOAD

An oral water load, in a dosage of 22 ml/kg, should be drunk by the subject within 30 min. The investigation is carried out in the morning, as far as possible in an isolated, quiet room. A small breakfast of a dry role or slice of bread with a cup of unsweetened tea can be allowed. At 7:00 or 8:00 AM the subject empties his bladder, thus starting the first collection period. Following bladder emptying, the water load (room temperature) is administered. To prevent any action of excessive hypotonicity on the gastric mucosa, the water load should be tap water, not distilled. The load is usually tolerated better if made up as unsweetened weak tea. Urine is then collected at 30 min intervals for the next 3–4 hours. It is usually best to have the subject seated (except for micturition) during the investigation and all urine samples are voided spontaneously. Reading of light literature is usually of advantage over the 3–4 hour period. If fluid retention (e.g. idiopathic oedema) is suspected, the investigation should be carried out twice at an interval of a few

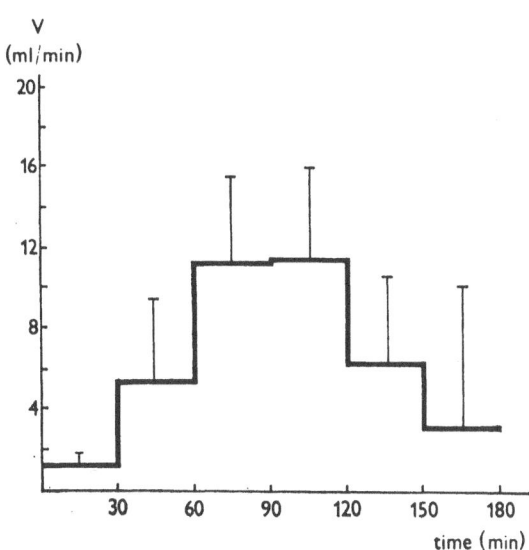

Fig. 48: Time course of urine flow rate (V) after water load (22 ml/kg) in healthy subjects.

145

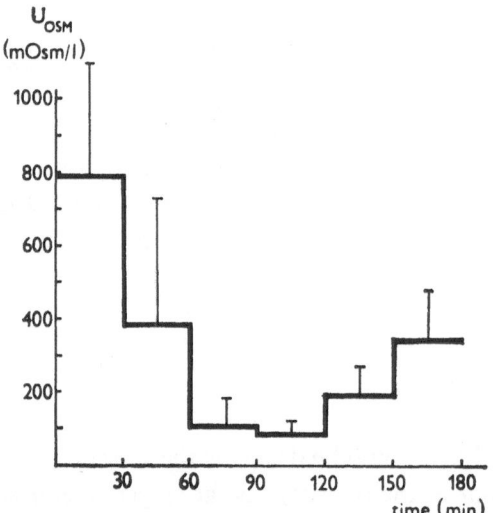

Fig. 49: Time-course of urine osmolarity (U_{osm}) after water load (22 ml/kg) in healthy subjects.

days — once in a reclining position and once again while walking about the room. The subject is weighed before and after the investigation. Each urine sample is measured, for purposes of orientation only, for changes in specific gravity. Otherwise, the osmolalities of all urine samples are measured and, if desired, also creatinine concentrations of both urine and serum from blood withdrawn at the height of the diuresis as estimated both by urine flow rate and minimal U_{osm}

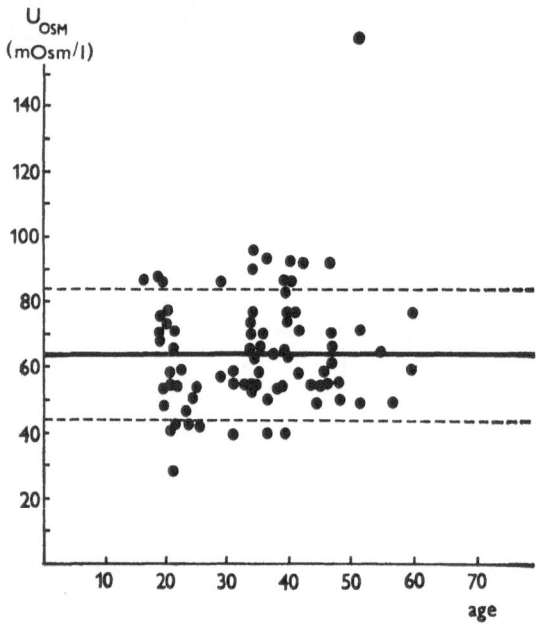

Fig. 50: Minimal values of urine osmolarity (U_{osm}) after water load (22 ml/kg) in healthy subjects of various age.

146

(specific gravity) in successive samples. This peak period usually occurs in the 3rd or 4th 30-min collection period.

The time course of changes in urine flow rate in healthy subjects on a normal diet is shown in Fig. 48. From this it is clear that maximal diuresis occurs between 60 and 120 min after the oral water load. The time course of changes in U_{osm}

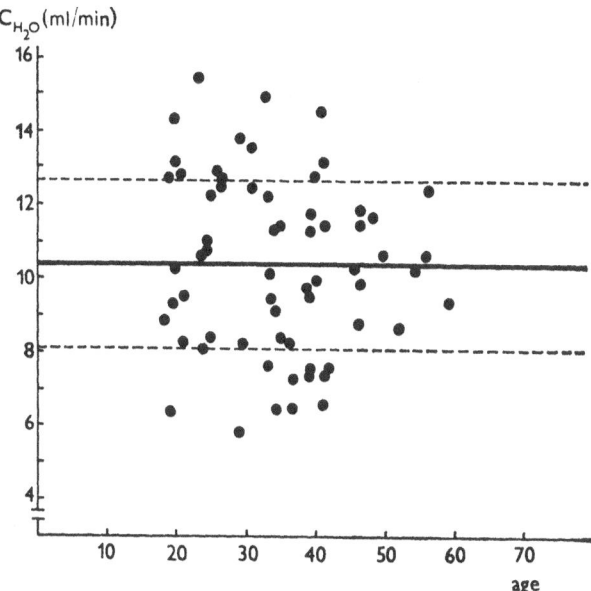

Fig. 51: Maximal values of solute-free water (C_{H2O}) after water load (22 ml/kg) in healthy subjects of various age.

shown in Fig. 49. The lowest values are attained between 90 and 120 min after the oral water load. Fig. 50 shows a comparison between age and minimum U_{osm} values in 86 healthy subjects from 17 to 59 years of age. In the given age range no relation between the two parameters could be seen. There is, however, published data that at age 70 or greater, peak diuretic urine specific gravity and osmolality values are higher than in young and middle-aged healthy subjects (Nádvorníková 1968, Dontas et al. 1972).

Values of $(C_{H_2O}/C_{cr}) \times 100$ also showed no relation to the age of the subject (Fig. 51). Mean values $\pm$ SD for parameters measured in this series of healthy volunteers aged 17 to 59 years (standard water load 22 ml/kg over 30 min) were as follows:

Table 1

U_{osm}	63 ± 20 mOsm/l
$V/C_{cr} \times 100$	$13.8 \pm 3.3\%$
$C_{osm}/C_{cr} \times 100$	$2.3 \pm 0.8\%$
$C_{H_2O}/C_{cr} \times 100$	$11.4 \pm 2.8\%$

The peak of maximal water diuresis at about 60 mOsm/l is equivalent to specific gravity measurements during the experiment of 1.000 to 1.002. The mean $U_{osm} +$ $+ 1$ SD equals, in this series, 83 mOsm/l. These values were achieved with values of $(C_{osm}/C_{cr}) \times 100$ about 2.3%. The lowest observed value of U_{osm} was about 40 mOsm/l.

For ordinary clinical evaluation, these values have the following approximate meaning:

In the age range between 17 and 59 years, with a normal diet and conditions as above, U_{osm} after a "bolus" oral water load of 22 ml/kg (over 30 min) should decrease in healthy subjects to below 100 mOsm/l. These findings are in agreement with those published elsewhere (Smith 1956).

Table 1 shows that at the height of maximal water diuresis fractional excretion of water attains an average values of 14%, in agreement with the views expressed above on maximal suppression of water reabsorption in the diluting segment of the nephron at peak diuresis. In a few cases this value reaches 20%. From the above results, healthy subjects under the given conditions of testing should show an FE_{H_2O} value of at least 10%.

Evaluation of a cumulative group of investigations of healthy subjects from 17–90 years of age (Nádvorníková 1968) showed that the volume of excreted water over 4 hr after the oral water load decreased significantly with age (Fig. 52). This volume relation with age was explained by an age-related decrease in GFR.

The clearance of solute-free water (per 100 ml C_{cr}) was about 11% in these healthy subjects. The lowest value which can be expected in healthy subjects would be 8.0%.

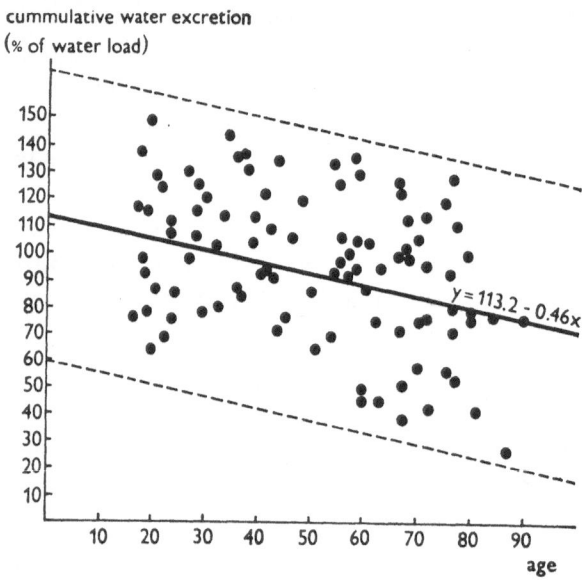

cummulative water excretion
(% of water load)

$y = 113.2 - 0.46x$

age

Fig. 52: Cummulative water excretion over 4 hr after water load (22 ml/kg) in healthy subjects of various age.

148

MAINTAINED MAXIMAL WATER DIURESIS

This variation of diuretic investigation is of use in studying the action of such factors as drugs on tubular reabsorption of Na in the distal nephron. Up to the end of the first 30-min period initiation of the investigation is the same as in the "bolus" experiment. When urine volume is measured after the first and as many subsequent 30-min periods as desired, the subject drinks the same volume as excreted as soon as that volume is measured, +1 ml for each minute elapsed in the collection period (i.e. + 30 ml in the case of 30-min periods) to cover insensible water loss. Thus the initial hypotonic load of 22 ml of extra water/kg body weight is maintained constant for the several hours required for an experiment. Urine is again collected by spontaneous voiding, and if very high urine flow rates are attained, the collection periods will have to be shortened to 20 or 10 min to prevent incomfortable bladder distension.

A stabilized maximal water diuretic state should be so reproducible that the flow rate of urine/min should not vary by more than 1.0–1.5 ml, provided that no other stimulus (drug) is administered.

INDUCTION OF WATER DIURESIS BY INTRAVENOUS INFUSION OF A HYPOTONIC SOLUTION

The most frequently used infusion solution is 1/2-normal, or 0.45% (w/v) NaCl, the osmotic concentration of which is 154 mOsm/l. In order to maximalize suppression of endogenous VP secretion, a small amount of ethyl alcohol can be added. Since this infusion is usually given at a high rate, it is wise first to test the osmotic resistance of the patient's erythrocytes from a blood sample in vitro, in order to prevent the possibility of haemolysis during a subsequent infusion investigation.

A water diuresis can be induced only by infusing 0.45% NaCl, but in actual practice it is wise to start with the same oral load as above (22 ml tap water/kg body weight over 30 min) and then to maintain the maximal water diuresis by infusion maintenance of the load. The infusion rate can vary from 10 to 20 ml/min. In children the rate of infusion is 1000 ml/1.73 m² of body surface area over 2 hr (Rodriguez-Soriano et al. 1980).

The infusion rate is adjusted in order to stabilize and maintain the maximal water diuresis state, by watching urine flow rates and osmolarity from the preceding period.

Maximal values of $(C_{H_2O}/C_{cr}) \times 100$ measured during infusion of 0.45% NaCl are usually somewhat higher than when the diuresis is induced and maintained by tap water alone. It would appear likely that the expansion of ECF volume due to the infusion of salt decreases tubular reabsorption of Na in the proximal nephron so that the diluting segment of the nephron receives a somewhat higher input load of isotonic luminal fluid. The result of this would be an increase in C_{H_2O}.

Indications for investigation

1. Normovolaemic hyponatraemia of unknown cause

This involves patients with hyponatraemia not associated with either oedema or signs of ECT volume depletion. Normovolaemic hyponatraemia can be associated with inappropriate ADH secretion syndrome (SIADH), hypopituitarism, hypothyroidism or the use of some drugs which have antidiuretic properties.

Clinical recognition of hypopituitary and hypothyroid states are based on clinical history and examination and the appropriate endocrinological workup — this does not belong in the context of the present monograph and is dealt with elsewhere.

Recognition of SIADH is not always a simple task. This possible diagnosis can be considered when normovolaemic hyponatraemia is associated with any pathology in the CNS or lungs or with neoplastic disease located anywhere, but particularly in the lungs. SIADH can involve not only unregulated excess production and secretion of VP, but also abnormal appreciation of a thirst afferent signal.

Clinical workup of SIADH candidates show no signs of abnormal cardiac or liver function, there are no signs of either dehydration or oedema or other signs of hypervolaemia. Of great importance, from the viewpoint of renal functional investigation, for establishing a diagnosis of SIADH are the following signs:

1) the patient continually forms urine of high osmolarity
2) the dilution capacity of the kidney is below normal — a water load is not followed by the expected decrease in U_{osm} and increase in urine flow rate
3) GFR, as estimated by C_{cr}, is in the normal range
4) Na excretion into the urine is above normal
5) P_{osm} is below normal.

A raised plasma level of VP can be measured by RIA. More detailed investigation of SIADH patients should involve measurement of plasma VP levels in relation to changes in P_{osm} (Robertson et al. 1977).

Some patients with normovolaemic hyponatraemia behave as if their "osmostat" were reset downward. Excretion of water load is normal, but low serum osmolarity is maintained. Patients with tuberculosis and cirrhosis appear to predispose to this disorder.

2. Idiopathic oedema

The clinician often meets with cases, particularly young females, with transitory oedema but no signs of organ disease (heart, liver or kidneys) which could explain retention of Na and water. Serum Na concentrations are normal.

These women often show an abnormal diluting capacity of the kidney when investigated in a vertical position. When reclining, the diluting capacity of the kidney is normal.

Such a finding has been explained as an increase in capillary permeability with transudation of ECF from the vascular compartment to the extravascular in the lower limbs in the upright position. The resulting decrease in circulating plasma volume gives rise to secretion of both aldosterone and VP. The upright position can also be associated with haemodynamic changes which decrease GFR.

3. The differential diagnosis of polyuric states

The most important diagnostic point to be decided is whether we are dealing with a water diuresis, an osmotic diuresis or a mixture of both.

"Water polyuria" is characterized by a combination of U_{osm} less than P_{osm} and FE_{osm} in the normal range (i.e. does not exceed 4%). As explained later (cf.p. 161) polyuria resulting from osmotic diuresis is associated with an FE_{osm} greater than 4% and U_{osm} is higher, or at the same levels as P_{osm}.

If the polyuria is the result of a water diuresis, then one must differentiate between the following three pathological states:
1. central DI
2. psychogenic polydipsia and
3. nephrogenic DI.

To do this, the patient must be taken off any drug administered to mitigate the polyuria, and time allowed until the polyuric state is reestablished. Investigation starts then by stopping fluid intake, emptying of the bladder and starting of collection of urine samples at hourly intervals. If a high rate of urine flow continues despite a lack of fluid intake, significant dehydration will develop within several hours. For example, if the initial urine flow rate is 10 ml/min, 1.8 l of urine will form in 3 hr and this will show up as an easily measurable weight loss.

Developing dehydration can also be measured as a rise in P_{osm}. If water respresents about 60% of body weight, then a 70 kg subject with an initial P_{osm} of 290 mOsm/kg will, after a loss of 1.5 l of water, show a P_{osm} of

$$(42 \times 290) / (42 - 1.5) = 301 \text{ mOsm/kg},$$

a measurable change.

If removal of fluid intake in this investigation is followed by a decrease in urine flow rate and a rise in U_{osm} to values $2 \times P_{osm}$ or higher, then central DI can be excluded and psychogenic polydipsia entertained as a diagnosis.

If absence of fluid intake is not accompanied by a decrease in urine flow rate and a rise in U_{osm}, we must further distinguish between central and nephrogenic DI by administering exogenous VP or a VP-like peptide.

After 4–5 collection periods without an endogenous antidiuretic reaction, either 5 IU of Pitressin tannate in oil i.m. or — 5 units of aquoeous vasopressin subcutaneously are given. If the patient has central DI, he will respond (within 2 hours with Pitressin, within 30 min with dDAVP) with a marked decrease in urine flow rate and a rise in U_{osm}.

Difficulties in differetinal diagnosis will arise with cases of partial central DI in whom VP secretion is not completely gone — i.e. the patient will respond to absence of fluid intake with some degree of VP release, but not to a sufficient degree to produce a full antidiuretic response. In such cases, the differential diagnosis will only be certain with measurements of plasma levels of VP by RIA.

In patients with nephrogenic DI, exogenous VP at the above doses will not produce a decrease in urine flow rate and a rise in U_{osm}. If there is no family history to suggest a congential defect, the investigation must then be shifted on to the next stage — does the patient have a primary renal disease which has resulted in a loss of tubular sensitivity to the antidiuretic action of VP? Patients with either central DI or psychogenic polydipsia will, provided no co-existing primary renal disease is present, usually show normal GFR values.

Patients with acquired nephrogenic DI will often show a decreased GFR as a result of the primary renal disease which produced the syndrome.

4. Thirst and osmolarity of residual urine in patients in the terminal stages of chronic renal failure

Patients in the terminal stages of chronic renal failure often experience thirst and increase their spontaneous water intake to levels which their diseased kidneys cannot compensate for. If the patients are on a regular dialysis maintenance programme, this increase in spontaneous water intake is seen as a weight increase between dialysis sessions. If NaCl intake is too high, these weight increases are more pronouced. Analysis of cause and mechanism of this effect is seldom simple, and changes in serum Na concentration are not usually very informative.

Since the dilution capacity of residual nephrons is, per nephron, usually intact, it should be expected that with excess water loading these nephrons should produce hypotonic urine. Hypotonicity of residual urine could also result from vasopressin resistance. Fig. 53 summarizes U_{osm} data (116 observations in 50 patients) in subjects in a regular dialysis maintenance programme (all with C_{cr} below 6 ml/min). The mean value was 286 ± 57 mOsm/l. In about 1/2 the cases U_{osm} was below

300, and in a significant portion U_{osm} was below 250 mOsm/l. In agreement with this, $(C_{H_2O}/C_{cr}) \times 100$ was also raised in these patients, with a mean value of $2.3 \pm 4.7\%$ (Fig. 54).

Follow-up of regular measurements of $(C_{H_2O}/C_{cr}) \times 100$ in regularly dialyzed patients who show weight gains between dialysis sessions will draw attention to

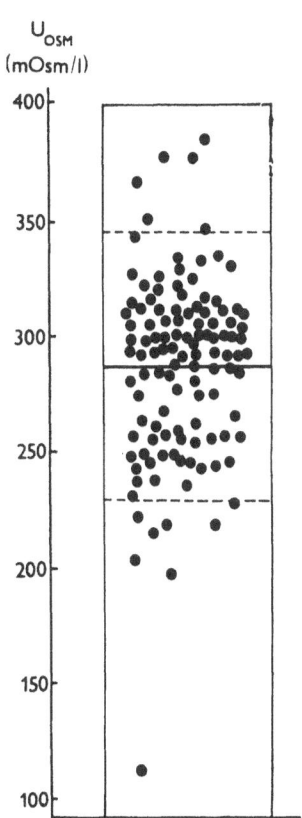

Fig. 53: Osmolarity of residual urine (U_{osm}) in patients with chronic renal failure on the regular dialysis maintenancs program

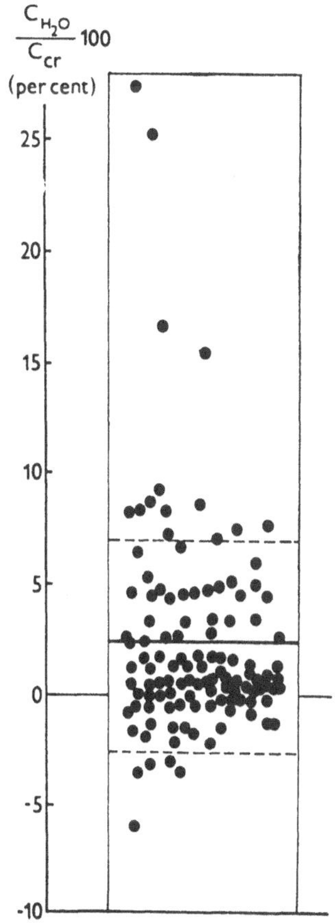

Fig. 54: Solute-free water clearance (calculated per 100 ml C_{cr}) in patients with chronic renal failure on the regular dialysis maintenance program.

abnormally high spontaneous water intake (Erben et al. 1981). Measurement of $(C_{H_2O}/C_{cr}) \times 100$ does not require quantitative collection of a urine sample and can be calculated from plasma and urine concentrations of creatinine and osmols, since the expression can be treated as follows:

$$(C_{H_2O}/C_{cr}) \times 100 = [(V - C_{osm})/C_{cr}] \times 100 = \frac{(1 - U_{osm}/P_{osm})}{U_{cr}/P_{cr}} \times 100 \qquad (3)$$

$(C_{H_2O}/C_{cr}) \times 100$ as a follow-up criterion is more useful than U_{osm} alone since, if a combination of water and osmotic diuresis exists, even a small decrease of U_{osm} below the level of P_{osm} can be related to a high degree of water diuresis.

5. Localization of changes in tubular reabsorption of Na based on measurement of C_{H_2O} or $(C_{H_2O}/C_{cr}) . 100$

As explained on p. 145, calculation of C_{H_2O} can give indirect evidence of changes in distal reabsorption of Na. This method has been widely applied in various physiological, pathophysiological and pharmacological studies. The subject should be in a state of maintained maximal water diuresis.

Contraindications to the investigation

Oral or i.v. water loading is contraindicated in patients with cardiovascular disease and in patients with renal insufficiency.

REFERENCES

Balment, R. J., Jones, I. C., Henderson, I. W. et al.: Effects of adrenalectomy and hypophysectomy on water and electrolyte metabolism in male and female rats with inherited hypothalamic diabetes insipidus. (Brattleboro strain). J. Endocrinol. *71*: 193, 1976

Anderson, B.: Regulation of body fluids. Ann. Rev. Physiol. *39*: 185, 1977

Berliner, R. W., Davidson, P. G.: Production of hypertonic urine in the abscence of pituitary antidiuretic hormone. J. clin. Invest. *36*: 1416, 1957

Bray, J. A.: Freezing point depression of rat kidney slices during water diuresis and antidiuresis. Am. J. Physiol. *199*: 15, 1960

Cohen, L. F., diSant'agnese, P. A., Taylor et al.: The syndrome of inappropriate antidiuretic hormone secretion as a cause of hyponatremia in cystic fibrosis. J. Pediatrics *4*: 574, 1977

Coscia, M., Brown, R. D., Miller,M . et al.: Ectopic production of antidiuretic hormone (ADH), adrenocorticotrophic hormone (ACTH) and beta-melanocyte stimulating hormone by an oat cell carcinoma of the lung. Am. J. Med. *62*: 303, 1977

Dontas: Mechanism of renal tubular defect in old age. Postgrad. med. J. *48*: 293, 1972

Dousa, T. P., Valtin, H.: Action of antidiuretic hormone in mice with inherited vasopressin-resistant urinary concentration defects. J. clin. Invest. *54*: 753, 1974

Dousa, T. P.: Cellular actions of vasopressin in the mammalian kidney. Kidney int. *10*: 46, 1976

Dunn, M. J., Hood, V. L.: Prostaglandins and the kidney. Am. J. Physiol. *2*: F 169, 1977

Erben, J., Schück, O., Zahradnik, J., Nádvorniková, H.: Osmolarita residuální moči nemocných v pravidelném dialysačním programu. Čas. Lék. Čes. *120*, 1206, 1981

Fanestil, D. D.: Hypoosmolar syndrome. In: Disturbances in body fluid osmolality. Ed. T. E. Andreoti, J. J. Grantham, F. C. Rector Jr. Bethesda, Am. Physiol. Soc. 1977, 267—284

Fichman, M. P.: Disorders of renal concentration and dilution: hyponatremia and hypernatremia. In: Current Nephrology, Vol. 2 Ed. H. C. Gonick Boston Houghton Mifflin Prof. Publ., 1978, 145–261

Gottschalk, C. W., Mylle: Micropuncture study of mammalian urinary concentrating mechanism: evidence for the countercurrent hypothesis. Am. J. Physiol. *196*: 927, 1959

Johnson, M. D., Malvin, R. L.: Stimulation of renal sodium reabsorption by angiotensin II. Am. J. Physiol. *1*: F 198, 1977

Leaf, A., Frazier, H. S.: Some recent studies on the action of neurohypophyseal hormones. Progr. Cardiovase. Dis. *4*: 47, 1961

Nádvorniková, H.: Konzentrations- und Dilutionsfähigkeit bei Erwachsenen und im Alter. Z. ges. inn. Med. *24*: 810, 1968

Nonnenbruch, W.: Über die Beurteilung der Nierenfunktion in der Praxis. Med. Welt 577, 1941

Orloff, J., Handler, J.: The role of adenosine 3', 5' — phosphate in the action of antidiuretic hormone. Am. J. Med. *42*: 757, 1967

Padfield, P. L., Morton, J. J., Brown, J. J. et al. Plasma arginine vasopressin in the syndrome of antidiuretic hormone excess associated with bronchogenic carcinoma. Am. J. Med. *61*: 825, 1976

Randall, R. V., Clark, E. C., Bahn, R. C.: Classification of the causes of diabetes insipidus. Proc. Mayo Clin. *34*: 299, 1959

Robertson, G. L., Athar, S., Shelton, R. L.: Osmotic control of vasopressin function. In: Disturbances in body fluid osmolality. Eds. T. E. Andreoti, J. J. Grantham, F. C. Rector Jr. Bethesda, Amer. Physiol. Soc. 1977, 125–148

Rodriguez-Soriano, J., Vallo, A., Castillo, G., Oliveros, R.: Renal handling of water and sodium in children with proximal and distal renal tubular acidosis. Nephron *25*: 193, 1980

Ross, L. S., Franki, N., Hays, R. M.: Independent control of water and urea transport. Kidney int. (abstr.) *10*: 597, 1976

Schafer, J. A., Andreoli, Th. E.: The effect of antidiuretic hormone on solute flows in mammalian collecting tubules. J. clln. Invest. *51*: 1279, 1972

Schrier, R. W., Berl, T., Anderson, R. J. et al. Nonosmolar control of renal water excretion. In: Disturbances in body fluid osmolality. Eds. T. E. Andreoti, J. J. Grantham, F. C. Rector Jr. Bethesda, Amer. Physiol. Soc. 1977, 149–178

Seif, S. M., Zenser, T. V., Huellmantel, A. B. et al.: Elevated plasma vasopressin in impaired renal cyclic nucleotide generation in myxedematous rats. Endocrine Society (Abstr.) 1977, p. 243

Smith, H. W.: The kidney; structure and function in health and disease. New York, Oxford Univ. Press, 1951

Smith, H. W.: Principles of renal physiology. New York, Oxford Univ. Press, 1956

Schwartz, I. L., Rasmussen, H., Schoessler, M. A., Silver, L., Fong, C. T. O.: Relation of chemical attachment to physiological action of vasopressin. Proc. nat. Acad. Sci *46*: 1288, 1960

Thibonnier, M. J., Marchetti, J. P., Corvoli, P. L., Menard, J. E., Sire, O. G., Milliez, P. L.: Influence of previous diuretic intake on the humoral and hormonal profile of idiopathic oedema. Europ. J. clin. Invest. *11*: 19, 1981

Thomas, T. H., Lee, M. R.: The specifity of antisera for the radioimmunoassay of arginine-vasopressin in human plasma and urine during water loading and dehydration. Clin. Sci. mol. Med. *51*: 525, 1976

Ullrich, K. J., Jarausch, K. H.: Untersuchungen zum Problem der Harnkonzentrierung und Harnverdünnung. Pflüger's Arch. ges. Physiol. *267*: 207, 1956

Urakabe, S., Takamitsu, Y., Shirai, D., Yuassa, S., Kimura, G., Orita, Y., Abe, H.: Effect of different prostaglandins on the permeability of the toad urinary bladder. Comp. Biochem. Physioi. *52*: 1, 1975

Verney, E. B.: Antidiuretic hormone and factors which determine its release. Proc. roy. Soc. Med. *135*: 25, 1947

Volhard, F.: Über defunktionelle Untersuchung der Schrumpfnieren. Verh. dtsch. Ges. inn. Med. *27:* 735, 1910

Walker, A. M., Bott, P. A., Oliver, J., McDowell, M. C.: The collection and analysis of fluid from single nephrons of the mammalian kidney. Am. J. Physiol. *134:* 580, 1941

Walker, L., Whorton, R., France, R. et al.: Antidiuretic hormone increased renal prostaglandin E_2 production in rats (Brattelboro) with hereditary hypothalamic diabetes insipidus. Fed. Proc. *36:* 402, 1977

Wirz, H., Hargitay, B., Kuhn, W.: Lokalisation des Konzentrierungsprozesses in der Niere durch direkte Kryoskopie. Helv. physiol. pharmacol. Acta *9:* 196, 1951

Wirz, H.: Der osmotische Druck der corticalen Tubuli der Rattenniere. Helv. physiol. pharmacol. Acta *14:* 353, 1956

Wohltmann, J., Halushka, P. V., Privitera, P. J. et al.: Effects of indomethacin on fluid intake, urine volume, urine prostaglandin E like material and kallikrein in vasopressin resistant diabetes insipidus. Pediatr. Res. *11:* 433, 1977

Zusman, R. M., Keiser, H. R.: Prostaglandin biosynthesis by rabbit renomedullary interstitial cells in tissue cultures: stimulation by angiotensin II, bradykinin, and arginine vasopressin. J. clin. Invest. *60:* 215, 1977

EXCRETION OF OSMOTICALLY ACTIVE SOLUTES

PHYSIOLOGY AND PATHOPHYSIOLOGY

Measurement of the urinary excretion of osmotically active solutes is an important part of investigation of both concentrating and diluting functions of the kidney. It stands by itself as a technique, in human subjects, of measuring tubular transport of these solutes, and is of particular importance in deciding whether osmotic diuresis has developed as a result of primary renal disease or not.

Under conditions of a balanced metabolic state with no significant extrarenal losses of water and electrolytes, the total elimination of osmotically active solutes is determined by the renal excretion mainly of Na, K, ammonia and urea. With some degree of simplification, the relation between total excretion of osmotically active solutes ($U_{osm}V$) and the above urinary components can be expressed as follows:

$$U_{osm}V = 2(U_{Na}V + U_{K}V + U_{NH_4}V) + U_{urea}V \qquad (1)$$

The factor of 2 is inserted for the cations to allow for accompanying anions. It is clear from this that total excretion of osmotically active solutes will be a function of their oral intake in the diet (i.e., intake of Na, K and protein).

Equation (1) is valid if no other osmotically active solutes, such as glucose in patients with diabetes mellitus or mannitol infused to induce osmotic diuresis, enter into the determination of $U_{osm}V$.

The total value of $U_{osm}V$ is also determined by the filtered load of osmotically active solute (GFR $\times$ P_{osm}) and the amount of reabsorbed solute in the tubules (T_{osm}), both in the same time unit. Therefore,

$$U_{osm}V = GFR \times P_{osm} - T_{osm} \qquad (2)$$

Equation (2) indicates that an increase in $U_{osm}V$ can occur either because of an increase in GFR $\times$ P_{osm} or a decrease in T_{osm}. The former case can be referred to as an **overflow osmotic diuresis**.

P_{osm} can be increased by a number of circumstances, e.g. increases in plasma levels of glucose or urea. An exogenous substance such as mannitol will give the same result.

An increase in GFR can play a role in producing overflow osmotic diuresis in patients with a reduced number of functioning glomeruli. In residual nephrons the single nephron GFR (SNGFR) can be increased even though total kidney GFR is decreased. In this case, it is the filtered osmotic load per nephron which increases.

If the increase in $U_{osm}V$ is due to a decrease in T_{osm}, the state is referred to as a **tubular osmotic diuresis.** This can occur 1) if the reabsorptive capacity for a given osmotically active solute is saturated, or 2) is decreased by virtue of a pathological process. An example of the above is osmotic diuresis in renal diabetes mellitus. The decrease in T_{osm} can also be deliberately induced by such drugs as diuretics (saluretics). Obviously, both overflow and tubular forms of osmotic diuresis can co-exist.

In practice, we usually calculate fractional excretions (FE_{osm}) indicating excretion of osmotically active solutes per nephron:

$$FE_{osm} = \frac{U_{osm}V}{GFR \times P_{osm}} \, 100 \tag{3}$$

Under normal conditions, FE_{osm} varies between 2 and 3%, i.e. FR_{osm} varies from 97 to 98%.

FE_{osm} should be calculated in order to evaluate excretion of osmotically active solutes in patients with a decreased GFR due to chronic renal disease. The absolute value of $U_{osm}V$ in such patients need not be increased (and can even be low) despite the fact that the residual nephrons are in a state of osmotic diuresis. In addition, the rate of urine flow need not be increased despite a significant decrease in the fractional reabsorption of water in residual nephrons.

A number of factors play a role in the development of osmotic diuresis in the residual nephrons of patients with chronic renal disease. Due to the factors listed above, this state can be characterized as a combination of overflow and tubular factors. Contributing to the overflow factor are both an increase in plasma urea concentration and increase of SNGFR in the residual nephrons. The tubular component is mainly the decrease in tubular reabsorption of Na. This decrease in FR_{Na} is adaptive in nature, allowing a maintenance of Na and volume homeostasis under conditions where most of the nephron population is out of function. In some cases, the decrease in FR_{Na} results from an abnormality of the tubular cells per se — this is dealt with in detail on p. 184.

Increased excretion of osmotically active solutes is usually associated with an increase in urine flow rate. To what degree the decrease in solute reabsorption determines urine flow rate depends upon a number of factors. Decreased proximal tubular solute reabsorption is accompanied by a proportional decrease in water reabsorption. In other words the ratio of solute to water in the ECF remains the same since the proximal tubular wall is freely permeable to water.

Such an effect in the proximal tubule results in an increased delivery of luminal

158

fluid to the distal nephron. The final product then depends upon the rate of reabsorption of osmotically active solutes in the distal nephron and the permeability of the latter to water. Unreabsorbed solutes and water from the distal nephron make up the final urine sample.

If distal reabsorption of osmotically active solutes is decreased, the change in water reabsorption depends upon water permeability in the same segment: if the starting value of distal water reabsorption is high, then a decrease in solute reabsorption decreases water reabsorption and urine flow rate increases.

If the starting level is low (e.g. the investigated subject is in water diuresis) then a decrease in distal solute reabsorption leaves the urine flow rate relatively unchanged.

These comments can be utilized, for example, to localize the site of action of diuretics on tubular reabsorption of Na.

METHODS OF INVESTIGATION

EXCRETION OF OSMOTICALLY ACTIVE SOLUTES PER 24 HOURS

This investigation involves no more than accurate collection of the total 24 hr urine volume and measurement of U_{osm} in the mixed sample. $U_{osm}V$ usually varies between 600 and 800 mOsm/24 hr, this value being dependent upon the rate of excretion of Na, K, ammonia, and urea, as presented above. When protein and salt intakes are high, $U_{osm}V$ can exceed 1000 mOsm/24 hr. It can be calculated that if $I_{Na} = 300$ mmol/24 hr, K intake = 90 mmol/24 h and $I_{Pr} = 100$ g/24 hr, $U_{osm}V$ — in a balanced state — should be about 1330 mOsm/24 hr.

THE OSMOLAR CLEARANCE (C_{osm})

This value is calculated by the classic clearance equation:

$$C_{osm} = \frac{U_{osm}V}{P_{osm}} \qquad (4)$$

Aside from determining $U_{osm}V$ as above, this measurement requires only one further sampling of venous blood. The duration of the measurement period can vary from several to 24 hr. In healthy adults on a normal diet, C_{osm} usually varies between 2 and 3 ml/min. Any value above 4 ml/min is abnormal. C_{osm} relates the rate of excretion of osmotically active solutes to plasma concentration. P_{osm} in normal subjects = 285–295 mOsm/kg.

An increase in P_{osm} in patients with renal disease is most usually the result of a rise in plasma urea concentration. In severely ill patients P_{osm} can be increased by 40–50 mOsm/kg. In water depletion Na will play the major role in an increase in P_{osm}, in diabetics the role is taken over by glucose.

A decrease in P_{osm} in patients with renal disease is usually conditioned by water retention and is associated with hyponatraemia.

Calculation of C_{osm} over a 24 hr period is of practical significance in patients in the advanced stage of chronic renal disease who are unable to form hypertonic urine. In patients with isosthenuria, urine volume per unit time varies with C_{osm}.

Knowledge of intake levels of Na, K and protein allows us to estimate the volume of isosthenuric urine which such patients must form if an external balanced state of osmotically active substances is to be maintained.

THE FRACTIONAL EXCRETION OF OSMOTICALLY ACTIVE SUBSTANCES (FE$_{osm}$)

Measurement of this parameter requires, in addition to the above, also measurement of urine and plasma creatinine levels. The collection period can vary — it should be stressed that for this calculation accurate urine collection is not necessary (for calculation see p. 262).

In healthy adults on a normal diet, our mean FE_{osm} values are $2.3 \pm 0.8\%$. The upper limit of normal is considered to be 4%.

Calculation of FE_{osm} enables us to judge whether osmotic diuresis exists in the investigated subject or not. It is not enough for this purpose to measure only V, $U_{osm}V$ and C_{osm}. The latter parameters can be used for this purpose only if GFR is within the normal range. With renal disease associated with a decrease in GFR and osmotic diuresis there occurs an increase in the fractional excretion of water (FE_{H_2O}). The latter parameter is calculated as:

$$FE_{H_2O} = \frac{V}{GFR} \times 100 = \frac{P_{cr}}{U_{cr}} \times 100 \qquad (5)$$

Healthy adults on a normal diet and fluids ad libitum show FE_{H_2O} levels about 1.0%. With a low water intake this parameter can decrease to about 0.4%. Any calculated value higher than 2.0% is considered abnormal.

With isosthenuria and U_{osm} approaching values of P_{osm}, levels of FE_{H_2O} and FE_{osm} are practically identical.

INDUCED OSMOTIC DIURESIS

Measurement of the reabsorption of solute-free water ($T^c_{H_2O}$) under conditions of induced osmotic diuresis can be used to test the concentrating capacity of the kidney. Mannitol is used for this purpose, and for details of the procedure cf.p. 126.

Indications for investigation

Differential diagnosis of polyuric states

Diagnosing the existence of an endogenous osmotic diuresis requires the measurement of FE_{osm}. In patients with polyuria on the basis of a water diuresis, FE_{osm} lies within a normal range. With a combined water and osmotic diuretic state, FE_{osm} is increased, but U_{osm} is lower than P_{osm}.

In patients with osmotic diuresis, U_{osm} is usually isotonic or slightly hypertonic to plasma, but in extreme cirumstances urine that is slightly hypotonic may be produced.

The differencial diagnostic criteria for evaluation of these polyuric states are shown in table 1.

Table 1

Parameter	Water diuresis	Osmotic diuresis	Combined diuresis
U_{osm}	$< P_{osm}$	$\gg P_{osm}$	$< P_{osm}$
FE_{H_2O}	increased	increased	increased
FE_{osm}	normal	increased	increased
$(C_{H_2O}/C_{cr}) \times 100$	> 0	$\leqslant 0$	> 0

Thus we can not only determine the existence of osmotic diuresis on the basis of polyuria, but also determine the cause or the mechanisms involved.

The first task is to determine the presence or absence of overflow or tubular osmotic diuresis — and P_{osm} values are of assistance here. If the latter parameter is raised, the contents of the increased solute concentration must be analyzed. First attention is given to Na, urea and glucose.

If P_{osm} is normal, an increased FE_{osm} is conditioned mainly by a decreased fractional reabsorption of osmotically active solutes. Further investigation will be required to establish all the chemical components of the osmotic substances which are not being adequately reabsorbed. Of practical importance is to determine whether Na plays a major role in the latter effect.

Differentiation between the two types of osmotic diuresis can be accomplished by calculating the ratio C_{Na}/C_{osm}. If Na plays a major role in the osmotic diuresis, this ratio should be significantly raised.

Investigation of 71 healthy volunteers gave a mean value of $(C_{Na}/C_{osm}) \times 100 =$ $= 32.2 \pm 8.5\%$.

When Na plays a significant role in producing the osmotic diuresis, this ratio can reach 90%. An example of this is the polyuria produced by diuretic drugs. For example, after administration of furosemide i.v. (20 mg) the ratio reached a mean value of 94%; ethacrynic acid administration (50 mg) yielded a ratio of 89%. Osmotic diuresis, produced by a load not involving Na, resulted mainly in the excretion of the substance (e.g. mannitol) used to induce the diuresis, so that the ratio $(C_{Na}/C_{osm}) \times 100$ was increased, but not to levels seen when Na was the main osmotic element of the diuresis. A high mannitol-induced diuresis will result in a ratio of 40% — values over 50% are seldom seen.

Evaluation of the degree of osmotic diuresis in chronic renal insufficiency

In patients in advanced stages of chronic renal disease osmotic diuresis is present in the residual nephrons. Both an increase in P_{osm} (urea) and a decrease in FR_{osm} (mainly Na) play roles in this. Total 24 hr urine volume in these patients can be raised, but normal or decreased values do not exclude the presence of osmotic diuresis in the residual nephrons.

A basic criterion for judging osmotic diuresis in residual nephrons is FE_{osm}. This parameter increases in hyperbolic relation to the decrease in GFR (Fig. 55). As can be seen in this Fig. extremely low values of GFR are associated with FE_{osm}

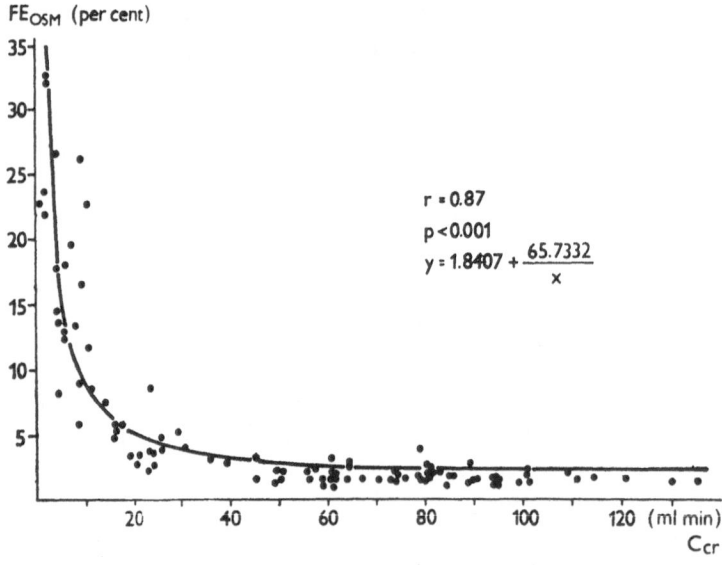

Fig. 55: Relationship between clearance of endogenous creatinine (C_{cr}) and fractional excretion of osmotically active substances (FE_{osm}) in patients with chronic renal diseases.

values about 30%. Stated otherwise, the fractional reabsorption of osmotically active solutes can decrease to values about 70% or even lower in some cases. Analogous to the increase in FE_{osm}, FE_{H_2O} also increases in hyperbolic relation to GFR (Fig. 56). With very low values of GFR, FE_{H_2O} can also reach 30%.

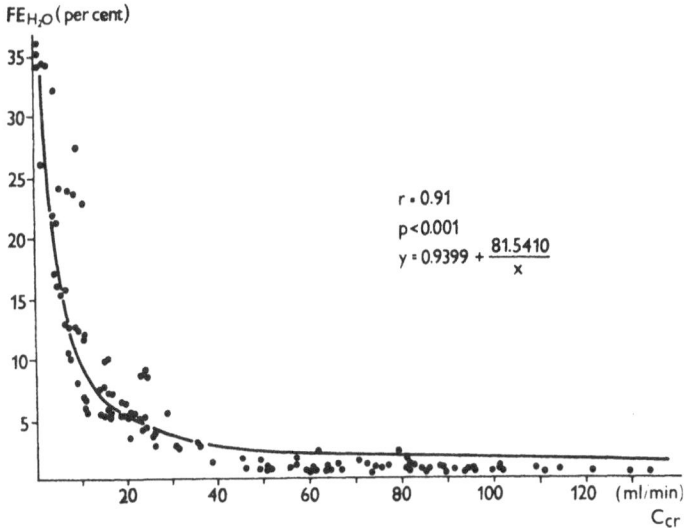

Fig. 56: Relationship between clearance of endogenous creatinine (C_{cr}) and fractional water excretion (FE_{H_2O}) in patients with chronic renal diseases.

Evaluation of the degree of osmotic diuresis when the latter is induced for therapeutic reasons

Mannitol-induced osmotic diuresis is often used in the management of various intexications. Normal clinical practice is to evaluate the effect only on the basis of the increase in urine flow rate. It is also of use to measure FE_{osm} since, particularly in patients with a low GFR, this shows whether a maximal osmotic diuretic state has been achieved (i.e. it tests whether the mannitol has been maximally effective). FE_{osm} values in the range of 30 to 35% can be considered to be sufficiently high for clinical purposes.

Contraindications of the investigation

This investigation has no contraindications. Induction of mannitol diuresis is, however, contraindicated in patients with congestive failure, oedema or other signs of ECF volume expansion.

EXCRETION OF POTASSIUM

PHYSIOLOGY AND PATHOPHYSIOLOGY

Potassium is mainly an intracellular cation. The total volume of ECF contains only about 2% of the organism's total K. Potassium is mainly excreted from the organism through the kidneys.

Micropuncture data have given the following picture of K excretion (Giebisch and Stanton 1979): K freely penetrates the glomerular membrane. K concentration in the glomerular filtrate is practically the same as that in the ECF. The small differences which exist are due to the Donnan equilibrium. In the proximal tubule (that part available for micropuncture) 50–70% of the filtered load is reabsorbed. K concentration in the lumen in this portion of the nephron remains about the same as in the glomerular filtrate. Under normal conditions K reabsorption in the proximal tubule is tightly coupled to that of Na and water. In principle, however, tubular K transport in this portion of the nephron can take place independently of Na transport (Beck et al. 1973).

In the loop of Henle here is further K reabsorption, so that the amount of K which reaches the start of the distal tubule is 5 to 10% of the filtered load. The fine regulation of K excretion occurs in the distal tubule and in the collecting ducts.

Transport of K in the distal tubule and in the collecting ducts depends upon the metabolic state of the organism. If K intake is very low, this portion of the nephron reabsorbs more K. On the other hand, if K intake is high, there is K secretion in the distal tubule. Under normal conditions, K excreted into the final urine is mainly due to distal tubular secretion.

Distal tubular K transport is heavily influenced by the size of the Na load and the volume of luminal fluid entering the distal segment of the nephron (Giebisch 1971, Wright 1974, 1976, Grantham 1976). The rate of delivery of Na into the distal nephron can influence the tubular transport of K probably in a number of ways.

The rate of distal Na reabsorption, and the resulting concentration of Na in the luminal fluid, can influence the trans-tubular potential difference. The greater the distal transport of Na, the greater the electrical gradient which stimulates K secretion (Giebisch et al. 1967). An increase in the delivery of tubular urine to the distal segment is associated with an increased flow of fluid in the same segment. The greater the flow of luminal fluid in the distal segment, the greater the K secretion (Khuri et al. 1975).

Tubular K transport in the distal segment depends upon the state of acid-base balance. Metabolic alkalosis stimulates K secretion, metabolic acidosis inhibits this process (Malnic et al. 1971, Gennari and Cohen 1975). There is an inverse relation between excretions of K and NH_4 (Tannen 1977).

Distal K transport is also influenced by mineralocorticoids. Deficiency of aldosterone decreases the capacity of the kidneys to excrete K. The stimulation by aldosterone of K excretion depends upon an adequate Na delivery to the distal nephron. If K intake is very low, aldosterone is not capable of increasing K excretion (Giebisch 1971).

The mechanism of tubular K transport is not completely clear, and there probably are differences from one tubular segment to the other.

Micropuncture data suggest that the distal mechanism of K transport is as follows (Giebisch and Stanton 1979): at the basal membrane of the tubular cells K transport is in exchange for Na. At the luminal membrane there is active K reabsorption. As a result of active K transport both from the blood (at the basal membrane) and from the tubular urine (luminal membrane) the intracellular K concentration increases. At the same time there is passive penetration of Na from the tubular fluid into cells. These processes form an electrochemical gradient which favours passive penetration of K from the cells into the tubule.

The micropuncture studies of Wright (1974) and Karlmark et al. (1979) suggest that K secretion in the cortical collecting ducts is an active process.

Abnormal renal function can alter K homeostasis and be a cause of very serious metabolic changes.

It is important, for functional diagnosis, to determine whether abnormal K excretion is determined by a primary pathology of the kidneys or whether it is primarily extrarenal, involving regulatory mechanisms of renal K excretion. The final K concentration in the ECF is the result of many factors, not only renal.

A sudden collapse of renal function (acute renal failure) results in a significant decrease or cessation of K excretion. The catabolic state and metabolic acidosis along with a decrease in renal K excretion, result in hyperkalaemia. A disturbance in K excretion in these cases results from the decrease in GFR.

In patients without complete anuria, so that a small amount of urine is being formed, it is possible that in addition to the decrease in GFR a decreased flow rate of luminal fluid will contribute to decreased K excretion. Since K excretion is a flow-dependent process, tubular transport can be altered.

Since the ECF K content is such a small fraction of the total, a small shift of

K from cells into the ECF can result in a large change in ECF concentration if GFR is absent or low.

Thus, for example, in an adult with 14 l of ECF and an ECF K concentration is 4 mmol/l the total amount of K in the ECF = 54 mmol. If K content is increased by 30 mmol (e.g. because of K loss from damaged muscle), the serum K concentration increases to 6 mmol.

In patients with chronic renal failure, urinary K excretion can be normal — i.e. the external K balance can be 0. Serum K can be normal, increased, or even decreased from the norm.

The rate of K excretion by residual nephrons in these patients is increased. Leaf and Camera (1949) and Kleeman et al. (1966) showed that in patients with chronic renal failure, urinary excretion can exceed the filtered K load. These findings suggest an intense tubular K secretion in the residual nephrons, but a patient with chronic renal failure cannot adequately excrete a K load (Keith and Osterberg 1947, Gonick et al. 1971).

Experimental reduction of the renal parenchyma (Schultze et al. 1971) results in an increase in fractional K excretion in the residual nephrons. Adaptation of K excretion in residual nephrons is sufficient to maintain K homeostasis despite a loss of 75% of renal parenchyma. It has not yet been made clear how residual nephrons make this adaptation. Increased K excretion by residual nephrons is not mediated by aldosterone because it occurs in animals, after adrenalectomy, which have been placed on constant exogenous dosing of mineralocorticoids.

Decreased renal K excretion and hyperkalaemia may occur in pathological states associated with decreased aldosterone production or with a decreased sensitivity of the tubules to this steroid. Hyperkalaemia caused by inadequate renal K excretion belongs to the characteristic clinical signs of Addison's disease.

In so-called selective hypoaldosteronism, only the formation of this steroid is abnormal. Present data suggest that most of such cases are the result of a decreased mobilization of renin, i.e. the stimulus for aldosterone production is less. These cases are termed hyporeninaemic hypoaldosteronism. A primary disturbance in aldosterone synthesis has been described (Jacobs and Posner 1964, Ulick et al. 1964) but this would appear to be very rare.

It is possible that various chronic renal diseases can damage the juxtaglomerular apparatus and thus decrease renin production with a resulting loss of aldosterone stimulation. Aminopeptidases in the adrenal zona glomerulosa produce angiotensin-III (A-III) (des-1-Asp-A-II), which binds to the cell membranes of the zona glomerulosa. A-III enables penetration of K into the glomerulosa cells, thus stimulating the production of aldosterone. The production of aldosterone is also stimulated by ACTH, and this also requires the presence of K.

Na plays a role in aldosterone production in terms of changes in ECF volume, but it is also possible that Na depletion stimulates conversion of corticosterone to aldosterone.

A disturbance in renal K excretion can result from a decreased sensitivity of tubular cells to aldosterone. This syndrome is called pseudo-hypoaldosteronism. There are two forms: classical pseudo-hypoaldosteronism (Type I) characterized by hyperkalaemia, salt-wasting and hypotension, and Type-II pseudo-hypoaldosteronism (Schambelan et al. 1981) characterized in a similar fashion but without signs of salt-wasting. As explained on p. 199, it is possible that Type-II is associated with increased Cl reabsorption in the distal nephron.

A decrease in renal K excretion and development of hyperkalaemia can result from administration of drugs with a K-retaining effect (K-sparing agents). Such drugs include antagonists of aldosterone, triamterenein and amiloride.

Some investigators believe (Paver and Pauline 1964, Arnold and Healy 1969, Spitzer et al. 1973) that hyperkalaemia can result from a primary defect in tubular K transport.

K homeostasis can be altered by excessive renal K excretion, with the development of hypokalaemia. Most pathological states involved here are associated with increased aldosterone production. This can be due to primary adrenal disease or increased renin stimulation.

Primary hyperaldosteronism (Conn 1955) is either related to an adrenal tumor or bilateral hyperplasia. Plasma renin activity (PRA) is markedly depressed. Primary hyperaldosteronism is characterized by hypokalaemia and metabolic alkalosis. Pathological states involving increased renin stimulation are referred to as secondary hyperaldosteronism. Such pathologies include the nephrotic syndrome, liver cirrhosis, congestive heart failure and so-called idiopathic oedema. There is a physiological rise in aldosterone production in pregnancy. This appears to be related to an increase in renin substrate — induced by estrogens and an antagonist action of progesterone on aldosterone receptor sites.

Increased renal K excretion can be secondary to a primary disturbance of tubular Na or Cl transport.

Bartter (1980) believes that "Bartter syndrome" involves a disturbance in Cl reabsorption in the thick ascending limb of the loop of Henle, with resulting changes leading to increased renal K excretion. Schematically, these processes are as follows (see schema on p. 168).

An increase in aldosterone production occurs in salt wasting due to various forms of interstitial nephritis and tubular defects. Increased urinary K excretion is related to both increased aldosterone production and increased bulk flow of luminal fluid in the distal segment due to osmotic diuresis.

Hypokalaemia occurs in patients with renal tubular acidosis (RTA). The pathological basis of increased renal K excretion in both types of RTA is probably not identical. In distal RTA (Type I) it can be assumed that decreased $Na^+ + H^+$

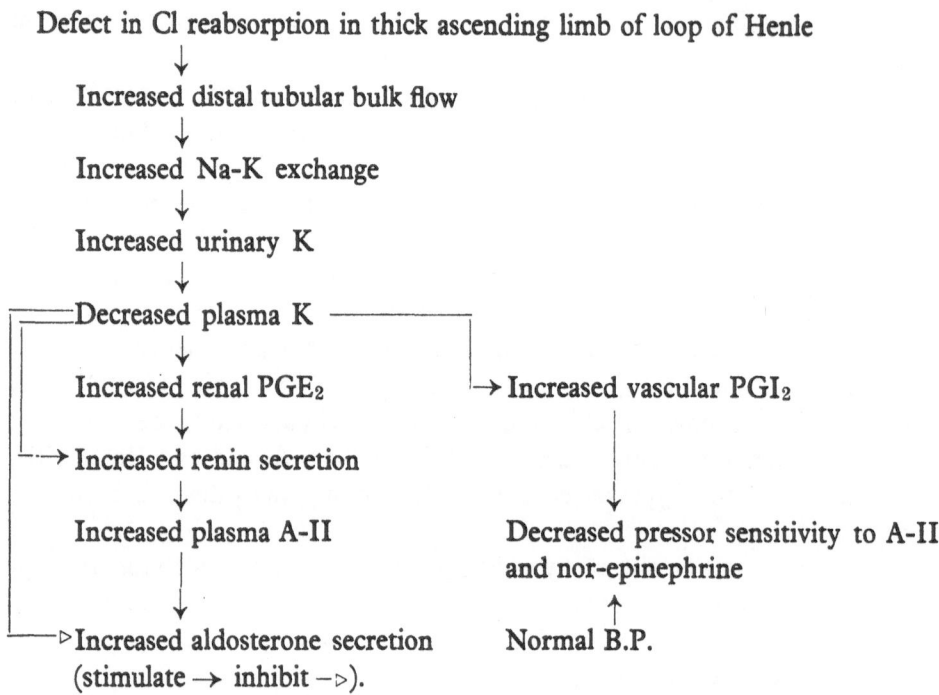

Defect in Cl reabsorption in thick ascending limb of loop of Henle
↓
Increased distal tubular bulk flow
↓
Increased Na-K exchange
↓
Increased urinary K
↓
Decreased plasma K ───────→ Increased vascular PGI$_2$
↓
Increased renal PGE$_2$
↓
Increased renin secretion
↓
Increased plasma A-II   Decreased pressor sensitivity to A-II and nor-epinephrine
↓   ↑
Increased aldosterone secretion   Normal B.P.
(stimulate → inhibit –▷).

exchange results in increased K$^+$ secretion. This would not be the only mechanism, and other factors most certainly play a role. Sebastian et al. (1971) have shown that in such patients urinary K excretion is far higher at any given level of serum K than one would expect. These investigators therefore believe that in patients with Type I RTA, changes in distal tubular membrane permeability for K play a role, these changes allowing increased diffusion of K from cells into the luminal fluid. Alkalinization therapy decreases renal K excretion in this type of RTA.

In patients with proximal RTA (Type II) the urinary K loss increases with base administration. As soon as plasma HCO$_3$ increases to a level above its renal threshold, there is increased delivery to the distal nephron. Since HCO$_3$ is poorly reabsorbed in the distal segment, intraluminal negativity increases, and this stimulates K secretion. In patients with RTA, aldosterone production is increased, which further stimulates K secretion.

Alteration of urinary K excretion occurs in patients with accelerated arterial hypertension. In these cases one can demonstrate increased aldosterone production as a result of increased renin production. Hypokalaemia associated with arterial hypertension can develop on the basis of various parenchymatous diseases of the kidney, and renovascular hypertension. Increased renin production, and the resulting increase in aldosterone production, hypokalaemia and arterial hypertension all result from a tumour arising in the juxtaglomerular apparatus (Robertson et al. 1967).

Hypokalaemia and arterial hypertension also result from the adrenogenital syndrome. With a deficiency of 11-hydroxylase there is a block in the formation of cortisol with a secondary increase in ACTH release and a subsequent stimulation of production of androgens and desoxycorticosterone. If the deficiency is in 17-hydroxylase (Biglieri et al. 1966), there is a deficit in androgen and cortisol synthesis. There is, however, a rise in ACTH release resulting in increased production of desoxycorticosterone, leading to hypokalaemia and arterial hypertension.

For clinical practice, hypokalaemia which results from diuretic therapy is of great importance. Thiazides, furosemide and ethacrynic acid all increase renal K excretion. On the other hand — aldosterone antagonists, triamterene and amiloride decrease urinary K excretion. The mechanism of this diuretic-induced K loss is not simple — a number of factors play a role.

Furosemide and ethacrynic acid inhibit tubular Cl transport in the thick ascending limb of the loop of Henle (Burg and Green 1973). Thiazides and chlorthalidone affect tubular Na transport in the cortical segment of the ascending limb of the loop of Henle and at the start of the distal tubule. Acetazolamide inhibits carbonic anhydrase in the proximal tubule, and thus also the reabsorption of HCO_3 which, along with Na, reach the distal segment.

Osmotic diuresis (e.g. due to mannitol infusion) decreases water reabsorption in the proximal tubule and loop of Henle because of the luminal osmotic effect of unreabsorbable solute. The decrease in water reabsorption dilutes the Na concentration in the proximal luminal fluid. Since the proximal tubular cells can transport Na only against a limited concentration gradient, total proximal Na reabsorption is decreased. Regardless of the mechanism of action of diuretics, there is an increased bulk delivery of luminal fluid to the terminal part of the distal tubule and the collecting ducts.

Increased Na delivery to the latter nephron segment increases its tubular reabsorption at the same site. Increased Na reabsorption in the terminal portion of the distal tubule and in the collecting ducts leads to increased secretion of K and protons. Distal K secretion is markedly stimulated by an increase in bulk flow of tubular fluid. It is further increased by the accumulation of poorly reabsorbed anions in the tubular fluid of the distal segment. This mechanism plays a role in the action of carbonic anhydrase inhibitors and the resulting increased distal load of HCO_3. The same mechanism is involved in decreased Cl reabsorption in the distal segment. Unreabsorbed anions in the distal tubule increase the transepithelial electrochemical gradient and are responsible for passive transfer of K^+ into the luminal fluid.

METHODS OF INVESTIGATION

URINARY K CONCENTRATION (U_K)

varies widely in relation to the load to be excreted and the rate of water flow. In a group of 45 healthy controls on a normal diet, U_K after 24 hr fluid deprivation was 93 ± 39 mmol. After a water load of 2% body weight U_K at the height of the diuresis was 4.9 ± 3.1 mmol. In clinical practice, U_K alone is of little use — rather its ratio to U_{Na} is of interest. The mean value of $U_{Na}:U_K$ in healthy controls on a normal diet was 2.4 ± 1.3. A decrease in this ratio to below 1.0 can be considered to be abnormal and usually occurs when distal Na reabsorption is increased. Micropuncture data suggest that a decrease in this ratio is the result of increased Na-for-K exchange in the distal segment. For this reason, low ratios are observed in patients with high aldosterone levels, e.g. with ECF volume restriction, or patients with the nephrotic syndrome.

URINARY K EXCRETION ($U_K V$)

shows wide variations in healthy adults, from 30 to 100 mmol/day depending upon K intake. In most cases the daily K excretion varies from 50 to 70 mmol. If the patient has haematuria, U_K can be distorted by erythrocyte K diffusing out of cells. Menstruating women will have this complication.

Measurement of $U_K V$ under conditions in which intake is not regulated or measured gives an orientational view of the intensity of urinary excretion. In patients with a very low GFR, $U_K V$ usually is decreased to less than 20 mmol/day. A sharp decrease in urinary K excretion also exists in patients with extrarenal K losses, usually from the gut. In such cases urinary K excretion also usually decreases to less than 20 mmol/day. In addition, a decreased $U_K V$ follows a decrease in intake (e.g. anorexia, pathological states affecting food intake, unconsciousness state). K-sparing diuretics also decrease $U_K V$.

As opposed to urinary Na excretion, $U_K V$ never decreases to practically nil values. The latter can be increased to over 100 mmol/day in various pathological states. Most frequently this involves osmotic diuresis produced by kaliuretic diuretics, patients with decompensated diabetes mellitus, infusion of hypertonic solutions (most frequently mannitol) and the polyuric stage after acute tubular necrosis.

All states of increased aldosterone production can also result in increased $U_K V$. For diagnostic purposes it is of importance that normal urinary K excretion does not exclude the presence of increased K secretion. In other words, even with unchanged urinary K excretion there may be hypokalaemia of renal origin. As explained below, increased tubular K secretion in such cases can be manifest only by an increase in fractional K excretion.

According to Narins et al. 1982 renal potassium waisting cannot be excluded unless low urinary K excretion (less than 20 mmol day) is accompanied by more than 100 mmol of sodium.

A detailed evaluation of urinary K excretion from the metabolic point of view requires measurement of the external balance. Oral K intake is usually calculated from tables. Very precise measurements require chemical analysis of aliquots of the same foods.

Fecal K excretion is usually insignificant in relation to intake. Under normal conditions, urine contains about 92% of the total excretion, the feces about 8%. With precise balance measurement, fecal excretion is also measured. Fecal excretion of K is increased in patients with chronic renal failure. In such patients, the fecal quantity assumes relatively greater importance if K intake is decreased.

THE RENAL CLEARANCE OF K(C_K)

(Calculation see p. 262). The investigation utilizes either a 24-hr urine sample or samples over only several hr of collection. Measurement of C_K also requires a blood sample. Various technical errors can cause artefacts. P_K can be increased because of improper sampling from the antecubital vein. The application of a tourniquet for sampling and exercising the arm can lead to K coming out from red blood cells. Evaluation of P_K with an improper sampling should be taken with reserve.

Blood samples should be processed within 1–2 hr. The sample should be carefully transported to the laboratory, otherwise K release from blood cells will cause artefacts.

C_K in healthy controls on a normal diet and ad libitum fluids shows a wide variation. In our own group of normal controls C_K (AM urine collection) was 13.0 ± 6.1 ml/min (i.e. 0.22 ± 0.10 ml/s). The upper limit of normal was 20 ml/min (0.32 ml/s), the lower limit was 6 ml/min (0.10 ml/s).

Interpretation of C_K involves the same factors listed for evaluation of $U_K V$. Both values change in the same direction in various pathological states, so that levels of clearance do not really give us any more information than urinary excretion levels.

FRACTIONAL K EXCRETION (FE$_K$)

gives the relation between urinary excretion and the filtered K load. (Calculation see p. 262).

In healthy adult controls on a normal and fluid intake ad libitum diet, FE$_K$ was $11.1 \pm 5.4\%$. Under the above conditions, FE$_K$ does not exceed 17% and does not fall below 5.5%. In patients with a low GFR, FE$_K$ can exceed 100%, which indicates that the excreted K is greater than the filtered load. These results indicate intense tubular secretion.

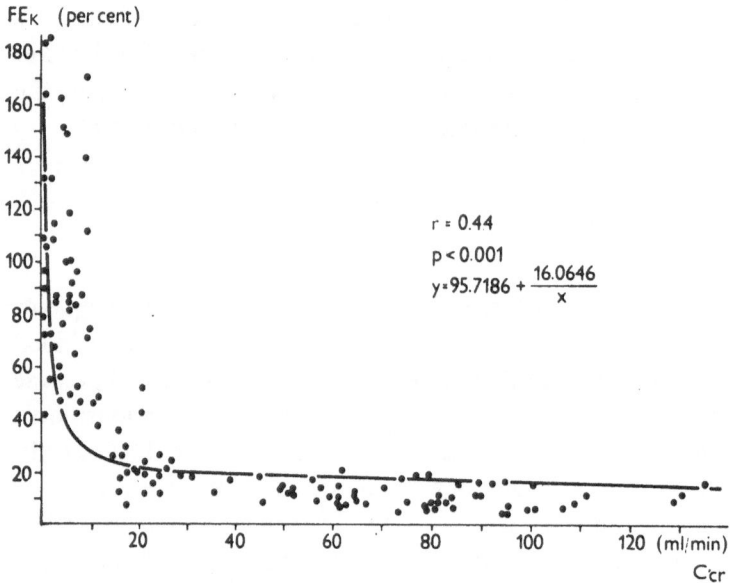

Fig. 57: Relationship between clearance of endogenous creatinine (C$_{cr}$) and fractional potassium excretion (FE$_K$) in patients with chronic renal diseases.

FE$_K$ increases in hyperbolic relation to a decrease in GFR. Fig. 57 shows this in 115 subjects with chronic renal diseases with various degrees of decrease in C$_{cr}$. The Fig. 57 shows that at very low GFR levels (below 6 ml/min or 0.1 ml/s) FE$_K$ can reach 150–200%, and even higher values in individual cases.

The concept of adequate FE$_K$

Clinical disorders of potassium homeostasis may be caused by alteration of renal excretion, inadequate intake, excessive extrarenal loss or by changes of distribution between intracellular and extracellular compartments.

Recognition of the renal origin of hypo- and hyperkalaemia can be difficult

172

because the daily urinary excretion of K need not be changed. Changes of urinary K excretion could have been transient and after this phase a new steady state (with normal urinary K excretion, but abnormal plasma K level) can follow.

Recognition that hypo- or hyperkalaemia in these cases is of renal origin can be made on the basis of the measurement of the fractional potassium excretion (FE_K) which is higher (in patients with hypokalaemia) or lower (in patients with hyperkalaemia) than it should be with respect to potassium intake (I_K), GFR and the metabolic state of the whole organism. The value of FE_K which corresponds to all the above conditions and which would guarantee a normal plasma potassium level, we denote as "adequate fractional potassium excretion" (FE_{K-adq}) (Schück 1982).

In the following part of this chapter we shall explain this method of investigation in detail.

From the physiological commentary it is clear that the values of FE_K can be clinically interpreted as an indicator of distal potassium secretion.

The relation between FE_K and some fundamental metabolic parameters of K can be derived from the formula for the calculation of FE_K.

Fractional potassium excretion (like FE of other substances excreted by the kidneys) is given by the ratio of its urinary excretion ($U_K V$) to the filtered load (GFR P_K).

$$FE_K = \frac{U_K V}{GFR\, P_K}\, 100 \tag{1}$$

Furthermore, the external K balance can be characterized by the following simple equation:

$$U_K V = I_K - EE_K \tag{2}$$

where EE_K denotes the extrarenal K excretion. If the extrarenal loss of K is not increased, and I_K is within normal limits, the value of EE_K can be neglected, because the renal excretion of K represents about 90% of its intake. If we accept this simplification, the equation (1) can be expressed as follows:

$$FE_K = \frac{I_K}{GFR\, P_K}\, 100 \tag{3}$$

The P_K value is also influenced by its distribution between intracellular and extracellular compartment — the so called internal K balance. As is known, the latter balance is significantly influenced by the acid-base and metabolic state of the organism.

The input of K into extracellular fluid is given by the sum of its oral intake (I_K) and the rate of penetration of K from the intracellular into extracellular compartment (M_{Ki}). The total output of K from ECF is given by the sum of $U_K V$, EE_K and the rate of the potassium transfer from ECF into ICF (M_{Ko}). Under conditions of a balanced metabolic steady state the following equation expresses the relation between the above parameters:

$$I_K + M_{Ki} = U_K V + EE_K + M_{Ko} \tag{4}$$

This equation can be rearranged as follows.

$$I_K - (U_K V + EE_K) = M_{Ko} - M_{Ki} \qquad (5)$$

The regulation of ihe K content of ECF is schematically shown in Fig. 58.

If we return to equation (3), we can make a further simplification for clinical use. If we substitute for P_K the average normal value (4,5 mmol/l) and if we further express I_K in mmol/24 hr and GFR (usually C_{cr}) in ml/min, we can calculate the value of FE_{K^-adq} on the basis of the following formula:

$$FE_{K-adq} = \frac{\dfrac{I_K}{1440}}{GFR \dfrac{P_K}{1000}} \; 100 \quad \text{or} \qquad (6)$$

$$FE_{K-adq} = 15 \frac{I_K \,(mmol/24\ hr)}{C_{cr}\,(ml/min)} \qquad (7$$

Formula (7) gives the value of FE_K which would guarantee a normal P_K unde conditions of a balanced metabolic steady state (external balance = 0, interna balance = 0), with respect to I_K and GFR. Furthermore the calculation of FE_{K-adq} according to formula (7) also includes the condition that EE_K is negligible with respect to I_K.

An example of application of this method of investigation can serve patient A.F., a 42 years old female with dg. Bartter's syndrome.

This patient was investigated for three weeks under balance conditions. I_K averaged 60 mmol/24 hr and $U_K V$ averaged 50 mmol/24 hr. P_K was stabilized at 2.5 mmol/l, C_{cr} was 50 ml/min, FE_K averaged 27%. Metabolic alkalosis was present (plasma bicarbonate concentration was 29 mmol/l).

The laboratory data indicate that in this patient, the urinary K excretion was

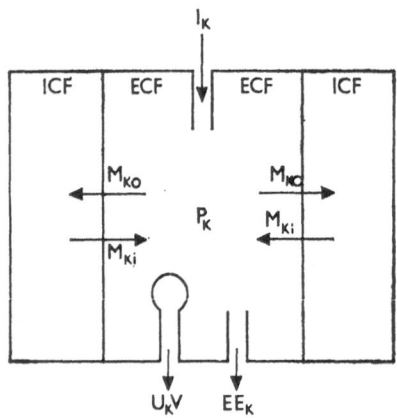

Fig. 58: Schematic presentation of the factors affecting external and internal potassium balance. I_K = potassium intake, $U_K V$ = urinary potassium excretion, EE_K = extrarenal potassium excretion. ECF = extracellular fluid, ICF = intracellular fluid. P_K = plasma potassium concentration, M_{Ko} = potassium transport from ECF into ICF, M_{Ki} = potassium transport from ICF into ECF.

inappropriately high with respect to the serum K level and therefore renal potassium waisting can be assummed. Such approach is clinically useful but it does not allow quantitative evaluation of the alteration of K tabular transport.

The renal contribution to the development of hypokalaemia in this case can be estimated as follows.

The calculated value of FE_{K-adq} in this case is $15 \times 60/50 = 18\%$. The measured value of FE_K was higher (27%) than FE_{K-adq} and therefore hypersecretion of K in the residual nephrons in this patient can be assumed, and that alteration of tubular function contributed to the development of hypokalaemia. Obviously, the metabolic alkalosis stimulated the tubular secretion of K in residual nephrons.

The hypokalaemia in this case was not due to increased extrarenal loss of K because the calculated extrarenal K excretion ($I_K - U_K V$) amounted to 10 mmol/24 hr. In cases where hypokalaemia is due to increased extrarenal loss of K, measured EF_K is significantly lower than calculated FE_{K-adq}.

Analogous, this method can be used in patients with chronic renal disease and metabolic acidosis.

Hyperkalaemia in these patients usually develops when GFR decreases to an extreme low level. As mentioned above (cf. p. 172), FE_K in patients with very low GFR (<6 ml/min) can reach values to 150–200%.

Inadequate increase of tubular secretion of K in residual nephrons can also significantly contribute to development of hyperkalaemia.

In patients with chronic renal failure, fecal K excretion need not be negligible with respect to its intake. Therefore in patients with normal values of P_K the measured values of FE_K are also rather lower than the calculated values of FE_{K-adq}. If, in a patient with chronic renal disease and hyperkalaemia, the measured FE_K is significantly lower than calculated FE_{K-adq}, it can be assumed that inadequate increase of K secretion contributes to the alteration of K homeostasis.

Provided I_K, $U_K V$ and P_K are stabilized as well as the acid-base status, it can be

I_K	$U_K V$	$I_K - U_K V$	P_K	P_{HCO_3}	C_{cr}	FE_K	FE_{K-adq}
	mmol/24 hr			mmol/l	ml/min	per cent	
50	31	19	5.8	19	12	30.9	38.7
44	25	19	6.0			24.1	31.2
52	35	17	5.9	20		34.3	43.7
40	20	20	5.6			20.6	25.0
50	28	22	6.1			26.5	35.0
48	22	26	5.7	18		22.3	27.5
45	29	16	5.9			28.4	36.2
Mean: 47	27	20	5.8			23.8	33.9

assumed that EE_K is also stabilized. An evaluation of the possible participation of the residual renal parenchyma in the disturbance of potassium homeostasis illustrates the following example. L.K. (a female 56 years old with dg chron. renal insufficiency, chron. glomerulonephritis) (see table on p. 175).

On the basis of these data it can be assumed that a balanced state of K metabolism in this patient was achieved, but P_K oscillated at an elevated level. The calculated extrarenal K excretion was 20 mmol/24 hr in average, corresponding to 42% of I_K. In this case the residual renal parenchyma had to excrete 27 mmol of K daily in average, to maintain the balanced state. As explained above, this quantity of K can be excreted at various P_K levels, depending on the value of FE_K (tubular secretion rate of K).

If the value of EE_K is not negligible, FE_{K-adq} can be calculated (under conditions of a balanced metabolic state) according to the formula:

$$FE_{K-adq} = 15 \frac{U_K V \, (\text{mmol/24 hr})}{C_{cr} \, (\text{ml/min})} \qquad (8)$$

The effect of acid-base status of ECF on tubular K secretion can be excluded, if FE_K is investigated after the normalization of blood pH and P_{HCO_3}.

Indications for investigation

Acute renal failure

Measurement of $U_K V$ should be made in both oliguric and polyuric stages of the disease. In oliguria there will be hyperkalaemia because of the decrease in renal K excretion and an increase in catabolism and development of metabolic acidosis.

A low U_{Na}/U_K ratio (below 1.0) in the oliguric phase suggests an increase in aldosterone secretion. This is found when there is a sudden ECF volume restriction.

In the polyuric phase there can be increased renal K losses related to the development of osmotic diuresis. In this phase there may be hypokalaemia. $U_K V$ should be measured if these losses are to be replaced.

Chronic renal failure

$U_K V$ and FE_K should be measured. In patients not in K homeostasis and with P_K not in the normal range, we try to determine the role of inadequate adaptation of residual nephrons with reference to K excretion.

From the nephrological point of view the most important pathology under this heading is the nephrotic syndrome. In such patients secondary hyperaldosteronism may result in K depletion. The rate of K excretion depends on GFR and the delivery of luminal fluid to the distal segment of the nephron. If GFR is low, U_KV need not be raised even if there is hypersecretion of aldosterone. K depletion is usually associated with metabolic alkalosis.

Biochemical data can be modified by diuretic therapy. A potent saluretic such as furosemide or ethacrynic acid increases urinary K loss as well and also increases, thereby, metabolic alkalosis. Diuretics with a K-sparing effect (aldosterone antagonists, triamteren, amiloride) decrease urinary K excretion, inhibit the development of metabolic alkalosis or can even result in the development of metabolic acidosis. Evaluation of the state of K metabolism should take into account I_K, including K supplementation in the diet. Administration of KCl has an acidifying effect; administration of $KHCO_3$ or K citrate has an alkalinizing action.

Arterial hypertension. Changes in K excretion in hypertensive patients are usually due to the use of diuretics in therapy. In patients with prolonged hypokalaemia which does not react to K supplementation, U_KV should be measured. Problems with correction of P_K can occur since the usual KCl doses need not be adequate.

Measurement of renal K excretion is of particular importance if GFR is low and K-sparing diuretics are used.

If we find hypokalaemia in patients with arterial hypertension who have not received diuretics, the investigation should try to determine if aldosterone or a different adrenocortical mineralocorticoid is raised. In such patients we should measure with plasma renin and aldosterone levels.

High renin activity and aldosterone level are seen in accelerated hypertension and juxtaglomerular apparatus tumours and can also be present in renovascular hypertension. A low PRA and high aldosterone level are seen in primary hyperaldosteronism. Normal PRA and aldosterone levels are found in Cushing's syndrome.

Low PRA and aldosterone levels are characteristic of adrenogenital syndrome, ectopic tumours which produce ACTH or licorice ingestion.

Hypokalaemia of unknown origin. If hypokalaemia is present without arterial hypertension, measurement of the state of acid-base balance is of diagnostic assistance. Hypokalaemia with metabolical alkalosis develops in repeated vomiting, Bartter's syndrome, after some diuretics (thiazide, furosemide, ethacrynic acid), and in periodic paralysis.

Hypokalaemia with metabolic acidosis develops with diarrhea, RTA, after ureterosigmoidostomy, after administration of acetazolamide, in diabetic ketoacidosis and during fasting.

Laboratory methods

Normal flame photometry is used to determine K concentrations in plasma and urine.

REFERENCES

Arnold, J. E., Healy, J. K.: Hyperkalemia, hypertension and systemic acidosis without renal failure associated with the tubular defect in potassium excretion. Am. J. Med. *47*: 461, 1969

Bartter, F. C.: Clinical problems of potassium metabolism. Contr. Nephrol. *21*: 115, 1980

Beck, L. H., Senesky, D., Goldberg, M.: Sodium independent active potassium reabsorption in proximal tubule of the dog. J. clin. Invest. *52*: 2641, 1973

Biglieri, E. G., Herron, M. A., Brust, N.: 17-hydroxylation deficiency in man. J. clin. Invest. *45*: 1946, 1966

Burg, M. B., Green, N.: Function of the thick ascending limb of Henle's loop. Am. J. Physiol. *224*: 659, 1973

Conn, J. W.: Primary aldosteronism: a new clinical syndrome. J. lab. clin. Med. *45*: 6, 1955

Gennari, F. J., Cohen, J. J.: Role of the kidney in potassium homeostasis: lessons from acid base disturbances. Kidney int. *8*, 1, 1975

Giebisch, G.: Renal potassium excretion. In: C. Reuiller and A. F. Müller (Eds.) The kidney. Vol. 3. New York and London Academia 1971, p. 329

Giebisch, G., Klose, R. M., Malnie, G.: Renal tubular potassium transport. Bull. Swiss Acad. Med. Sci. *23*: 287, 1967

Giebisch, G., Stanton, B.: Potassium transport in the nephron. Ann. Rev. Physiol. *41*; 241, 1979

Gonick, H. C., Kleeman, C. R., Rubini, M. E., Maxwell, M. H.: Functional impairment in chronic renal disease III. Studies of potassium excretion. Am. J. Med. Sci. *261*: 281, 1971

Grantham, J. J.: Renal transport and excretion of potassium. In: B. M. Brenner and F. C. Rector Jr. (Eds.) The kidney. Philadelphia, Saunders 1976, p. 299

Jacobs, D. R., Posner, J. B.: Isolated analdosteronism II. The nature of the adrenal corticolenzymatic defect on the influence of diet and various agents on the electrolyte balance. Metabolism *13*: 225, 1964

Karlmark, B., Jaeger, Ph., Giebisch, G.: Micropuncture study of tubular acidification and NH_3 — NH_4 transport during chronic potassium depletion quoted by Giebisch, G. and Staton, B. Ann. Rev. Physiol. *41*: 241, 1979

Keith, N. M., Osterberg, A. E.: Tolerance for potassium in severe renal insufficiency. A study of 10 cases. J. clin. Invest. *26*: 773, 1947

Khuri, R. N., Wiederholt, M., Strieder, N., Giebisch, G.: Effects of flow rate and potassium intake on distal tubular potassium transfer. Am. J. Physiol. *228*: 1249, 1975

Kleeman, C. R., Okun, R., Heller, R. J.: Renal regulation of sodium and potassium in patients with chronic renal failure (CRF) and the effect of diuretics on the excretion of these ions. Ann. N. Y. Acad. Sci. *139*: 520, 1966

Leaf, A., Camara, A. A.: Renal tubular secretion of potassium in man. J. clin. Invest. *28*: 1526, 1949

Malnic, G., Mello-Aires, M., Giebisch, G.: Potassium transport across renal distal tubules during acid-base disturbances. Am. J. Physiol. *221*: 1192, 1971

Narins, G. N., Jones, E. R., Stom, M. C., Rudnick, M. R., Bastl, Ch. P.: Diagnostic strategies in disorders of fluidelectrolyte and acid-base homeostasis. Am. J. Med. *72*: 496, 1982

Paver, W. K. A., Pauline, G. J.: Hypertension and hyperpotassemia without renal disease in a young male. Med. J. Aust. *2*: 305, 1964

Robertson, T. W., Klidjian, A., Harding, L. K., Walters, G., Lee, M. R., Robb-Smith, A. H. T.: Hypertension due to a renin secreting renal tumor. Am. J. Med. *43*: 963, 1967

Schampelan, M., Sebastian, A., Rector, F. C. Jr.: Mineralocorticoid-resistant renal hyperkalemia without salt wasting (type II pseudohypoaldosteronism). Role of increased renal chloride reabsorption. Kidney int. *19*: 716, 1981

Schück, O.: Recognition of tubular hypersecretion of potassium in patients with hypokalemia. Min. Electrolyt. Metabol. *7*: 54, 1982

Schultze, R. G., Taggart, D. B., Shapiro, H., Pennell, J. P., Caglar, S., Bricker, N. S.: On the adaptation in potassium excretion associated with nephron reduction in the dog. J. clin. Invest. *50*: 1061, 1971

Sebastian, A., McSherry, E., Morris, R. C. Jr.: Renal potassium waisting in renal tubular acidosis. J. clin. Invest. *50*: 667, 1971

Spitzer, A., Edelman, C. M. Jr., Goldberg, L. D., Henneman, P. H.: Short stature, hyperkalemia, and acidosis, a defect in renal transport of potassium. Kidney int. *3*: 251, 1973

Tannen, R. L.: Relationship of renal ammonia production and potassium homeostasis. Kidney int. *11*: 453, 1977

Ulick, S., Gantrer, E., Vetter, K. K., Amrkello, J. R., Yaffe, S., Lowe, C. V.: An aldosterone biosynthetic defect in a salt losing disorder. J. clin. Endocrinol. Metabolism *24*: 669, 1964

Wright, F. S.: Potassium transport by the renal tubule. In: MTP Intern. Rev. of Sci., Kidney and Urinary Tract Physiology, ed. K. Thurau, *6*: 273, 1974

Wright, F. S., Strieder, N., Fowler, N. B., Giebisch, G.: Potassium secretion by distal tubule after potassium adaptation. Am. J. Physiol. *221*: 437, 1971

EXCRETION OF SODIUM

PHYSIOLOGY AND PATHOPHYSIOLOGY

The regulation of the renal excretion of Na plays a fundamental role in the regulation of ECF volume. Maintenance of a constant ECF volume requires a balanced state of intake and output. Under normal conditions — without abnormal losses in sweat or from the gut — the urinary excretion of Na corresponds to its intake.

Changes in ECF volume or oral intake produce quite rapid responses in the excretion rate.

Abnormalities of external Na balance can be a function of:

1. abnormalities in regulatory mechanisms which are reflected in the excretion rate (renal function is otherwise intact)

2. a primary abnormality in tubular Na transport. In such cases we may be dealing either with secondary functional changes in tubular transport or a primary defect.

Differential diagnosis here is important in order to select the correct management and therapy.

Na^+ penetrates freely into the glomerular filtrate, with practically no change (vs plasma) in concentration.

The small differences which are found are due to the Gibbs-Donnan equilibrium. (The Gibbs-Donnan factor for monovalent cations is 0.95.) Plasma Na concentration is further influenced by proteins since the latter make up part of the circulating solution and this will slightly change the concentration per unit volume, depending upon whether one is on one side of the capillary endothelium or the other.

The factor (f) which corrects for the above can be calculated as follows (Rieder, 1963):

$$f = 100/[100 - (0.75 \times \text{plasma prot. conc.})].$$

With normal concentrations of plasma proteins, f ranges about 1.05.

For clinical purposes, the above correction need seldom be carried out, because the Gibbs-Donnan factor cancels out f.

The fact that the concentration of Na in the glomerular filtrate is practically the same as that in plasma has been repeatedly confirmed by micropuncture studies. With normal GFR and P_{Na} values, about 24,000 mmol Na penetrate the glomeruli each day. The final urine contains, however, only 100–300 mmol/day. In other words, almost all the filtered Na load is reabsorbed by the tubules; only about 1% is excreted.

Thus it appears that relatively small changes in tubular reabsorption of Na can result in large changes in urinary excretion. A decrease in reabsorption of only 1% can increase urinary excretion by 100%. On the other hand, a small increase in reabsorption can have a considerable effect in decreasing excretion.

The mechanism of this tubular transport is still not completely clear. A large part of it is due to active transport, requiring metabolic energy. There is a significant relation between O_2 uptake in the kidney and the amount of Na transported by the tubules (Deetjen and Kramer 1961). Micropuncture studies have shown, however, that not all reabsorption of Na is active (Ullrich 1966). It is estimated that about 40% of the total reabsorbate is active, the remainder being passive.

In the proximal tubule 2/3rds to 7/8ths of the total filtered load of both Na and water is reabsorbed. This is an iso-osmotic process, so that the concentration of Na in the lumen does not change. Micropuncture studies have shown that in the proximal tubule Na penetrates passively from the lumen into the tubular cells. It has been argued that this is facilitated diffusion with carrier assistance. It has been demonstrated that Na is co-transported in the proximal tubule along with phosphate glucose and amino acids (Ullrich 1979). Part of the reabsorbed Na ions are exchanged for protons. The accompanying anion is mainly Cl.

Active transport of Na in the proximal tubule occurs at the basal membrane of tubular cells to get the cation back out of cells into the peritubular interstitial fluid (ISF). There may also be transport from the lateral membranes into intercellular spaces in the proximal tubule. This active expulsion of Na has been attributed to a "sodium pump". The metabolic substratum of the Na pump is still not clear. It is probable that the process is associated with the function of Na-K-ATPase (Skou 1957). The extrusion of Na back out of the proximal tubular cells allows more Na to enter passively from the luminal side.

The rate of proximal reabsorption of Na and water changes in direct relation to GFR. This is referred to as "glomerular-tubular balance". The mechanism of the latter is not yet clear. It is probable that the rate of iso-osmotic absorption by the tubules is a function of the rate at which the same iso-osmotic fluid is removed from the peritubular ISF into peritubular capillaries and transported out of the proximity of the tubules. This latter mechanism is in turn a function of the hydrostatic and oncotic pressure differences in the capillary vs the interstitial fluid. Oncotic pressure in the postglomerular peritubular capillaries is high because of glomerular ultrafiltration. If the filtration fraction (FF) (i.e. FF = GFR/RPF) increases, the oncotic gradient also increases.

The next site of changes in Na transport in the kidney is the loop of Henle. As detailed elsewhere (p. 110) in discussion of the countercurrent system of the renal medulla, the wall of the descending limb of the loop is relatively impermeable to Na, but allows diffusion of water. In the thin portion of the ascending limb Na can penetrate from the lumen into the surrounding interstitium, but this wall is relatively impermeable to water. In the thick ascending limb of the loop of Henle Na accompanies actively transported Cl. The rate of absorption of Na and water in the loop of Henle also depends on the rate of luminal loading of isotonic fluid from the end of the proximal tubule. Total absorption of Na in the loop is greater than that of water, so that the luminal fluid which enters the distal convolutions is hypotonic with regard to Na. Micropuncture measurements of Na concentration in the tubular lumen at the start of the distal convolutions range about 60 mmol. This concentration is further reduced along the distal tubule. The total Na reabsorbate in the distal tubule is about 10–15% of the filtered load.

Distal tubular Na transport is active against a concentration gradient. Reabsorption of Na is to a large degree accompanied by Cl. Some micropuncture findings suggest that reabsorption of Cl in parts of the distal tubule is per se an active process. A minority of Na reabsorption in the distal tubules and in the collecting ducts is exchanged for protons and K.

Total reabsorption of Na along the tubule under normal conditions ranges about 99% of the filtered load. The rate of Na reabsorption is finely regulated to maintain Na and volume homeostasis of the internal milieu. These regulatory mechanisms are only partly understood.

One of the most studied humoral regulatory mechanism is the renin-angiotensin--aldosterone system.

Aldosterone can influence only about 2% of the total Na reabsorbed. Nevertheless, this regulation which determines the final urine composition is of quantitative importance. Micropuncture data suggest that aldosterone affects tubular Na transport in the collecting ducts (Hierholzer et al. 1965, Wiederholt et al. 1964). Aldosterone also affects tubular K transport and proton secretion. The effect of aldosterone on Na can be differentiated from its effect on K and H by actinomycin--D (Lifschitz et al. 1973). The mechanism of the cellular action of aldosterone is not yet clear. Edelman (1968) believes that aldosterone stimulates tubular Na transport by an action on nuclear receptors and increases DNA-directed synthesis of RNA which coats a specific protein. Sharp et al. (1963) believe that a protein, the synthesis of which is induced by aldosterone, is a "permease" which influences the apical membrane.

The action of aldosterone on tubular transport depends to a large degree on the presence of other steroids. Progesterone inhibits aldosterone effects (Landau et al. 1955). Antagonists of aldosterone have been synthetized (Kagawa et al. 1957).

Other humoral factors than aldosterone also play a role in Na transport. In recent years prostaglandins have been actively studied. Kidney homogenates contain all groups of prostaglandins (Lee et al. 1965). These substances influence the activity of adenylcyclase and stimulate the formation of cAMP (Ramwell and Shaw 1970). Prostaglandins A and E increase RBF in man, and also cause natriuresis and diuresis (Herzog et al. 1967, Murphy et al. 1970). The mechanism of this effect is not clearly understood. Prostaglandins also influence renin release and in this manner also play a role in regulating renal Na excretion.

The role of kallikrein is still not clear in the regulation of renal Na excretion. Animal experiments have shown repeatedly an action of vasopressin on Na excretion and on Na transport by a number of membranes (Brunner et al. 1956, Herken et al. 1957, Jard and Morel, 1963). In man, however, vasopressin does not play an important role in regulating renal Na excretion.

A great deal of attention has been devoted to research on a "natriuretic hormone" (Cort 1965, Lichardus 1980, de Wardener et al. 1961, Burgoigne et al. 1974, Fine et al. 1976, Favre| 1978). This problem has been studied from two aspects: 1) the mechanism by which isotonic expansion of ECF volume increases Na excretion by the kidneys and 2) the mechanism of increased Na excretion by residual nephrons in patients with chronic renal failure or in animals after surgical reduction of the renal parenchyma.

Expansion of the ECF volume by isotonic saline results in natriuresis even under conditions of adrenalectomy (and a constant dosage of mineralocorticoids given exogenously) and GFR is either unchanged or decreased. The evidence for a humoral factor involves experiments with crossed-circulation in dogs, in which the non-expanded partner also experienced natriuresis. These findings support the view that the expanded dog partner supplied a humoral substance to the circulation of the non-expanded partner (de Wardener et al. 1961). Natriuresis from residual nephrons after reduction of the parenchymal mass of the kidney can also be explained by the presence of such a hormone. There has been no success so far in attempts to identify this hormone chemically despite two decades of research. The site of production of this hormone is also unknown. It is striking, however, that after hypophysectomy ECF volume expansion does not result in natriuresis (Lichardus and Ponec 1972). Micropuncture data suggest that such a hormone affects tubular Na transport in the proximal tubule. Other biological actions of this factor have not yet been described. De Wardener et al. (1980) believe that the hormone influences Na transport extra-renally as well, and can serve as a partial explanation of Na abnormalities in essential hypertension.

Renal Na excretion is also influenced by neural regulation.

Recent histochemical and electron microscopical findings (Barajas and Mueller 1973) show direct innervation of tubular cells in the rat and monkey renal cortex. The adrenergic nerve terminals are separated from the proximal and distal tubular cells only by the basal membranes. DiBona (1977) has confirmed these findings in the dog. These findings are in agreement with the data of Gill (1969), Schrier and de Wardener (1971), Takacs et al. (1971, 1978) and Bello-Reuss (1978) which indicate that the sympathetic nervous system can directly affect tubular reabsorption of Na.

Present data suggest that efferent impulses to the kidney can produce increased Na and water reabsorption. The precise mechanism of this effect is not clear, but it can be suggested that it is mediated by neurotransmitters (Gottschalk 1979).

The excretion of Na in pathological states, including renal pathology, has yet to be explained. Abnormal Na excretion can involve changes in GFR and in tubular reabsorption. A sudden decrease in GFR to practically nil values of course decreases excretion of Na and water and expands ECF volume. Such a state is represented by acute renal failure with oliguria.

A slow decrease in GFR, as in chronic renal failure, usually does not result in decreased Na excretion. The decrease in filtered load is compensated by an adaptive decrease in tubular reabsorption of Na in residual nephrons (Platt 1950, 1952, Bricker et al. 1965. Slatopolsky et al. 1960).

A number of investigators feel that this adaptive change in tubular Na reabsorption in residual nephrons is due to the action of "natriuretic hormone".

Investigation of patients allows these changes to be evaluated as a function of the fractional excretion of Na (FE_{Na}). In some patients this adaptation in tubular reabsorption is not adequate biologically, and increased Na losses occur (renal salt wasting). This syndrome can be seen under conditions in which Na intake is low, but the kidneys do not conserve Na to the required level. The causes of renal salt wasting are not completely clear.

In some cases, renal salt wasting may be associated with a decreased tubular production of protons and NH_4. Since acid metabolites must be accompanied by a cation, a decreased production of H and NH_4 can result in an increased Na loss, as well as loss of other cations.

A primary disturbance in tubular Na reabsorption may also be involved. This occurs in patients with various forms of interstitial nephritis (Cove-Smith and Knapp 1973) and some congenital diseases of the kidney such as hereditary cystic disease of the medulla (Strauss 1962, Gardner 1971) and Fanconi syndrome.

Abnormal Na conservation has been described in distal forms of RTA (Sebastian et al. 1976).

Renal salt wasting can also result from a tubular resistance to mineralocorticoids. This state is termed pseudo-hypoaldosteronism (Cheek and Perry 1958, Donnell et al. 1959, Roesler et al. 1977).

Renal salt wasting occurs when too little aldosterone is produced, as in Addison's disease, after bilateral adrenalectomy, in various forms of congenital disturbances of steroidogenesis and decreased aldosterone secretion due to a low renin production.

Some chronic renal diseases are, to the contrary, associated with Na retention despite the fact that GFR is normal or only slightly decreased. In such cases, increased tubular reabsorption is at fault.

All factors influencing Na reabsorption have not yet been elucidated. The role of aldosterone has been most studied in salt retention in patients with the nephrotic syndrome. The latter lose considerable plasma protein into the urine, are hypoproteinaemic and the volume of circulating plasma is not adequate. This latter serves as a volume stimulus which increases aldosterone secretion.

Cardiac failure can also play a role in Na retention in patients with chronic renal disease.

METHODS OF INVESTIGATION

URINE Na CONCENTRATION (U_{Na})

Measurement of urine Na concentration is simple and can give us useful information. In healthy adults on a normal diet, urine Na concentration ranges widely depending upon salt and water intake. U_{Na} measured during dehydration of varying duration in 29 healthy controls are given in table:

Duration of dehydration (hr)	12–16	16–20	20–24	24–28	28–32	32–36
Mean U_{Na} (mmol/l)	158	162	177	177	173	183
$\pm$SD	(56)	(65)	(61)	(58)	(56)	(51)

This table shows that in the course of prolonged dehydration, U_{Na} increases fairly little. Mean U_{Na} values exceed plasma Na concentrations (135 ± 5 mmol/l), but U_{Na} — 1SD ranges from 102 to 132 mmol. In other words, in healthy controls on an ad libitum diet, U_{Na} increases at least to 100 mmol after fluid withdrawal.

If a water load is drunk, U_{Na} decreases to low values. With a 2% body weight load (drunk over 30 min) U_{Na} decreases over the next 4 hr to 16.7 ± 5.3 mmol/l.

A decrease in Na intake is followed by a decrease in U_{Na}, but water intake determines the actual level.

When water diuresis is combined with a low Na intake, U_{Na} falls in healthy subjects to very low values, about 1–2 mmol (Coleman et al. 1966). Under these conditions U_{Na} is more or less stabilized and does not change if the urine flow rate increases, which would appear to be related to the attainment of a maximal transepithelial concentration gradient for Na in the distal nephron. In patients with abnormal Na transport in the distal nephron, such low values of U_{Na} are not attained.

During osmotic diuresis unrelated to a salt load (e.g. hypertonic mannitol infusion) U_{Na} decreases to values about 40–80 mmol/l.

The finding that U_{Na} can decrease to levels markedly lower than plasma concentration shows that a fraction of Na reabsorbed was not accompanied by an equivalent amount of water (for isotonicity).

Since very low Na concentrations in the tubular urine can be achieved only in the distal nephron, such a finding suggests that in such cases it is the distal segment which is responsible. In oedematous patients U_{Na} is very low and tubular Na reabsorption high. U_{Na} can fall to unmeasurable values, but, in general, values less than 10 mmol/l are routine in such cases.

Transport of Na in the distal nephron is subject to the action of aldosterone. If the latter is in overabundant supply, U_{Na} is low (along with $U_{Na}V$). At the same time K secretion is raised in the distal nephron, so that the U_{Na}/U_K ratio decreases.

Measurement of U_{Na} can assist the differential diagnosis of oliguric states. If oliguria is associated with a low concentration (U_{Na} less than 20 mmol/l), it can be taken that severe damage to the tubular cells has not occurred, since a considerable transepithelial gradient for Na can still be maintained. The aldosterone response to contraction of the ECF volume will produce such a situation.

URINARY EXCRETION OF Na ($U_{Na}V$)

In clinical practice we usually measure Na excretion per 24 hr. Na concentration is measured in a mixed sample.

If the test is not part of a balance study, $U_{Na}V$ varies from day to day in relation to intake. Intake on an ad libitum diet can vary from 100 to 300 mmol/day. (Since 1 g NaCl = 17 mmol Na, this represents an NaCl intake of about 6–18 g).

Under normal conditions, fecal excretion of Na is small — negligible in relation to intake levels (usually not greater than 5 mmol/day). Significant extrarenal Na loss may occur with excessive sweating.

If the subject does not have abnormal salt loss through the gut or skin, the approximation can be accepted that $U_{Na}V$ = total excretion.

Even if Na intake is not followed in balance studies, measurement of $U_{Na}V$ can still offer valuable information. For example, in patients in the polyuric phase of chronic renal failure or of acute tubular necrosis, $U_{Na}V$ can serve as the basis for quantitative loss replacement.

In patients with oedema, measurement of $U_{Na}V$ can show the effects of therapy.

Measurement of $U_{Na}V$ under balance conditions.

This test involves measurement not only of total urinary excretion of Na, but measuring intake as well. Precise measurements on a low-Na diet also requires measurement of fecal Na content.

The test usually requires the cooperation of a dietician. Separate foodstuffs are measured, and the Na content is calculated on the basis of tables. In very precise metabolic studies, aliquot amounts of the same foodstuffs are analyzed. Careful measurement of Na intake from tabular values (Watt and Merrill 1963) can achieve the precision of chemically measured values. For example, Sebastian et al. (1976) found in balance studies with low-Na diets only 1.4 ± 1.4 mmol Na as the difference between tabular and directly measured values of intake. Individual differences ranged from -0.9 to $+4.7$ mmol.

Urine is collected by spontaneous voiding over 24 hr. Stools are collected with precision for analysis. The patient is weighed daily.

Investigation of renal function here involves measurement of the external Na balance in cases where we wish to determine whether the patient has renal salt wasting. Most cases will be those in which ordinary measurements are not diagnostic, and a low-Na intake must test whether the kidneys are able to decrease excretion proportionately and set up a new balanced state.

The investigation involves 3–5 days of a diet of known Na content ranging about 150 mmol/day. Over the following 7–8 days, a very low-Na diet is given. Technically, one can prepare a diet with a Na content of 20–10 mmol/day.

On the very low-Na diet there is a rapid antinatriuretic response. By the second day on the diet $U_{Na}V$ is clearly depressed, and after several days should correspond to the intake level. This can occur within 3–4 days. $U_{Na}V$ usually stabilizes at levels about 2–3 mmol/day lower than intake (Crabbé et al. 1958, Leutcher and Axelrod 1954).

Balance studies of Na excretion on a very low Na diet requires us to follow the condition of the patient carefully — pulse and BP should be measured several times a day in both horizontal and vertical positions. If the kidneys cannot react adequately to decreased Na intake, ECF volume would decline with haemodynamic sequelae which might be dangerous to the patient. Rapid loss of ECF volume can be measured by weighing the patient.

If the negative Na balance can be observed to have clinical effects, the study must be interrupted and, according to the state of the subject, it may be necessary to infuse isotonic saline or, in lesser cases, increase salt intake. The clinical answer to the ability of the kidneys to retain Na adequately is clear, however. In slight forms of renal salt wasting, only the balance calculations will reveal the state.

In patients with renal salt wasting, renal losses are greater than intake, and a new balanced state is not attained during the test.

Diagnosis of renal salt wasting requires further investigation to differentiate the cause. The first subsequent measurement is the adequacy of mineralocorticoid secretion. If inadequacy is found, this may be due to malfunction of the adrenal cortex or inadequate adrenal stimulation by renin. This involves RIA measurement of circulating A-II, PRA and aldosterone and measurement of the renal response to mineralocorticoid administration. Usually we administer DOCA or fluorocortisone in therapeutic doses and the degree of the antinatriuretic response is followed. In pseudo-hypoaldosteronism the tubules are resistant to aldosterone.

Renal salt wasting may accompany various primary parenchymatous diseases of the kidney. The decrease in tubular Na reabsorption can also be secondary to other functional changes, such as decreased secretion of protons in RTA. Further, in some cases, there may be a primary defect in tubular Cl transport, as is assumed in Bartter's syndrome (Bartter 1979).

In patients in positive Na balance, the reason should be found. If the patients are not end-stage cases of renal failure, further investigation must determine whether nephrotic syndrome or cardiac failure is present.

The relation between Na balance and body weight can be simplified for clinical purposes. If there do not appear to be extrarenal losses, the following equation applies:

$$I_{Na} - U_{Na}V = \Delta BW \times P_{Na} \tag{1}$$

where I_{Na} = Na intake in mmol/day, ΔBW = change in body weight in kg/day and P_{Na} = plasma Na concentration in mmol/l.

Equation (1) further assumes that the change in ECF volume is isotonic. With a negative Na balance, ΔBW is negative. With a balanced state $\Delta BW = 0$ and $I_{Na} = U_{Na}V$.

Diurnal rhythm of Na excretion

In healthy adults more Na is excreted during the day than during the night. Under various pathological conditions this rhythm can be reversed.

The investigation is usually carried out by having the subject collect his own urine separately from 6 to 18 hr and from 18 to 6 hr.

In 17 healthy adult controls on a normal diet we found the following values: (Stříbrná et al. 1976):

Daily excretion: 133 ± 37 mmol/12 hr

Night excretion: 102 ± 41 mmol/12 hr

Changes in the diurnal Na rhythm can be related to changes in the diurnal GFR rhythm, as is the case in patients with cardiac failure (Fejfar and Fejfarova 1961) or as a result of changes in tubular Na reabsorption, as in patients in the advanced stages of chronic renal failure (Jirka et al. 1964) or in patients with essential or renovascular hypertension (Stříbrná et al. 1976).

THE RENAL CLEARANCE OF Na (C_{Na})

Since P_{Na} remains more or less constant, C_{Na} is mainly determined by the rate of excretion. With external balance of Na and ad libitum Na intake, C_{Na} varies from 0.51 to 1.53 ml/min, or 0.085 to 0.255 ml/s. (for calculation see p. 262).

Since C_{Na} is influenced mainly by $U_{Na}V$, calculating the clearance value does not really give us more information than only knowing $U_{Na}V$.

FRACTIONAL EXCRETION OF Na (FE_{Na})

FE_{Na} tells us the fraction of the filtered Na load which is excreted in the final urine.

The usual manner of collecting this data is from a 24-hr urine sample and plasma concentration from one sample of venous blood taken at any time during the day. We also measure the levels of endogenous creatinine in the same urine and blood samples.

In a group of healthy adult volunteers on a normal diet, FE_{Na} was $1.05 \pm 0.89\%$. As a rule, we take 2.0% as the upper limit of normal.

In patients with chronic renal disease, FE_{Na} increases in hyperbolic relation

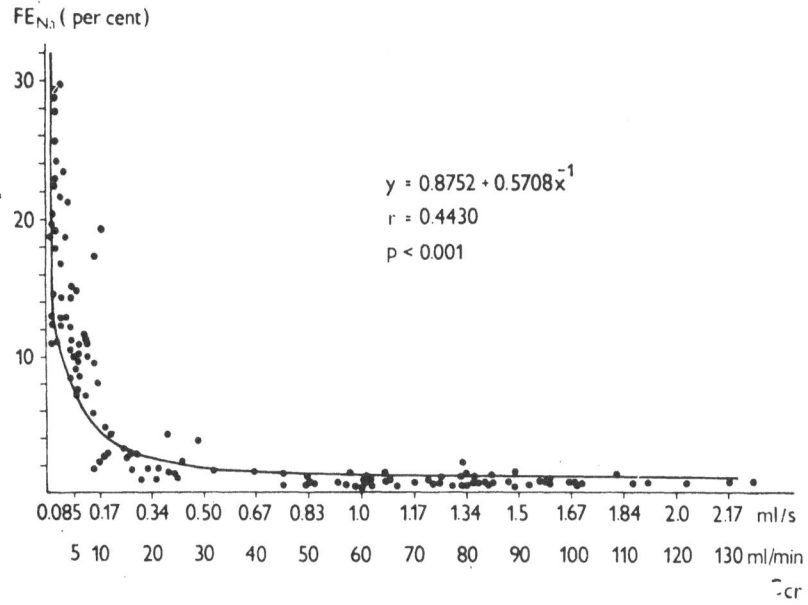

Fig. 59: Relationship between clearance of endogenous creatinine (C_{cr}) and fractional sodium excretion (FE_{Na}) in patients with chronic renal diseases.

189

to GFR. This is shown in Fig. 59. This Fig. shows clearly that when C_{cr} decreases to below 10 ml/min (0.17 ml/s), FE_{Na} can attain values of 25 to 30%.

The increase in FE_{Na} with a decrease in C_{cr} in chronic renal disease is usually a manifestation of adaptive functional changes in the residual nephrons. In other words, this is compensation for the decrease in the number of functional nephrons. The function of residual nephrons can be considered as adequately adapted if body weight is stable, P_{Na} is normal and the external Na balance is 0.

The value of FE_{Na}, which allows a 0 external Na balance to exist will be referred to as "adequate" value — i.e. $FE_{Na\ adq}$ if we can be allowed to introduce a new concept. (See also p. 172).

$FE_{Na\ adq}$ is calculated as follows (Schück, 1982): under conditions of a balanced state of Na metabolism the external Na balance can be expressed as

$$I_{Na} = U_{Na}V + EE_{Na} \qquad (2)$$

where EE_{Na} = external elimination. If EE_{Na} is negligible in relation to $U_{Na}V$, equation (2) can be simplified:

$$I_{Na} = U_{Na}V$$

If external balance of Na = 0, equation for FE_{Na} calculation can be re-arranged:

$$FE_{Na}(\%) = \frac{\dfrac{I_{Na}}{1440}}{\dfrac{GFR \cdot P_{Na}}{1000}} \, 100 \qquad (3)$$

where I_{Na} is in mmol/day, GFR in ml/min and P_{Na} in mmol/l. The factor of 1440 is the number of min/day.

If we substitute for P_{Na} the normal mean value (135 mmol and GFR is based upon C_{cr},) we re-arrange:

$$FE_{Na-adq} = 0.5 \, \frac{I_{Na}\,(mmol/24hr)}{C_{cr}\,(ml/min)} \qquad (4)$$

If, for example, a patient with $C_{cr} = 8$ ml/min has an intake of 150 mmol Na, his residual renal parenchyma can maintain 0 external Na balance if FE_{Na} is: $0.5 \times 150/8 \doteq 9.4\%$. This value for the patient is "adequate" to maintain him compensated with his given GFR and Na intake. $FE_{Na} = 9.4\%$ is not a difficult task for residual nephrons, since with extreme limitation of GFR, FE_{Na} can reach (as mentioned above) values as high as 25–30%.

If a patient with $C_{cr} = 2$ ml/min had an intake of 150 mmol Na, his adequate FE_{Na} would have to be: $0.5 \times 150/2 = 37.5\%$. This value exceeds the maximum FE_{Na} and this patient very likely would not be in an externally balanced state.

In aedematous states FE_{Na} decreases to very low values. In patients with the nephrotic syndrome and marked oedema, FE_{Na} can be lower than 0.2% and in severe cases this value can be even lower.

DISTAL Na REABSORPTION

As explained on p. 145, it is possible on the basis of the clearance of solute-free water (C_{H_2O}) indirectly to estimate the rate of reabsorption of Na in the distal tubule. The measurement must be carried out under conditions of maximal water diuresis (cf. p. 142).

Interpretation of C_{H_2O} as an index of Na reabsorption in the distal (dilution) segment of the nephron requires us to take into account a number of factors (Danowitch and Bricker 1976). C_{H_2O} or C_{H_2O}/GFR is a measure of distal Na reabsorption only if: 1) formation of solute-free water occurs only because of distal NaCl reabsorption, 2) water reabsorption in the diluting segment is completely suppressed, both because VP secretion has disappeared and because there is no reabsorption of water independent of VP.

On the basis of studies by Wallin et al. (1973) it would appear that the diluting segment during maximal water diuresis is not completely impermeable to water, so that C_{H_2O}/GFR is rather an approximation of Na reabsorption in the diluting segment, but nevertheless clinically useful.

Evaluation of distal Na reabsorption also requires knowledge of the rate of Na delivery from the "proximal" tubule (i.e. proximal to the diluting segment) into the diluting segment.

The load of isotonic fluid transferred to the diluting segment is evaluated in three ways:

1. With the assumption that water reabsorption in the diluting segment in maximal water diuresis is negligible in relation to the final rate of urine formation, it can be taken that the distal osmotic load corresponds to the rate of final urine flow (Eknoyan et al. 1967, Stein et al. 1967, Bennett 1973, Martinez-Moldonado et al. 1974).

The value of V ceases to be an index of the distal Na load if the tubular urine contains non-Na osmotically active substances, e.g. glucose or mannitol.

2. The distal Na load can be estimated on the basis of values of $(C_{H_2O} + C_{Na})$/ /GFR (Barton et al. 1972, Kahn et al. 1972).

The expression of distal load does not take into account reabsorption of Na by exchange for H or K.

3. Finally, the distal NaCl load can be characterized by values of $(C_{H_2O} + C_{Cl})$/ /GFR (Seldin and Rector, 1972). With this approach distal transport of Na is evaluated in terms of Cl reabsorption, so that the result is not influenced by the amount of Na exchanged in the distal tubule.

In healthy adult controls on a normal diet, $[(C_{H_2O} + C_{Na})/GFR]\,100 = = 12.5 \pm 4.3\%$ and $[C_{Na}/(C_{H_2O} + C_{Na})]\,100 = 8.1 \pm 2.9\%$.

The latter gives the distal excretion fraction of Na (i.e. that part of the distal load excreted into the final urine).

The value of the ratio $[C_{H_2O}/(C_{Na} + C_{H_2O})]\,100 = 91.3 \pm 2.9\%$ and gives us the distal Na reabsorption in relation to its distal load. Values based upon C_{Cl} are given, along with their meaning, on p. 200.

Indications for investigation

Acute oliguric states

The differential diagnosis of acute oliguric states must decide between functional changes and acute damage to the renal parenchyma. If oliguria is related to increased tubular reabsorption of Na and water, as with aldosterone secretion after ECF volume depletion, U_{Na} decreases to very low values, usually below 20 mmol and FE_{Na} decreases to less than 1 %. In acute oliguric states resulting from severe damage to tubular cells, isosthenuric urine is formed with U_{Na} higher than 40 mmol usually about 50–70 mmol and FE_{Na} is higher than 2 %. (Miller et al. 1978, Vertel and Knochel 1967.

As soon as the patient is given an infusion of mannitol or an injection of furosemide, these criteria are no longer valid. Investigation of renal function is also important in the polyuric stage of acute renal failure conditioned by tubular necrosis. In such cases a large amount of isosthenuric urine is formed, and Na depletion can occur with a resulting loss of ECF volume. Daily measurements of $U_{Na}V$ gives us the basis for quantitative replacement of Na losses.

Chronic renal failure

Measurement of daily Na excretion allows us to judge the excretion capacity of the residual tubular parenchyma for Na. Measurement of FE_{Na} tells us whether the excretion capacity is exhausted or not. In advanced states of chronic renal failure, FE_{Na} can reach 25–30 %.

Measurement of Na excretion is also of practical use in patients who are in a regular dialysis programe and still have a residual urine flow. Correction of Na intake or administration of furosemide, if indicated, can maintain body weight constant. This is of particular importance in the presence of arterial hypertension which is volume-dependent, and in patients with signs of cardiac failure.

Renal salt wasting

The causes of this syndrome may be related to a number of pathologies. We see the syndrome quite frequently as a result of **excessive diuretic therapy** in the treatment of moderate oedema. This can be associated with tachycardia and orthostatic hypotension. In some cases, convulsion can occur. The data suggest a contraction of ECF volume. The plasma protein concentration and Hct are increased. (This, of course, depends upon baseline values before administration of diuretic drugs). Na concentration in the plasma can be normal — in severe cases hyponatrae-mia can exist.

Renal salt wasting can result from a deficiency of aldosterone. The classical example is Addison's disease. General clinical findings and measurement of a 24-hr urine excretion of aldosterone — 18-glucuronide, plasma levels of aldo-sterone and renin after a night's rest in the horizontal position and after 4 hr in a vertical position, all help to establish the diagnosis. If salt wasting can be related to aldosterone, further endocrine tests are necessary. The latter should assist in distinguishing between inadequate renin release or whether aldosterone secretion is low despite adequate renin stimulation.

Attention is, of course, paid to a diagnosis of salt wasting on the basis of primary parenchymatous renal disease. Detailed functional tests are therefore needed.

Oedematous states

These mainly involve the nephrotic syndrome. In such cases we measure urinary Na excretion to estimate external Na balance. Follow-up of urinary excretion of Na and water, and body weight, are helpful in judging the effectiveness of therapy.

Arterial hypertension

In patients with arterial hypertension, limitation of Na intake is usually indicated. Measurement of Na excretion/day in ambulant patients allows us to judge whether the recommended diet is being maintained or not. If the daily Na excretion is higher than 200 mmol, it is hard to believe that the patient is restricting salt intake. If the patient does not sufficiently cooperate so that one cannot depend upon the precision of urine collection, FE_{Na} should be used as a criterion. If GFR is normal, FE_{Na} on a salt-poor diet should be less than 1%. Patients with arterial hyperten-sion can have a reversed diurnal rhythm of Na excretion. In renovascular hyperten-sion, there should be assymmetry in both Na excretion and FE_{Na}. The kidney with a stenosed artery has a lower FE_{Na} value than the contralateral normal organ. This investigation has been of great assistance in the differential diagnosis of arterial hypertension. At present we have methods which enable us to eliminate ureteral catheterization (cf.p. 79).

The transplanted kidney

Interpretation of Na excretion and FE_{Na} in a transplanted kidney is complex. Immediately after surgery, the renal excretion of Na is influenced by ischaemic effects in the transplanted organ before insertion. The degree of tubular damage suffered by the organ during transplantation is important. The course of changes in Na excretion and FE_{Na} can show a similar pattern to that after the onset of acute tubular necrosis. Na excretion and FE_{Na} immediately after transplantation can be further affected by the state of water and electrolyte metabolism in the receiver. If during transplantation there was an ECF volume expansion, it is possible that the regulatory mechanisms in the receiver can alter the function of the freshly attached organ.

The later course of events with Na excretion and FE_{Na} depends upon the changes in GFR and on immunobiological processes.

A rejection reaction can be manifest by a decrease in $U_{Na}V$ and FE_{Na} (Hamburger et al. 1964, 1965, Starzl 1964). Evaluation of these parameters must ignore absolute values and concentrate on the dynamics of change.

It is further necessary in such interpretation to take into account whether the results are influenced by the residual function of the remaining diseased kidney of the receiver. Finally one must remember that Na excretion can be affected by the drugs used.

Laboratory methods

Measurement of urine and plasma Na is simple and very precise. Small samples are required (0.1–1.0 ml). Routine flame photometry is all that is required.

REFERENCES

Barajas, L., Müller, J.: The innervation of the juxtaglomerular apparatus and surrounding tubules: A quantitative analysis by serial section electron microscopy. J. Ultrastruct. Res. *43*: 107, 1973

Bartter, F. C.: Clinical problems of potassium metabolism. Contr. Nephrol. *21*: 115, 1980

Barton, L. J., Lackner, H. L., Rector, F. C., Seldin, D. W.: The effect of volume expansion on sodium reabsorption in the diluting segment of the dog kidney. Kidney int. *1*: 19, 1972

Bello-Reuss, E., Trevino, P. L., Gottschalk, C. W.: Effect of renal sympathetic nerve stimulation on proximal water and sodium reabsorption. J. clin. Invest. *57*: 1104, 1976

Bennett, C. M.: Effect of extracellular volume expansion upon sodium reabsorption in the distal nephron of dogs. J. clin. Invest. *52*: 2548, 1973

Bourgoignie, J., Hwang, J., Ipaskehi, E., Bricker, N. S.: The presence of a natriuretic factor in urine of patients with chronic uremia. The absence of the factor in nephrotic uremic patients. J. clin Invest. *53*: 1559, 1974

Bricker, N. S., Klahr, S., Parkenson, M., Schultze, R. G.: Renal function in chronic renal disease. Medicine *44*: 263, 1965

Brunner, H., Kushinsky, G., Peters, G.: Die Wirkung von Vasopressin auf die renale Wasser- und Salzausscheidung der Ratte bei Veränderungen der Salzkonzentration des Trinkwassers und nach Nierenparenchymresektion. Naunyn-Schmiedeberg's Arch. exp. Path. Pharmacol. *228*: 434, 1956

Cheek, D. B., Perry, J. W.: A salt wasting syndrome in infancy. Arch. Dis. Child. 33: 252, 1958

Coleman, A. J., Arias, M., Carter, N. W., Rector, F. C. Jr., Seldin, D. W.: The mechanism of salt wastage in chronic renal disease. J. clin. Invest. 45: 1116, 1966

Cort, J. H.: Electrolytes, fluid dynamics and the nervous system Prague. Publ. House Czechoslov. Acad. Sci. 1965

Cort, J. H., Lichardus, B.: The natriuretic activity of jugular vein blood during carotid occlusion. Physiol. bohemoslov. 12: 497, 1963

Crabbé, J., Ross, E. J., Thorn, G. W.: The significance of the secretion of aldosterone during dietary sodium deprivation in normal subjects. J. clin. Endocrinol. Metabol. 18: 1159, 1958

Cove-Smith, J. R., Knapp, M. S.: Sodium handling in analgesic nephropathy. Lancet 2: 70, 1973

Danowitch, G. M., Bricker, N. S.: Influence of volume expantion on NaCl reabsorption in the diluting segments of the nephron: A study using clearance methods. Kidney int. 10: 229, 1976

DeWardener, H., McGregor, G.: The natriuretic hormone and essential hypertension. In: Hormonal regulation of sodium excretion (Eds. B. Lichardus, R. W. Schrier and J. Ponec) Amsterdam Elsevier/North-Holland Biomed. Press 1980, pp. 387–392

Deetjen, P., Kramer, K.: Die Abhängigkeit des O_2-Verbrauchs der Niere von der Na-Rückresorption. Pflüger's Arch. ges. Physiol. 273: 636, 1961

DeWardener, H. E., Mills, I. H., Clapham, W. F., Hayter, C. J.: Studies on the efferent mechanism of the sodium diuresis which follows the administration of intravenous saline in the dog. Clin. Sci. 21: 249, 1961

DiBona, G. F.: Neurogenic regulation of renal tubular sodium reabsorption. Am. J. Physiol. 233: F 73, 1973

Donnell, G. N., Litman, R., Roldan, M.: Pseudohypo-adrenalcorticism. Am. J. Dis. Child. 97: 813, 1959

Edelman, I. S., Fimongari, G. M.: On the biochemical mechanism of action of aldosterone. Recent Progr. Horm. Res. 24: 1, 1968

Eknoyan, G., Suki, W. N., Rector, F. C., Seldin, D. W.: Functional characteristics of the diluting segment of the dog nephron and the effect of extracellular volume expansion on its reabsorptive capacity. J. clin. Invest. 46: 1178, 1967

Favre, H.: An inhibitor of sodium transport in the urine of dogs and humans with normal renal function: A study of chronically expanded subjects. In: Natriuretic Hormone. Kramer, H. J., Krück, F. (Eds.) Berlin, Springer 1978, pp. 11–23

Fejfar, Z., Fejfarová, M.: Hämodynamische Veränderungen der Kreislaufströmungen. Berlin Volk und Gesundheit 1961

Fine, C. G., Bourgoignie, J. J., Hwank, K. H.: On the influence of the natriuretic factor from patients with chronic uremia on the bioelectric properties and sodium transport of its isolaetd mammalian collecting tubule. J. clin. Invest. 58: 590, 1976

Gardner, K. D.: Evolution of clinical signs in adult-onset cystic disease of renal medulla. Ann. intern. Med. 74: 47, 1971

Gottschalk, C. W.: Renal nerves and sodium excretion. Ann. Rev. Physiol. 41: 229, 1979

Hamburger, J.: A reappraisal of the concept of organ rejection based on the study of homotransplanted kidneys. Transplantation 5: 870, 1967

Hamburger, J., Richet, G., Crosnier, J., Funck-Bretano, J. L., Antoine, B., Durrot, H., Mery, J. P., DeMontera, H., Royer, P.: Nephrology. Co. Philadelphia, London, Toronto, W. B. Saunders 1968

Herken, H., Senft, G., Schaper, J.: Die Beteiligung des Vasopressins an der Entstehungs des Ödems. Naunyn-Schmiedeberg's Arch. exp. Path. Pharmacol. 230: 284, 1957

Herzog, J. P., Johnston, H. H., Lauler, D. P.: Effects of prostaglandins E_1, E_2 and A_1 on renal hemodynamics, sodium and water excretion in the dog. In: Prostaglandin Symposium of the Worcester Foundation for Experimental Biology, P. W. Ramwell, J. E. Shaw (Eds.). New York Interscience 1967 p. 147

Hierholzer, K. M., Wiederholt, H., Holzgrene, G., Giebisch, R. M., Klose, E., Windhager, E. E.: Micropuncture study of renal transtubular concentration gradients of sodium and potassium in adrenalectomized rats. Pflüger's Arch. ges. Physiol. *285*: 193, 1965

Jard, S. Morel, F.: Actions of vasotocin and some of its analogues on salt and water excretion by the frog. Am. J. Physiol. *204*: 222, 1963

Jirka, J.: Funkce ledvin při aktivním stoji a svalové námaze vleže u lidí se zdravými ledvinami a u nemocných chronickou glomerulonefritidou. Prague – Disseration thesis 1958

Kagawa, C. M., Cella, J. A., van Arman, C. G.: Action of new steroids in blocking effects of aldosterone and desoxycorticosterone on salt. Science *126*: 1015, 1957

Kagawa, C. M., Sturlevant, F. M., van Arman, C. G.: Pharmacology of a new steroid that blocks salt activity of aldosterone and desoxycorticosterone. J. Pharmacol. exp. Ther. *126*: 123, 1959

Kahn, T., Mohammad, G., Stein, R. M.: Alterations in renal tubular sodium and water reabsorption in chronic renal disease in man. Kidney int. *2*: 164, 1972

Landau, R. L., Bergenstal, D. M., Lugibihl Kascht, M. E.: The metabolic effects of progesterone in man. J. clin. Endocrinol. Metabol. *15*: 1194, 1955

Lee, J. B., Covino, B. G., Takman, B. H., Smith, E. R.: Renomedullary vasodepressor substance, medullin: Isolation, chemical characterization and physiological properties. Circulat. Res. *27*: 57, 1965

Leutcher, J. A. Jr., Axelrod, B. J.: Increased aldosterone output during sodium deprivation in normal man. Proc. Soc. exp. Biol. Med. *87*: 650, 1954

Lichardus, B., Ponec, J.: Effect of hypophysectomy on sodium excretion in rats without blood dilution during blood volume expansion. Experientia *28*: 471, 1972

Lifschitz, M. D., Schrier, R. W., Edelman, I.: Effect of actinomycin D on aldosterone-mediated changes in electrolyte excretion. Am. J. Physiol. *224*: 376, 1973

Martinez-Moldonado, M., Eknoyan, G., Suki, W. N.: Influence of volume expansion on renal diluting capacity in the rat. Clin. Sci. Mol. Med. *46*: 331, 1974

Miller, T. J., Anderson, R. J., Linas, S. L., Hendrick, W. L., Berns, A. S., Gabon, P. A., Schrier, R. W.: Urinary diagnostic indices in acute renal failure. A prospective study. Ann. intern. Med. *89*: 47, 1978

Murphy, G. P., Hesse, V. E., Evers, J. L., Hobika, G., Mosteret, J., Szolnoky, A., Schoonees, P., Abramczyk, J., Grace, J. Jr.: The renal and cardiodynamic effects of prostaglandins (PGE₁, PGA₁) in renal ischemia. J. Surg. Res. *10*: 533, 1970

Platt, R.: Sodium and potassium excretion in chronic renal failure. Clin. Sci. *9*: 367, 1950

Platt, R.: Structural and functional adaptation in renal failure. Brit. med. J. *1*: 1313, 1952

Ramwell, P. W., Shaw, J. E.: Biological significance of the prostaglandins. Recent Progr. Hormone Res. *26*: 139, 1970

Rieder, J.: Physikalisch-chemische und biologische Untersuchungen an Sulfonamiden. Arzneimittelforschung *13*: 81, 1963

Rösler, A., Theodor, R., Biochis, H., Gerty, R., Ulick, S., Alagem, M., Tabachnik, E., Cohen, B. Rabinowitz, D.: Metabolic responses to the administration of angiotensin II, K and ACTH in two salt-wasting syndromes. J. clin. Endocrinol. Metabol. *44*: 292, 1977

Sebastian, A., McSherry, E., Morris, R. C.: Impaired renal conservation of sodium chloride during sustained correction of systemic acidosis in patients with Type I, classic renal tubular acidosis. J. clin. Invest. *58*: 454, 1976

Seldin, D. W., Rector, F. C.: Evaluation of clearance methods for localizatin of site of action of diuretics. In: Modern diuretic therapy in the treatment of cardiovascular and renal disease. Amsterdam, Excerpta Medica 1972, p. 97

196

Schrier, R. W., DeWardener, H. E.: Tubular reabsorption of sodium ion influence of factors other than aldosterone and glomerular filtration rate. New Engl. J. Med. *285*: 1231, 1971

Schück, O.: Fractional sodium excretion in patients with chronic renal failure with respect to the therapy. Nephron *30*: 95, 1982

Schück, O., Stříbrná, J.: Renal clearance of sodium and solute-free water. Physiol. bohemoslov. *15*: 210, 1966

Sharp, G. W. G., Coggino, C. H., Lichtenstein, N. S., Leaf, A.: Evidence for a mucosal effect of aldosterone on sodium transport in the toad bladder. J. clin. Invest. *45*: 1640, 1966

Sharp, G. W. G., Leaf, A.: Studies on the biological action of aldosterone in vitro. J. clin. Invest. *42*: 978, 1963

Skou, J. C.: The influence of some cations on adenosintriphosphatase from peripheral nerves. Bioch. biophys. Acta *23*: 394, 1957

Slatopolsky, E., Elkan, I. O., Weerts, C., Bricker, N. S.: Studies on the characteristic of the control system governing sodium excretion in uremic man. J. clin. Invest. *47*: 521, 1968

Starzl, T. E.: Experience in renal transplantation. Philadelphia, Saunders 1964

Stein, R. M., Abramson, R. G., Kahn, T., Levitt, M. F.: Effects of hypotonic saline loading in hydrated dog: Evidence for a saline induced limit on distal tubular sodium transport. J. clin. Invest. *46*: 1205, 1967

Strauss, M. B.: Clinical and pathological aspects of cystic disease of the renal medulla. Ann. intern. Med. *57*: 373, 1962

Stříbrná, J., Růžičková, O., Schück, O., Firt, P., Dráb, K., Cholinský, K.: Changes in circadian sodium excretion in patients with essential hypertension and with renal artery stenosis. Cor Vasa *18*: 11, 1976

Takacs, L., Benosath, P., Demeczky, L.: Renal sodium and water excretion after unilateral splanchnitocomy in the dog. Acta physiol. Acad. Sci Hung. *39*: 289, 1971

Takacs, L., Benosath, P., Szalay, L.: Depressed proximal tubular transport capacity after renal sympathectomy. Proc. VIIth int. Congr. Nephrol. Montreal 1978 Basel, Karger 1978, pp. 553–558

Thurau, K.: Nature of autoregulation of renal blood flow. Proc. 3rd intern. Congr. Nephrol. Vol. 1 Basel, Karger New York 1967

Ullrich, K. J.: Sugar, aminoacid and Na+ cotransport in the proximal tubule. Ann. Rev. Physiol. *41*: 181, 1979

Ullrich, K. J.: Renal transport of sodium. Proc. 3rd Int. Congr. Nephrol. Vol. 1 Lasel, New York, Karger, 1966

Vertel, R. M., Knochel, J. P.: Nonoliguric acute renal failure. J. am. med. Assoc. *200*: 598, 1967

Wallin, J. D., Brennan, J. P., Long, D. L., Aronoff, S. L., Rector, F. C., Seldin, D. W.: Effect of increased distal bicarbonate delivery on free water reabsorption in the dog. Am. J. Physiol. *224*: 209, 1973

Watt, B. K., Merrill, A. L.: In: Composition of foods. Raw. Processed. Prepared. Consumer and food economics Research Division. Agricultural research service. Washington United States Dept. of Agriculture, (revised) 1963

Wiederholt, M., Hierholzer, K., Rumrich, G., Holzgreve, H.: Transtubuläre Natriumströme im proximalen und distalen Tubulus adrenalektomierter Ratten. Pflüger's Arch. ges. Physiol. *281*: 95, 1964

EXCRETION OF CHLORIDE

PHYSIOLOGY AND PATHOPHYSIOLOGY

Chloride changes usually follow Na changes in the urine, but they are not merely an electrostatic partner — in some cases there may be dissociation of the two.

Micropuncture studies (Walker et al. 1937, 1941) show that Cl freely penetrates the glomerular membrane, i.e. $[Cl]_{glom\ filtrate} = [Cl]_{plasma}$. The Gibbs-Donnan factor for univalent anions $= 1.05$.

In the proximal tubule most of the filtered Cl load is reabsorbed. This is a passive process, following electrochemical gradients. In the loop of Henle there is recirculation of Cl, and a medullary Cl gradient is formed (Ullrich et al. 1956). The findings of Burg and Green (1971) and Kokko (1974) suggest that tubular transport of Cl in the thick ascending limb of the loop of Henle is an active process.

Cl is also reabsorbed in the distal tubules and collecting ducts. The mechanism of the latter is not yet known. The earlier micropuncture studies of Rector and Clapp (1962) suggested active transport here as well.

Only 1% of the total filtered Cl load is excreted into the urine. Cl, and for that matter Na ions as well, are excreted from the organism almost exclusively by the kidneys. Excessive sweating can add to these losses.

Physiologically, Cl and HCO_3 are the main electrochemical partners for Na in the ECF.

Under various situations the Cl/HCO_3 ratio can change (sodium and osmolality remaining unchanged) and this reflects changes in the pH of the ECF.

Cl losses after thiazide diuretics are usually not great, and hypochloraemic alkalosis is not exaggerated. On the other hand, following furosemide therapy and the use of ethacrynic acid, Cl losses can be striking and hypochloraemic alkalosis can develop. Since the latter diuretics also increase renal K losses, the alkalosis also involves hypokalaemia.

Increased renal Cl losses can be a primary cause of Bartter's syndrome (Bartter, 1980). It is possible that decreased tubular Cl transport in the distal nephron is a cause of the increased tubular K secretion.

Increased distal tubular Cl reabsorption is assumed to play an aetiological role in some of electrolyte imbalances. Schambelan et al. (1981) described a patient with hyperkalaemia who was resistant to mineralocorticoids and did not lose Na. This is called type II pseudohypo-aldosteronism. The cause of the inadequate K secretion appeared to be increased distal Cl reabsorption, because with increased loading with un-reabsorbable anions into the distal nephron (e.g. SO_4) there was a significant increase in distal K secretion.

Urinary Cl excretion significantly decreases if there are large extra-renal Cl losses, e.g. repeated vomiting or suction drainage of the gastric contents. In unclear cases, when the quantities of Cl loss are not known, the urinary Cl concentration gives valuable information.

In pathological states involving HCO_3 losses into the urine (RTA) and a decrease in plasma levels, plasma Cl increases. Since proximal Cl reabsorption is passive, the rate of transport is significantly affected by the rate of proton secretion and the rate of HCO_3 reabsorption.

METHODS OF INVESTIGATION

URINARY EXCRETION OF Cl

This value shows a great degree of scatter as a function of oral intake. A healthy adult control will excrete into the urine 100 to 300 mmol/day. It is of greater significance to compare the excretions of Na and Cl.

In healthy adult controls on a normal diet the mean ratio U_{Na}/U_{Cl} was 0.89 ± 0.30. Differences are of greater significance clinically than absolute data (i.e. the Na-Cl difference).

THE RENAL Cl CLEARANCE (C_{Cl}) and fractional excretion of Cl (FE_{Cl})

In healthy adult subjects on normal diet, C_{Cl} ranges from 0.7 to 2.1 ml/min = $= 0.012 - 0.036$ ml/s.

The C_{Na}/C_{Cl} ratio was, on the average, 0.66 ± 0.14. The clearance data on their own do not give us more information than urinary excretion.

FE_{Cl} gives the fraction of the filtered Cl load excreted into the urine (for calculation see p. 262).

In healthy adult controls on a normal diet, FE_{Cl} was $1.20 \pm 0.50\%$. A value greater than 2% is considered abnormal.

DISTAL Cl REABSORPTION

As explained on p. 191, one can consider distal Cl reabsorption under conditions of maximal water diuresis as a function of C_{H_2O}. The amount of Cl which can be considered as a load for the distal nephron can be evaluated (Seldin and Rector, 1972) as:

$[(C_{H_2O} + C_{Cl})/GFR]$ 100. This value in our healthy subjects was 13.3 ± 2.5 ml/min/100 ml C_{cr}.

The relation between excretion of Cl into the final urine and the distal Cl load is given by:

$[C_{Cl}/(C_{H_2O} + C_{Cl})]$ 100. This ratio in healthy subjects was $10.1 \pm 6.9\%$. To express the rate of reabsorption of Cl in the distal nephron, we also use the ratio:

$[C_{H_2O}/(C_{H_2O} + C_{Cl})]$ 100. The latter value was $88.7 \pm 7.4\%$. This latter ratio gives us the fraction of the distal Cl load reabsorbed in the distal nephron.

Measurement of these ratios requires us to induce a maximal water diuresis during which we measure simultaneously the concentrations of Cl and cr and all osmotically active substances. Interpretation of these findings requires us to take into account all factors important for complete inhibition of tubular water reabsorption under conditions of maximal water diuresis (cf. p. 142).

Indications for investigation

Diuretic therapy

During therapy with furosemide or ethacrynic acid, or with prolonged use of hydrochlorothiazide, one should follow plasma Cl levels and urinary excretion. Diuretic therapy is the commonest cause of Cl depletion.

States associated with increased extrarenal Cl losses

Repeated vomiting or suction drainage of gastric contents will produce Cl depletion. In such cases the urinary concentration and excretion of Cl can decrease markedly.

Acid-base disturbances of unknown cause

In various pathological states, in which the acid-base balance is disturbed, it is necessary to investigate (in addition to direct parameters of acid-base balance), also renal Cl excretion. Such patients include: abnormalities of adrenal production of mineralocorticoids and glucocorticoids, Bartter syndrome, pseudohypo-aldosteronism, malignant tumours producing hormonally active peptides, severe K deficiency, excessive use of licorice.

Laboratory methods

Simple mercury titrations will give an accurate measure of Cl in urine and plasma (Schales 1941, 1953). Potentiometry (Seligson et al. 1958) as well as colorimetric methods (Kim et al. 1972) can be recommended.

REFERENCES

Bartter, F. C.: Clinical problems of potassium metabolism. Contr. Nephrol. *21*: 115, 1980

Burg, M., Green, N.: Effect of mersatyl on the thick ascending limb of Henle's loop. Kidney int. *4*: 245, 1973

Kim, E. K., Wadell, L. D., Logan, J. E.: Observation on diagnostic kits for the determination of chloride. Clin. Biochem. *5*: 214, 1972

Kokko, J. P.: Membrane characteristics governing salt and water in the loop of Henle. Fed. Proc. *33*: 25, 1974

Rector, F. C. Jr., Clapp, J. R.; Evidence for active chloride reabsorption in the distal tubule of the rat. J. clin. Invest. *41*: 101, 1962

Schales, O.: Chloride. Stand. Meth. clin. Chem. *1*: 37, 1953

Schales, O., Schales, S. S.: A single and accurate method for the determination of chloride in biological fluids. J. biol. Chem. *140*: 879, 1941

Schambelan, M., Sebastian, A., Rector, F. C. Jr.: Mineralocorticoid-resistant renal hyperkalemia without salt wasting (type 1 pseudohypoaldosteronism): Role of increased renal chloride reabsorption. Kidney int. *19*: 716, 1981

Seldin, D. W., Rector, F. C.: Evaluation of clearance methods for localization of site of action of diuretics. In: Modern diuretic therapy in the treatment of cardiovascular and renal disease. Amsterdam Excerpta Med., 1972, p. 97

Seligson, D., McCormick, G. J., Sleeman, A.: Electrometric method for determination of chloride in serum and other biologic fluids. Clin. Chem. *4*: 159, 1958

Ullrich, K. J., Jarausch, K. H.: Untersuchungen zum Problem der Harnkonzentrierung und Verdünnung über die Verteilung der Elektrolyten (Na, K, Ca, Mg, Cl, anorgan Phosphat), Harnstoff, Aminosäuren und exogenes Kreatinin in der Rinde und Mark der Hundniere bei verschiedenen Diuresezuständen. Pflüger's Arch. ges. Physiol. *262*: 537, 1956

Walker, A. M., Bott, P. A., Oliver, J., McDowell, M. C.: The collection and analysis of fluid from single nephrons of the mammalian kidney. Am. J. Physiol. *134*: 580, 1941

Walker, A. M., Hudson, C. L., Findley, T. Jr., Richards, A. N.: The total molecular concentration and the chloride concentration of fluid from different segments of the renal tubule of amphibia. Am. J. Physiol. *118*: 121, 1937

EXCRETION OF CALCIUM AND PHOSPHATE

Investigation of the excretion of Ca and phosphates, as well as measurements of plasma concentrations, has taken on momentum in recent years. This is because: a) many patients with lithiasis also have hypercalciuria. The latter can have many metabolic causes but there may also be a primary defect in the renal excretion of Ca. b) Since in recent years there has been considerable progress in the management of chronic renal failure, abnormalities of Ca and bone metabolism complicate the state of such patients. Therefore the nephrologist must not only concentrate his attention on purely renal disease, but also on wider metabolic problems.

Measurement of plasma concentrations of Ca and inorganic phosphates (iP), and their renal excretion, is only a small part of a workup of Ca and bone metabolism. The renal defects which the nephrologist measures often serve as the initial stimulus for a more complex metabolic workup. The latter will include measurements (RIA) of parathormone levels in the plasma (PTH), determination of urinary excretion of cyclic AMP (cAMP) and hydroxyproline, and histological evaluation of bone biopsies.

PHYSIOLOGY AND PATHOPHYSIOLOGY

Ca and iP are excreted from the organism through the gut and kidneys. Renal excretion of these substances is finely regulated, since the concentrations of Ca and iP in the ECF are maintained quite constant, and the biologically allowable range of plasma Ca values is particularly narrow.

Renal excretion of Ca and iP has been intensively studied in recent years by micropuncture studies in animals. These studies can be concisely summarized as follows (Lassiter and Gottschalk 1963, Ullrich et al. 1976, Suki 1980, Lang 1980).

Ca concentration in the GF is 50–70% of plasma values, the mean being about 60%. In the proximal segment of the nephron, about 75% of the filtered amount is reabsorbed. Of this, about 60% is reabsorbed in the convoluted tubule and 15% in the pars recta. Fifteen percent is reabsorbed in the thick ascending limb of the loop of Henle, a further 15% is reabsorbed in the convoluted distal tubule and in the granulated part of the collecting ducts a further 9% is reabsorbed. Only 1% of the filtered Ca load reaches the final urine.

Approximately 2/3r of the total reabsorption of Ca in the proximal tubule takes place passively, while 1/3 is transported actively. Active Ca transport appears to involve the following mechanism: Ca^{++} penetrates the luminal membrane into tubular cells passively and is actively pumped out of the cells at the basal membrane in exchange for Na^+. Transport of Ca in the distal convoluted tubule is only active.

The concentration of iP in glomerular filtrate is about 90% of the plasma level. 2/3r of the filtered load is reabsorbed in the proximal tubules. The precise roles of the loop of Henle and the distal tubule have not yet been defined. There are many discrepancies between published results, which is perhaps related to the fact that superficial and deep nephrons behave in this regard quite differently. Some findings suggest that iP is secreted by the tubules.

Penetration of the luminal membrane by iP in the proximal tubular cells is uphill and is driven by coupling with two sodium ions, whereas exit at the basal membrane may be entirely passive. Tubular transport of iP is saturated with increased plasma P levels (Pitts and Alexander 1944).

Tubular transport of Ca and iP is influenced by a number of factors. Tubular reabsorption of Ca is stimulated by PTH, 1.25-$(OH)_2$-D_3 and alkalosis. The process is inhibited by calcitonin, growth hormone, thyroid hormone, insulin, acidosis, prolonged exposure to glucocorticoids and mineralocorticoids. Tubular reabsorption of iP is stimulated by P depletion, thyroxin, growth hormone, metabolic acidosis, acute administration of 1.25-$(OH)_2$-D_3, hypocalcaemia, metabolic alkalosis and respiratory acidosis.

From the above list it would appear that factors which affect tubular transport of Ca and iP also affect tubular transport of Na. The interrelation between renal excretion of Ca and Na (Walser 1961) has been demonstrated in many different situations. Increased Na excretion is usually associated with increased Ca excretion. It is therefore necessary to measure both cations. On the other hand, changes in plasma concentration of Ca affect tubular Na transport. Hypercalcaemia is associated with a decrease in tubular reabsorption of Na and results in natriuresis (Harrington and Cohen 1973). As an example of relations between renal excretion of Na and Ca in man, mention should be made of the reaction to natriuretic drugs (Sotornik et al. 1969) (Fig. 60).

The kidneys play a role in Ca homeostasis not only by excretion but also by virtue of their non-excretory metabolic function. The kidneys hydroxylate D_3. This vitamin is first metabolized in the liver to 25-(OH)-D_3, and the latter in the kidneys is converted to the dihydroxy derivative, the second -OH being placed at position 1 or 24.

If renal function is normal and Ca and iP metabolism unaltered, the renal tubules produce 24.25-$(OH)_2$-D_3. If plasma Ca is low and iP increased, 1.25-$(OH)_2$-D_3 is formed, which is the active form of vitamin D. This substance acts along with PTH on bone, the gut and the renal tubules to increase plasma Ca levels. The formation of active D_3 is stimulated by PTH. Hypophosphataemia also stimulates this conversion, independently of PTH.

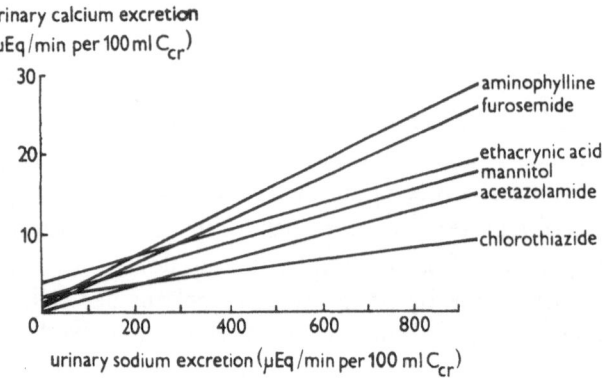

urinary calcium excretion
(μEq/min per 100 ml C_{cr})

aminophylline
furosemide
ethacrynic acid
mannitol
acetazolamide
chlorothiazide

urinary sodium excretion (μEq/min per 100 ml C_{cr})

Fig. 60: Relationship between urinary sodium and calcium excretion in healthy subjects after the administration of diuretics.

Urinary excretion of Ca and iP can be disturbed by primary kidney disease, or secondarily by damaged renal function which affects Ca and P metabolism.

Hypercalciuria produced by a decrease in tubular reabsorption of unknown cause was previously termed idiopathic hypercalcuria. Recent work has shown that such patients, previously thought to have a primary renal abnormality instead, could suffer from hyperabsorption of Ca in the gut (the absorptive type) or increased delivery of Ca from bone (osteoresorptive type). In the latter cases hypercalciuria would be a secondary change.

Metabolic studies of urolithiasis patients have shown that hypercalciuria is a pure finding in patients with Ca stones (Yendt 1970) and that this disturbance plays a significant role in stone formation.

For these reasons methods have been worked out to make the differential diagnosis clinically of the various causes of hypercalciuria (Pak et al. 1975). Here we shall only go over the principal highlights. Hypercalciuria on the basis of delivery from bone may result from a variety of pathologies. Most frequently this involves:

Hyperparathyroidism
Chronic immobilization
Cushing's syndrome and disease
Malignant tumours
Paget's Disease
Hyperthyroidism

Hypercalciuria on the basis of increased gut delivery of Ca occurs with excessive Ca intake, sarcoidosis and excessive vitamin D administration. If the cause are increased tubular losses, then we must take into account metabolic acidosis, medullary sponge kidney, primary hyperaldosteronism and excessive dosage with furosemide.

Research has shown (Bordier et al. 1977, Gray et al. 1977) that in some cases the primary defect may be in tubular iP reabsorption. This results first in hypophosphataemia, with secondary decrease in tubular reabsorption of Ca.

Patients with nephrotic syndrome often have abnormal Ca metabolism, even if the stage of renal failure has not been reached. Hypocalcaemia is often found in such cases, which is attributed to the loss of plasma proteins binding Ca. This defect occurs as a result of the urinary protein loss due to the increased glomerular permeability. In addition, such patients may show hypocalciuria and decreased gut Ca absorption.

Recent findings (Schmidt-Gayk et al. 1977) suggest that patients with nephrotic syndrome have plasma levels of 25-OH-D_3 lower than the norm. These investigators reported that plasma protein is low for active D_3 binding (a "binding protein" is thought to exist) and the urinary protein in such patients contained a fraction which could bind active D_3.

A decreased level of 25-OH-D_3 in nephrotic patients has also been demonstrated by other investigators (Barragry et al. 1977). Significant changes in Ca and iP metabolism also occur in chronic renal failure. This may be conditioned by iP retention, abnormal renal production of the 1.25 dihydroxy form of D_3 and decreased bone sensitivity to PTH.

The decrease in GFR in chronic renal disease is associated with a decrease in fractional reabsorption of iP (Better et al. 1967, Kleeman et al. 1967, Popovtzer et al. 1969, 1970). This enables plasma iP to be maintained at normal levels as long as GFR does not decrease to values lower than 20–30 ml/min.

The mechanism of decreasing tubular reabsorption of iP in residual nephrons is not yet completely clear. A number of findings suggest that to decrease this reabsorption one requires an increase in PTH production (Slatopolsky et al. 1966, 1968, 1972). Plasma PTH levels in patients with chronic renal failure, however, show a wide scatter (Massry et al. 1972). Infusion of parathyroid extract results in an increase in the excretion fraction of iP in healthy controls and in patients with a normal or moderately decreased GFR. In patients in an advanced state of renal failure the action of PTH on the excretion fraction of iP is not clearcut (Massry et al. 1973).

In addition to PTH, other factors also decrease the excretion fraction of iP. The findings of Popovtzer et al. (1969) showed that patients with chronic renal failure continue to have a high excretion fraction for iP even after complete removal of the parathyroids. An increase in ECF volume may play a role in this (Wen et al. 1976). The plasma iP level does not appear to have a great effect on excretion of iP in residual nephrons (Popovtzer et al. 1969).

Plasma Ca levels decrease in patients with advanced renal failure. The rise in plasma iP levels plays a role in this, along with the decrease in gut Ca absorption. A decrease in the renal production of "active" dihydroxy-D_3 may be responsible for the latter gut effect. Since metabolic acidosis is also present, the level of ionized Ca decreases more slowly than the total plasma level.

Fractional reabsorption of Ca in residual nephrons decreases, but despite this total Ca excreted into the urine in advanced renal failure also decreases.

Chronic renal failure is associated with a decreased sensitivity of bone to PTH. Some investigators feel that this factor is important and responsible for hypocalcaemia and secondary hyperparathyroidism.

This complex of metabolic and endocrine changes in chronic renal failure leads to the development of bone changes which are fairly varied in nature. In most cases there is a combination of osteitis fibrosa, osteomalacia, osteosclerosis and osteoporosis.

METHODS OF INVESTIGATION

URINARY EXCRETION OF Ca

A basic clinical test is measurement of total Ca excretion into the urine over 24 hr. Evaluation of the findings must also take into account Ca intake in the diet. The investigatory procedures are as follows:

1. Urinary excretion on a normal diet

The upper limit of normal ranges about 300 mg/24 hr. Hodgkinson and Pyrah (1959) report as upper limits: 300 mg for males, 250 mg for females. Pak et al. (1980) found in healthy controls a mean daily excretion level of 197 $\pm$ 81 mg/24 hr. In other words, the mean + 1 SD = 278 mg/hr. In our own group of controls in Prague, we found a similar value of 190 $\pm$ 65 mg/24 hr., so that the mean + + 1 SD = 255 mg/24 hr.

This data suggests that the upper limit of daily Ca excretion in healthy adults on a normal diet ranges about 250–300 mg/24 hr. The value of 250 mg is taken by a number of investigators (e.g. Suki 1980) as the upper limit of normal. Coe (1977) has reported that even lower values for Ca excretion/24 hr may be of diagnostic significance, and he introduced the concept of "marginal" hypercalciuria, set at 150 mg/g urinary creatinine, as the limiting value.

Some patients with Ca urolithiasis and only marginal hypercalcuria can, according to this investigator, show improvement during therapy which decreases urinary Ca excretion. Investigation of the Ca excretion per 24 hr is usually carried out several days in succession, and the scatter is taken note of. In nephrological tests, daily excretion is usually followed for 2–4 days.

2. Urinary excretion on a low Ca intake

With a decrease in Ca intake in healthy controls there is a decrease in urinary excretion. This reaction is usually rapid and occurs over the first 24 hr. By a decrease in Ca intake we understand a diet which excludes milk and all milk products. A more detailed investigation may require measurements of Ca in the separate foodstuffs ingested. This, however, can usually be accurate enough if Ca intake is calculated from tables of food Ca content.

This Ca-poor diet should contain 400 mg Ca or less/24 hr (Pak et al. 1980, Bordier et al. 1977). Nordin and Peacock (1972) have given diets of 150–200 mg Ca/day. Since renal excretion of Ca is influenced by the rate of Na excretion, and thus also by the level of Na intake, the diet should also be salt-poor. Adequate to the investigation would be a diet containing about 100 mmol Na/day (Pak et al. 1978).

Urine is collected over several days. Nordin and Peacock (1972) give a Ca-poor diet for 3 days and urine Ca excretion is measured on the 3rd day. Pak et al. (1980) give a Ca-poor diet for a week and measure Ca excretion on the 7th day. Obviously, during such a period the subject must not take any drugs which have an action on renal Ca excretion. If possible, all drug therapy should be interrupted.

On a diet containing 400 mg Ca and 100 mmol Na, according to Pak et al. (1980), there is a decrease in urinary Ca excretion to 118 ± 58 mg/day. In other words, the mean + 1 SD = 176 mg/day. In practise it is usually required that under these conditions there should be a decrease in urinary excretion to below 200 mg//day (Suki 1980).

The Ca/Cr ratio in fasting urine samples

The above ratio can diagnose hypercalciuria, In practise, it is important because the test is simple and quantitative urine collection is not necessary. The diet is normal in the preceding days. A morning, pre-breakfast, sample of urine is taken for Ca and creatinine analysis, and Ca excretion is expressed per 1 mg creatinine. Some investigators present Ca excretion data per 100 ml glomerular filtrate. This requires a sample of venous blood. According to Muldowney (1979) the mean Ca/Cr ratio is: 0.068 ± 0.044. The upper limit of normal is considered to be 0.11 mg Ca/mg creatinine (Suki 1980). When Ca excretion is expressed per 100 ml glomerular filtrate, the mean value of the ratio, according to Pak et al. (1975) is 0.053 ± 0.027 and according to Muldowney (1979) 0.07 ± 0.051.

Urinary Ca excretion after loading

Ca excretion on an empty stomach and after a Ca load is measured. Pak et al. (1975) carry out this test after a week of investigation of Ca excretion under conditions of a Ca-poor diet. Urine is collected in the morning over a 2-hr period, after which 1 g of elemental Ca (e.g. 2.5 teaspoons of $CaCO_3$ in Titralac or 2 tablets of Oscal-500, or as instructed in Calcitest Doyle) is given. Urine is then collected for a further 4 hr.

After this load there is an increase in Ca excretion to 0.131 ± 0.035 mg/mg creatinine (Pak et al. 1975). The mean value + 1 SD = 0.166 mg Ca/mg cr. As an upper limit of normal we can take 0.2 mg/mg cr (Suki 1980).

This Ca load test also measures the function of the parathyroid glands. In specialized laboratories measurements are also made of whether the Ca load decreases the secretion of PTH and the urinary excretion of cAMP.

SERUM Ca CONCENTRATION

The differential diagnosis of hypercalciuria requires a precise measure of serum Ca.

The limits presented in the literature of 9 to 11 mg% would appear to be too wide, so that cases of marginal hypercalaemia can escape detection. This assumption is also clear from the following argument: maintenance of Ca homeostasis is important to the organism and significant changes in concentration are dangerous. If, for simplicity's sake, we were to calculate that the normal mean value of total serum Ca = 10 mg%, an increase by 1 mg% = a 10% change — this degree of change goes beyond the boundaries of physiology. If we compare this to the sensitivity of the organism to changes in ECF osmolality or pH, we can see that a far greater precision of regulation is required. For example, changes in P_{osm} of 2% are a stimulus for a regulative response.

The range of physiological values of iP is greater than for Ca, and the same diagnostic problems do not arise. We must also distinguish between total and ionized Ca concentrations. Published reports give some scatter for total serum Ca concentratons in the fasting state. The following table gives reported values:

	Mean	+ 1 SD	+ 2 SD	+ 3 SD
Pak et al. (1975)	9.65	9.86	10.07	10.28
Muldowney (1979)	9.25	9.66	10.07	10.48

From this table it is clear that mean + 2 SD is about 10 mg%. Muldowney (1979) considers all values between 10 and 11 mg% as marginal hypercalcaemia. Serum ionized Ca in the fasting state is, on the average, 5.02 ± 0.29 mg%.

Because this measurement is so critical for differential diagnosis, each laboratory should know its own range of normal values from its own normal control population.

THE RENAL CLEARANCE OF Ca (C_{Ca})

Calculation of C_{Ca} on the basis of average rate of excretion and serum Ca does not usually offer more useful information than measurement of urinary excretion alone. Under normal conditions, in adult healthy controls, C_{Ca} calculated from total plasma Ca and average rate of Ca excretion/day ranges about 0.7–2.1 ml/min.

FRACTIONAL EXCRETION OF Ca (FE_{Ca})

This value tells us how much of filtered Ca from the glomerulus is excreted into the urine. To calculate this values, we must know the concentration of ionized Ca in plasma and GFR. In healthy adult controls on an empty stomach, this value of FE_{Ca} is $1.87 \pm 0.87\%$ (Muldowney 1979). Calculation of FE_{Ca} is made out on the basis of the standard equation (p. 262).

URINARY EXCRETION AND PLASMA CONCENTRATION OF PHOSPHATES

Urinary excretion of inorganic phosphates (iP) shows a great deal of scatter, depending upon intake, and varies from 700 to 1200 mg/day. Pak et al. (1978) reported a mean value of 1012 ± 274 mg/day.

Serum iP under normal conditions varies about 3 mg% in fasting healthy adults. The scatter here is greater than that with Ca. In our laboratory the interval of normal values is: 2.5–4.5 mg%. Muldowney (1979) reported from his series 2.6–4.2 mg%. Pak et al. (1978) gave 3.03 ± 0.25 mg%.

In healthy adult controls, FE_{iP} ranges from 13 to 17% and does not exceed 20%. In other words, FR_{iP} ranges from 83 to 87% and does not fall below 80%.

MAXIMAL TUBULAR REABSORPTION OF PHOSPHATES (Tm_{iP})

Tubular reabsorption of iP (T_{iP}) increases in relation to an increase in plasma concentration. After reaching a critical plasma concentration, T does not further increase, plateauing at a fairly constant level (Pitts and Alexander 1944). This latter value is the Tm_{iP}. Tubular reabsorption of iP thus resembles tubular glucose transport. However, Tm_{iP} is not such a constant as $Tm_{glucose}$ because tubular transport of iP is affected by a number of factors. One of the most important of these factors is PTH.

The measurement begins by comparing urinary excretion and plasma concentration of iP. The basic condition is that plasma concentration must be continuously raised (Anderson 1955, Bijvoet 1969, Stamp and Stacey 1970).

After P_{iP} reaches the saturation concentration, there is a linear relation between it and $U_{iP}V$. This means that

$$\Delta(U_{iP}V) / \Delta(P_{iP}) = GFR$$

In rat experiments it has been observed that during gradual increase of P_{iP}, there is a decrease in Tm_{iP} (Oberleithner et al. 1979). This decrease does not occur if the decrease in plasma Ca concentration which occurs automatically during infusion of iP (Frick et al. 1978 is prevented.

Tm_{iP} depends to a large measure on GFR, but the ratio Tm_{iP}/GFR is usually constant. For this reason Bijvoet (1969) and Stamp and Stacey (1970) both recommend the measurement of the Tm_{iP}/GFR ratio in clinical investigation, labelling this as the theoretical renal iP threshold (TRPT). As shown from the relation of $U_{iP}V$ vs P_{iP} in Fig. 61, TRPT is given by the intersection of the regression line with the abscissa. A further advantage of this approach is that Tm_{iP} need not be calculated per 1.73 m² body surface area, particularly since patients with abnormal phosphate metabolism and excretion may have skeletal deformities which distort surface area measurements. Finally, measurement of TRPT does not involve errors from incomplete bladder emptying, and if the rate of urine flow is high enough, bladder catheterization is not necessary.

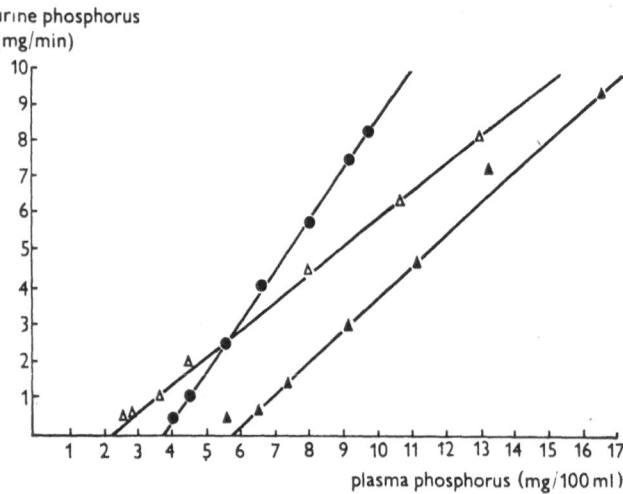

urine phosphorus (mg/min)

plasma phosphorus (mg/100 ml)

Fig. 61: Relationship between plasma concentration and urinary excretion of phosphate during phosphate infusions designed to produce a linear rise of plasma phosphorus with time (Stamp and Stacey 1970).

The procedure for measuring Tm_{iP} and TRPT is as follows (Bijvoet 1969, Stamp and Stacey 1970):

The subject is without food and drink from the evening of the preceding day. After 12–14 hr of fasting, the test is started in the A. M. First we give water to ensure an adequate rate of urine flow (400–600 ml distilled water each hr).

After spontaneous bladder emptying, the control urine collection period starts and lasts for 30–60 min. Following this, an infusion is set up containing iP (antecubital vein). The infused solution contains bufferred Na phosphate (pH 7.4). More concentrated solutions can be used, allowing a slower rate of infusion. The more concentrated solution (Bijvoet 1969) contains:

65.7 g $Na_2HPO_4 . 2.H_2O$
11.5 g $NaH_2PO_4 . 2H_2O$
to 1.0 liter water.

The more dilute solution (Stamp and Stacey, 1970) is:

13.8 g $Na_2HPO_4 . 2H_2O$
 3.6 g $NaH_2PO_4 . 2H_2O$
to 1.0 liter water.

The initial rate of infusion with the concentrated solution is 0.7 ml/min, and every 19th min this rate is increased by 0.1 ml/min. The infusion lasts for 3 hr., so that the final infusion rate is 1.6 ml/min. This stepwise increase is maintained with an infusion pump. The total volume of infused solution is small — about 200 ml — and the total amount of infused iP is about 2.8 g.

Urine is collected by spontaneous voiding at 30-min intervals. At the midpoint of each period a blood sample is drawn from the antecubital vein.

The data are graphed, plasma concentration vs rate of urinary excretion. By the time Tm is attained, both parameters are linear. The position of this straight line is best determined by calculating a regression curve in the usual manner. The intersect of this regression line with the abscissa $= Tm_{iP}$/GFR. The slope of the regression curve $=$ GFR.

This measurement involves attaining plasma iP values of about 8 mg%. No side-effects from this increase have been reported.

Stamp and Stacey (1970) have reported for healthy controls the following normal values:

TRPT: 3.4 ± 0.4 mg%
Tm_{iP}: 3.8 ± 0.9 mg/min/1.73 m^2

Indications for investigation

Urolithiasis

Recent clinical studies have shown that the most frequent form of urolithiasis is associated with Ca salts and about 40% of these subjects have abnormalities of Ca metabolism with hypercalciuria.

Each patient with clear urolithiasis, either by X-ray or by examination of the composition of a passed stone, should be investigated to determine the possible metabolic substrate of the disease.

The first investigation is a measurement of the possible presence of hypercalcuiria. The upper limit of normal on a normal diet is considered to be a Ca excretion of 250 mg/day. In patients who cannot guarantee quantitative urine collection for 24 hr, we measure U_{Ca}/U_{cr} in a fasting urine sample. If this ratio is higher than 0.11, hypercalciuria can be diagnosed and a further workup is indicated. The type of hypercalciuria should be determined.

Absorption hypercalcuiria can be diagnosed when decreasing Ca intake is followed by a decrease in excretion. On a low-Ca diet, the daily Ca excretion should go below 200 mg.

If the syndrome is not absorptive, we must distinguish between renal causes and primary hyperparathyroidism (reabsorptive hypercalciuria). The so-called hypophosphataemic form can be excluded if plasma iP levels are normal. If iP levels are decreased (and FR_{iP} is decreased as well) the diagnosis is not clear as to the existence of hypophosphataemic hypercalciruia.

Repeated and precise measurements of plasma Ca are made (at least 3 values). If some total Ca values are marginally high, one can suspect primary hyperparathyroidism if no other pathology is present which could explain change in Ca metabolism (e.g. prolonged immobilisation, vitamin D excess, Paget's disease, sarcoidosis, the milk-alkali syndrome, hyperthyroidism, Cushing's disease and syndrome, malignant tumors).

Some investigators (Muldowney 1979) recommend repeated measurements of ionized Ca since cases exist in whom this latter value was above the upper limit of normal, but total plasma Ca not at all.

If serum Ca is repeatedly normal, we can consider a renal form of hypercalciuria or some other primary renal disease associated with hypercalciuria.

The differential diagnosis between renal hypercalciuria and primary hyperparathyroidism is often complex, requiring further specialized tests. Of these, the most important is measurement of plasma PTH, urinary excretion of cAMP and hydroxyproline, under baseline conditions and after Ca loading. These data should also assist in determining whether hyperparathyroidism, if present, is primary, secondary or tertiary.

Increased PTH levels in plasma under baseline conditions cannot per se distinguish between renal hypercalciuria and primary hyperparathyroidism. In both forms of hypercalciuria, plasma PTH is raised. In the renal form, the urinary losses can lead to secondary hyperparathyroidism.

If plasma PTH levels and urinary excretion of cAMP are both raised, further investigation must determine whether these findings are reversible after Ca-loading. In other words, is the overproduction of PTH autonomous (with primary or tertiary hyperparathyroidism) or are we dealing with secondary hyperparathyroidism?

In the latter form, plasma PTH levels can be decreased by Ca loading, along with the rates of excretion of cAMP and hydroxyproline. Plasma PTH in absorptive hypercalciuria is normal or decreased during both baseline conditions and Ca loading.

The presence of signs of secondary hyperparathyroidism indirectly suggest the presence of renal hypercalciuria. If the increases in PTH levels in the plasma and cAMP and hydroxyproline in the urine cannot be altered by Ca loading, the suggestion is that the subject has primary or tertiary hyperparathyroidism. The tertiary form can develop in renal hypercalciuria when continuous stimulation of the parathyroids is transformed into autonomous hyperactivity.

Further metabolic tests in patients with urolithiasis

The formation of Ca-oxalate stones can be associated with increased excretion of uric acid (Coe 1978). This type is labelled *hyperuricosuric-Ca urolithiasis*. Plasma and urine levels of uric acid must be determined, not only in cases of urolithiasis without X-ray contrast stones but even in patients with Ca present in their stones (cf. p. 245).

A detailed workup also requires determination of the urinary excretion of oxalate. Oxalate stones may be associated with increased intake of oxalate precursors, a deficiency of pyridoxine or an inborn metabolic error.

Recent studies (Williams 1978) show that increased gut absorption of oxalate can play a role in the formation of Ca-oxalate stones. This syndrome is called enteric hyperoxaluria.

In healthy subjects, oxalates are poorly absorbed in the gut. If we give an oral load, 2.3–4.5% is absorbed (Archer et al. 1957). Pak et al. (1980) have reported that in healthy controls, average excretion of oxalate = 28.9 ± 7.4 mg/day.

We further investigate whether patients with urolithiasis have RTA in the usual manner. If metabolic acidosis is present with urolithiasis, with a normal or slightly decreased GFR, one should suspect this syndrome.

In all cases, urine bacteriology should be investigated. The presence of $Mg . NH_4, PO_4 . 6H_2O$ concrements is associated with urinary tract infection with a strain which contains urease to form NH_4 and alkalinizes the urine (Griffith 1978). The organisms involved include: Proteus vulgaris, mirabilis morgagni and rettgeri, Providencia alcaligenes and stuarti, Klebsiella pneumoniae, Pseudomonas aeruginosa and Serratia morcescens.

Finally, in uncertain cases we should exclude cystinuria on the basis of amino acid analysis of the urine (cf. p. 256).

Chronic renal failure

A decrease in GFR below 20–30 ml/min is usually associated with an increase in plasma iP levels. The latter change is slower that the former because there is a decrease in fractional reabsorption of iP in residual nephrons. A decrease in FR_{iP} in residual nephrons is clear from the hyperbolic relation between C_{in} and FE_{iP} (Fig. 62).

From fig. 62 it is clear that FE_{iP} can reach values close to, or exceeding, 100% with a decreased C_{in}. In our own group of patients, such high levels of FE_{iP} were found in 3 cases (110–135%). Therapy, and in particular prevention of bone pathology, requires maintaining plasma iP levels within normal limits (primarily by giving aluminum hydroxide which decreases gut absorption of iP).

The total level of plasma Ca in such patients is usually decreased. If plasma iP and proteins are normal, but Ca is decreased, one should consider a deficiency of the active form of vitamin D.

The level of ionized Ca in plasma decreases more slowly than the level of total Ca, because with metabolic acidosis less Ca is bound to plasma protein.

Measurement of plasma levels of Ca and iP in patients with chronic renal disease is of diagnostic significance. The Ca × iP product should also be calculated and

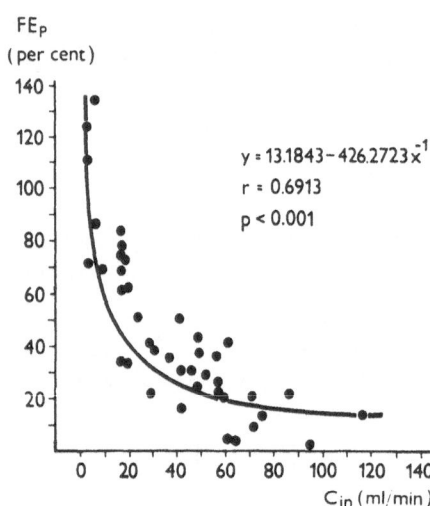

$$y = 13.1843 - 426.2723 x^{-1}$$
$$r = 0.6913$$
$$p < 0.001$$

Fig. 62: Relationship between inulin clearance (C_{in}) and fractional excretion of inorganic phosphorus (FE_P) in patients with chronic renal diseases.

recorded. If the latter value is greater than 40, solubility is decreased. If Ca × iP is greater than 70–75, the salt starts to be deposited.

Measurement of urinary Ca shows low values in patients with chronic renal failure.

Measurement of plasma levels of Ca and iP, and FE_{iP}, is part of the workup of patients with chronic renal failure to evaluate changes in bone metabolism. We also measure plasma alkaline phosphatase (bone iso-enzyme) and the skeleton is observed by X-ray and isotopes. RIA measurement of plasma PTH, estimates of metabolites of vitamin D and the urinary excretions of cAMP and hydroxyproline should all be measured.

To what degree osteodystrophy plays a role in the observed skeletal changes, as well as osteomalacia, osteoporosis and osteosclerosis, can be decided from a bone biopsy (from the iliac crest).

Laboratory methods

An atomic absorption flame photometer is necessary for Ca analysis. Ion-specific flow-through electrodes are used to estimate ionized Ca. iP is determined by the method of Gomori (1942), adapted for an auto-analyser, or the methods described by Kallner (1975) and Anner and Moosmayer (1975) can be recommiended.

REFERENCES

Anner, B., Moosmayer, M.: Rapid determination of inorganic phosphate in biological systems by a highly sensitive photometric method. Analyt. Biochem. *65*: 305, 1975

Anderson, J.: A method for estimating Tm for phosphate in man. J. Physiol. (London) *130*: 268, 1955

Archer, H. E., Dormer, A. E., Scowen, E. F., Watts, R. F.: Studies on the urinary excretion of oxalate by normal subjects. Clin. Sci. *16*: 405, 1957

Barragry, J. M., Carter, N. D., Beer, M. et al.: Vitamin D metabolism in nephrotic syndrome. Lancet *2*: 629, 1977

Better, O. S., Kleeman, C. R., Gonic, H. C., Varady, P. D., Maxwell, M. H.: Renal handling of calcium, magnesium, and inorganic phosphate in chronic renal failure. Isr. J. med. Sci *3*: 60, 1967

Bijvoet, O. L. M.: Relation of plasma phosphate concentration to renal tubular reabsorption of phosphate. Clin. Sci. *37*: 23, 1969

Bordier, P., Ryckewart, A., Gueris, J., Rassmussen, H.: On the pathogenesis of so-called idiopathic hypercalciuria. Am. J. Med. *63*: 298, 1977

Coe, F. L.: Treated and untreated recurrent calcium nephrolithiasis in patients with idiopathic hypercalciuria, hyperuricosuria or metabolic disorder. Ann. Intern. Med. *87*: 404, 1977

Coe, F. L.: Hyperuricosuric calcium exalate nephrolithiasis. Kidney int. *13*: 418, 1978

Epstein, F. H., Rivera, M. J., Carone, F. A.: The effect of hypercalcaemia induced by calciferol upon renal concentrating ability. J. clin. Invest. *37*: 1702, 1958

Frick, A., Durasin, I.: Maximal reabsorptive capacity for inorganic phosphate (TmiP) in the absence of parathyroid hormone in the rat: decrease of the PmiP during prolonged administration of phosphate and the role of calcium. Pflüger's Arch. ges. Physiol. *377*: 9, 1978

Gray, R. W., Wilz, D. R., Caldar, A. E., Lemann, J. Jr.: The importance of phosphate in regulating plasma 1.25 (OH)$_2$-vitamin D level in humans: studies in healthy subjects, in calcium stone formers and in patients with primary hyperparathyroidism. J. clin. Endocrinol. Metab. *45*: 299, 1977

Gomori, G.: A modification of the colorimetric phosphorus determination for use with the photo-electric colorimeter. J. lab. clin. Med. *27*: 955, 1942

Griffith, D. P.: Struvite stones. Kidney int. *13*, 372, 1978

Harrington, J. T., Cohen, J. J.: Clinical disorders of urine concentration and dilution. Arch. interm. Med. *131*: 810, 1973

Hodgkinson, A., Pyrah, L. N.: The urinary excretion of calcium and inorganic phosphate in 344 patients with calcium stone of renal origin. Brit. J. Surg. *46*: 10, 1958

Kallner, A.: Determination of phosphate in serum and urine by a single step malachite-green method. Clin. chim. Acta *59*: 35, 1975

Kleeman, C. R., Better, O. Massry, S. G., Maxwell, M. H.: Divalent ion metabolism and osteodystrophy in chronic renal failure. Yale J. Biol. Med. *40*: 1, 1967

Lang, F.: Renal handling of Calcium and Phosphate. Klin. Wochenschr. *58*: 985, 1980

Lassiter, W. E., Gottschalk, C. W., Mylle, M.: Micropuncture study of renal tubular reabsorption of calcium in normal rodents. Am. J. Physiol. *204*: 771, 1963

Massry, S. G., Coburn, J. W., Lee, D. N. B., Jowsey, J., Kleeman, C. R.: Skeletal resistance to parathyroid hormone in renal failure. Study in 105 human subjects. Ann. intern. Med. *78*: 357, 1973

Massry, S. G., Coburn, J. W., Peacock, M., Kleeman, C. R.: Turnover of endogenous parathyroid hormone in uremic patients and those undergoing hamodialysis. Trans. am. Soc. artif. intern. Organs *18*: 416, 1972

Muldowney, F. P.: Diagnostic approach to hypercalciuris. Kidney int. *16*: 637, 1979

Nordin, B. E. C., Peacock, M.: Hypercalciuria. Proc. int. Symp. on renal stone research Madrid. Basel, Karger, 1972 pp. 119–129

Oberleithner, H., Lang, F., Greger, R., Sporer, H.: Influence of calcium and ionophore 23187 on tubular phosphate reabsorption. Pflüger's Arch. ges. Physiol. *379*: 37, 1979

Pak, Ch. Y. C., Britton, F., Peterson, R. Ward, D., Northcutt, Ch., Breslau, N. E., McGuire, J., Sakhall, K., Bush, S., Nicar, M., Norman, D. A., Peters, P.: Ambulatory evaluation of nephrolithiasis. Am. J. Med. *69*: 19, 1980

Pak, C. Y. C., Kaplan, R. A., Bone, H., Townsend, J., Walters, O.: A simple test for diagnosis of absorptive, resorptive and renal hypercalciuria. N. Engl. J. Med. *292*: 497, 1975

Pitts, R. F., Alexander, R. S.: The renal reabsorptive mechanism for inorganic phosphate in normal and acidotic dogs. Am. J. Physiol. *142*: 648, 1944

Popovtzer, M. M., Massry, S. G., Makoff, D. L., Maxwell, M. H., Kleeman, C. R.: Renal handling of phosphate in patients with chronic renal failure. Isr. J. med. Sci *5*: 1018, 1969

Popovtzer, M. M., Schainack, L. I., Massry, S. G., Kleeman, C. R.: Divalent ion excretion in chronic kidney disease: relation to degree of renal insufficiency. Clin. Sci. *38*: 297, 1970

Schmidt-Gayk, H., Schmitt, W., Grauwunder, C. et al.: 25-hydroxy-vitamin D in nephrotic syndrome. Lancet *2*: 105, 1977

Slatopolsky, E., Gradowska, L., Kashemsant, C. et al.: The control of phosphate excretion in uremia. J. clin. Invest. *45*: 672, 1966

Slatopolsky, E., Robson, M., Elkan, I., Bricker, N. S.: Control of phosphate excretion in uremic man. J. clin. Invest. *47*: 1865, 1968

Slatopolsky, E., Rutherford, E., Hoffsten, P. E. et al.: Nonsuppressible secondary hyperparathyroidism in chronic progressive renal disease. Kidney int. *1*: 38, 1972

Sotornik, I., Schück, O., Stříbrná, J.: Influence of diuretics on renal calcium excretion. Experientia *25*: 591, 1969

Stamp, T. C. B., Stacey, T. E.: Evaluation of theoretical renal phosphorus threshold as an index of renal phosphorus handling. Clin. Sci. *39*: 505, 1970

Suki, W. N.: Renal handling of calcium. Contr. Nephrol. *23*: 1, 1980

Suki, W. N.: Hypercalciuria: Diagnosis and management. Contr. Nephrol. *23*: 21–33, 1980

Summer, J. B.: A method for the colorimetric determination of phosphorus. Science *100*: 413, 1944

Ullrich, K. J., Rumrich, G., Klass, S.: Active Ca^{++} reabsorption in the proximal tubule of the rat kidney. Pflüger's Arch. ges. Physiol. *364*: 223, 1976

Walser, M.: Calcium clearance as a function of sodium clearance in the dog. Am. J. Physiol. *200*: 1099, 1961

Wen, S. F., Boynar, J. W., Stoll, R. W.: Effects of volume expansion on phosphate transport in uremic dogs. Proc. Am. Soc. Nephrol. *9*: 7, 1976

Williams, H. E.: Oxalic acid and hyperoxaluric syndromes. Kidney int. *13*: 410, 1978

Yendt, E. R.: Renali calculi. Can. Med. Ass. J. *102*: 479, 1970

ACIDIFYING CAPACITY

PHYSIOLOGY AND PATHOPHYSIOLOGY

Non-volatile acid metabolites are excreted from the organism through the kidneys. Endogenous production of acid in the organism ranges about 1 mmol/kg/day. This means that for a normal person on a normal diet, the kidneys must excrete daily about 70 mmol acid.

Transfer of acid metabolites from tissues to the kidney is not a direct mechanism, since this would seriously disturb acid-base balance. Acid metabolites during such transport to the kidneys must be neutralized. This latter process is in large measure due to "borrowing" of HCO_3^- from the ECF into the circulation. After transport of Na salts of these acid metabolites to the kidneys, the HCO_3^- is "returned", because this anion is synthetized in the renal tubules. Acid metabolites are to a large degree phosphates, sulphates and some organic acids.

The mechanism of formation of HCO_3^- in the tubular cells is directly related to the excretion of protons and acidification of the urine. HCO_3^- synthesis starts in tubular cells, along with proton secretion, in the following manner:

$$H_2O + CO_2 \xrightarrow[CA]{} H_2CO_3 \, , \quad \text{where}$$

CA = carbonic anhydrase which accelerates or catalyzes the reaction. The resulting H_2CO_3 is partly dissociated to $H^+ + HCO_3^-$. This latter reaction is expressed as:

$$H_2CO_3 \longrightarrow H^+ + HCO_3^- \, .$$

The resulting protons are actively secreted into the tubular urine. Na ions exchange in equipotential quantity into cells for the excreted protons. In the proximal tubule Na penetration of the luminal membrane is a passive process. In this segment of the nephron protons in the tubular urine are associated with bicarbonate and H_2CO_3 is again formed — this time outside of the tubular cells. This again dehydrates into H_2O and CO_2. CO_2 penetrates into tubular cells and combines with water to form carbonic acid, which again dissociates. Bicarbonate penetrates the basal membrane of the tubular cell along with Na.

This mechanism results in the reabsorption of bicarbonate anion. It would appear from the above that bicarbonate is not reabsorbed as such, but CO_2 is re-absorbed resulting from the breakdown of carbonic acid, and this is then used for re-synthesis of carbonic acid.

Secreted cations can associate with urinary buffers, mainly phosphate. Thus, $HPO_4^=$ is transformed into $H_2PO_4^-$ ions. This occurs mainly in the distal segment of the nephron. Protons associated with urinary buffers are measured as "titratable acidity".

It is clear that the formation of titratable acidity in the distal segment of the nephron is dependent upon the supply of phosphate anion. This latter parameter is, of course, a function of the degree of phosphate reabsorption in the proximal tubule.

Na ion balancing this phosphate anion is replaced by protons. Protons secreted into the urine can also associate with NH_3 to form NH_4^+.

This resulting ammonium cation is exchanged for Na^+. NH_3 arises in the tubular cells mainly by desamination of glutamine. This process is catalyzed by glutaminase.

Formation of titratable acidity and ammonium ion can only occur if tubular urinary pH decreases, which in turn is a function of adequate proton secretion.

Since the permissible concentration of free protons (or hydroions H_3O^+) in the luminal urine is negligibly small, and since loss of each bicarbonate anion from the urine means retention of an equivalent amount of protons, the "net excretion" of protons is given as:

$$U_{TA}V + U_{NH_4}V - U_{HCO_3}V .$$

Tubular reabsorption of bicarbonate has a maximal limit which is not given by the amount of maximal bicarbonate reabsorption itself but by the ratio between total tubular reabsorption (T_{HCO_3}) and GFR, i.e. T_{HCO_3}/GFR.

With low plasma bicarbonate concentrations, all filtered anion is reabsorbed in the tubules. Urinary excretion of bicarbonate starts when the threshold concentration is exceeded. In healthy adults this value is 24–26 mmol/l. In children there is a lower threshold. About 85% of all filtered HCO_3 is reabsorbed in the proximal segment of the nephron — the remainder in the distal segment.

In healthy adults, tubular reabsorption of HCO_3 has a limiting value of about 2.5 mmol/100 ml GFR.

Renal regulation of acid-base balance can be altered by kidney pathology in a number of ways. The development of renal metabolic acidosis in kidney disease is probably due to two factors:

1. inability of the kidney to excrete sufficient acid catabolites, with resulting retention, because of a decrease in GFR (uremic acidosis)

2. as a result of abnormal tubular function: a) inability to reabsorb sufficient bicarbonate (bicarbonate wasting), b) inadequate secretion of NH_3, c) inability to

form or maintain an adequate gradient of protons between the tubular urine and the peritubular ECF (in the distal segment of the nephron).

These mechanisms can, of course, operate in combinations.

Comments on the above mechanisms

So-called **uraemic acidosis** develops in patients in advanced stages of chronic renal disease. A marked decrease in plasma bicarbonate occurs when GFR is decreased to about 20–30 ml/min. In some cases it can be observed that metabolic acidosis develops when GFR decreases to values about 10 ml/min.

A decrease in GFR results in retention of acid metabolites, mainly phosphates, sulphates and some organic acids. Such retention results in the development of an "anion gap". The latter term refers to the amount of anions given by the difference:

$$Na - (Cl + HCO_3).$$

The concentration of anions given by the above difference is about 12 mmol/l (± 2) under normal conditions. In patients with advanced renal failure, the anion gap increases.

A decrease in GFR has the further result that the filtered phosphate load — i.e. the most important urinary buffer — is decreased and thus the formation of titratable acidity can be compromised. A decrease in the amount of filtered phosphate is compensated by an increase in plasma levels and also by the fact that proximal fractional reabsorption is also decreased, so that the phosphate load which reaches the start of the distal segment of residual nephrons need not be decreased drastically.

The development of uraemic acidosis cannot, however, be explained only as the result of a decrease in GFR. The findings of Schwartz et al. (1959) suggest that in some patients in advanced stages of renal failure, tubular reabsorption of bicarbonate can also be decreased. In such cases the patients form a final urine from residual nephrons, the pH of which is relatively high despite the fact that marked metabolic acidosis is present. Detailed measurements in such cases show a decreased renal threshold for bicarbonate excretion and a decrease in T_{HCO_3}/GFR (Schwartz 1959, Muldowney 1979).

Furthermore, a decrease in the renal formation of ammonium cation plays a role in the formation of metabolic acidosis in patients with advanced renal failure. The total amount of ammonium ion excreted/24 hr is usually decreased. The inability of the residual parenchyma of diseased kidneys to form adequate amounts of ammonium cation is probably due to a metabolic defect in the tubular cells, the mechanism of which is not yet detailed (Lyons 1977). Perhaps a further factor here will be a decrease in the ability of tubular cells to extract glutamine from the circulation.

It is clear from the above that the development of uraemic metabolic acidosis has

220

a complex set of causes, and that changes in tubular function play a role in addition to the decrease in GFR. There will probably be a large degree of variation in the partition of tubular causes of acidosis from patient to patient.

Renal metabolic acidosis can also develop in patients who are either normal or who have only a slightly decreased GFR. This type of acidosis is termed **renal tubular acidosis (RTA).** This type of metabolic acidosis is characterized by a normal anion gap and the decrease in plasma bicarbonate is associated with an increase in plasma Cl concentration (hyperchloraemic acidosis).

There are a number of forms of RTA. **So-called classical RTA,** also referred to as **the distal form, or type I RTA,** is characterized by an inadequacy of the distal segment of the nephron to form or maintain an adequate proton gradient between the luminal fluid and the peritubular ECF. This results in an inability to form a final urine with a low pH. Urinary pH cannot be decreased even in the presence of increasing metabolic acidosis, e.g. administration of NH_4Cl. Urinary bicarbonate excretion is small in this form of RTA, and the excretion fraction usually does not exceed 5% (Sebastian and Morris, 1979). After a bicarbonate load urinary bicarbonate excretion increases only slowly. The difference between urinary CO_2 and blood CO_2 in HCO_3 rich urine (urinary pH > blood pH) is less than 20 torr. A defect in urine acidification in the distal segment of the tubule carries with it a number of serious metabolic consequences.

As a result of a decrease in the exchange of protons for Na^+ in the distal segment of the nephron there is a relative increase in urinary Na loss. This stimulates the adrenals to produce more aldosterone. The latter results in an increase in distal secretion of K^+ and the production of hypokalaemia.

Metabolic acidosis created by a defect in distal tubular function results in a freeing up of Ca from bone and this results in hypercalciuria. An increase in ionized Ca in plasma can also contribute to this.

Abnormal Ca metabolism in adults results in osteomalacia, in children it results in rickets. Hypercalciuria associated with an alkaline urine can lead to nephrocalcinosis and urolithiasis. A decrease in citrate excretion also contributes to lithiasis.

The distal form of RTA occurs as an isolated syndrome (primary or idiopathic) or in association with other disease (secondary).

Primary RTA can occur as a sporadic event or as an hereditary disease.

Secondary forms of distal RTA have been described in association with the following diseases:

1. hypergammaglobulinaemia
2. medullary sponge kidney
3. primary hyperparathyroidism with nephrocalcinosis
4. hyperthyroidism with nephrocalcinosis
5. liver cirrhosis
6. renal transplantation

7. tubulo-interstitial nephritis
8. drug effects due to, e.g., amphotericin B
9. hereditary elliptocytosis
10. Fabry's disease
11. Ehlers-Danlos syndrome
12. galactosaemia
13. hereditary fructose intolerance with nephrocalcinosis.

So-called **proximal RTA,** also called **type II RTA,** is characterized by abnormal bicarbonate reabsorption in the proximal tubules. This syndrome is manifest by a decrease in the bicarbonate threshold.

As a result of this decrease in reabsorption in the proximal tubules, there is an increased load in the distal segment of the nephron. Even with normal secretion of protons in the distal segment, urinary pH cannot be markedly decreased. If this distal tubular bicarbonate load is decreased, normal proton secretion occurs and urinary pH decreases. This latter effect can be achieved by deepening the degree of metabolic acidosis (e.g. by administration of NH_4Cl) and decreasing plasma bicarbonate concentration, with a pathological decrease in threshold values. Under such conditions the majority of filtered bicarbonate is reabsorbed proximally so that the distal situation becomes more normal.

Fractional bicarbonate excretion in proximal RTA is increased, usually greater than 15% (Sebastian and Morris 1979). A small sodium bicarbonate load results in a marked increase in urinary bicarbonate excretion. The difference between urinary CO_2 and blood CO_2 in HCO_3 rich urine is more than 20 torr. As with patients with distal RTA, hypercalciuria results. As opposed to distal RTA, however, there is no decrease in urinary citrate excretion.

Proximal RTA occurs as a primary (idiopathic) disease (sporadic or hereditary), or as a secondary one. The latter has been observed in association with:
1. secondary hyperparathyroidism
2. vitamin D deficiency
3. amyloidosis
4. kidney transplantation
5. multiple myeloma
6. medullary cystic disease
7. nephrotic syndrome
8. cystinosis
9. Wilson's disease
10. Lowe syndrome
11. tyrosinosis
12. Sjögren's syndrome
13. effect of heavy metals
14. hereditary fructose intolerance.

Further, there have been described forms of RTA which have been characterized as mixed or hybrid. In such cases the signs of both types of RTA are present.

Finally, in recent years there has been description of so-called type IV RTA, characterized by metabolic acidosis and hyperkalaemia. The pathophysiological basis of this form of RTA is a decreased proton secretion and K^+ secretion. Patients in this grouping usually have decreased values of GFR, but the degree of metabolic acidosis and hyperkalaemia is far greater than one would expect from the GFR deficit. A number of such patients have low renin secretion, and thus, as a result, a decreased secretion of aldosterone, although other adrenocortical functions are normal. Such cases are labelled hyporeninaemic hypoaldosteronism.

During spontaneous metabolic acidosis, the urine is acid without bicarbonate. However, with normalization of plasma bicarbonate values (sodium bicarbonate administration) the proximal reabsorption of bicarbonate decreases. The bicarbonate excretion fraction is usually less than 10%. Urinary excretion of ammonium is very low. The main pathophysiological basis of this form of RTA is a defect in the exchange of Na^+ for $(H^+ + K^+)$.

According to Sebastian and Morris (1979) this form of RTA occurs mainly in all pathological states associated with a decreased production of aldosterone, in tubulo-interstitial nephritis, in patients with a transplanted kidney, renal involvement with systemic lupus erythematosus and amyloid disease.

METHODS OF INVESTIGATION

A defect in the acidification capacity of the kidneys can in some cases be detected without any loading experiments. In many cases, however, loading tests must be carried out to produce or increase metabolic acidosis, or to follow the renal reaction to correction of the metabolic acidosis.

For investigatory purposes, it is frequently necessary to increase metabolic acidosis, but it should be realised that any induced change in acid-base balance will have many metabolic effects which might not be irrelevant to the subject. Thus, for instance, the state of acid-base balance significantly influences transport of K^+ between the ICF and the ECF, and the concentration of ionized Ca in the ECF. Equilibration of the bicarbonate concentration between the ECF and the cerebrospinal fluid is not immediate, and stimulation of the respiratory center might not be adequate to the acid-base state in the ECF.

Investigation of the acidification capacity of the kidney does not require detailed preparation. The subject should be in a balanced state of water and electrolyte metabolism. Activation of aldosterone during dehydration has an effect on distal secretion of protons. Expansion of the ECF volume decreases proximal reabsorption of bicarbonate. Proximal bicarbonate reabsorption further influences plasma Ca and phosphate levels. The subject should be in a balanced state of K metabolism.

For these reasons, before any test of acidification capacity of the kidney, serum electrolytes should be measured.

Since urine is collected by spontaneous voiding, an adequate level of urine flow rate must be induced. To this end, a small water diuresis is induced, maintained by replacement of water losses.

It is important that both urine and blood samples should be taken under anaerobic conditions. Ordinarily, urine is collected directly into a volumetric cylinder containing liquid paraffin. Blood samples are collected through an indwelling needle flushed with slightly heparinized saline.

The investigation is carried out in the morning. A diurnal rhythm of proton excretion must be counted with. Dosetor et al. (1973) have shown that with 4 days on a normal diet, and urine sampling in 6 hr intervals, the highest proton excretion is at night — between midnight and 6:00 AM. Proton excretion is inversely related to K^+ excretion (Mills and Stanbury, 1954).

According to the findings of Adler et al. (1968) and Agarwal and Cabebe (1960), there is a decrease in the acidification capacity of the kidneys in older subjects (demonstrable with an ammonium chloride load).

Urine infection plays a critical role. Proteus and other similar kidney infections which cleave urea to ammonia will have a significant effect on urinary pH. Investigation of the urine sediment and bacterial content are therefore important.

SPONTANEOUS ACIDIFICATION

This includes measuring the pH of the spontaneous morning urine in relation to the level of acid-base balance in the ECF. In our own normal control group (age range 23–44 years) this values was 5.36 ± 1.21. Agarwal and Cabebe (1980) reported for subjects aged less than 35 years: 5.69 ± 0.35, in the age range 35–65 years: 5.30 ± 0.27 and in the age range above 65 years: 5.90 ± 0.27.

If urinary pH decreases spontaneously to 5.3 or less, it can be concluded that the distal nephron is capable of secreting protons against a concentration gradient and further that this segment can maintain such a gradient between the luminal urine and the peritubular ECF. This finding exludes the presence of distal RTA.

If the morning urine pH is above 5.3, we must take into account the state of acid-base balance of the ECF.

If there are signs of metabolic acidosis and the kidneys do not form a really acid urine, we are probably dealing with a defect in the acidification capacity of the kidney. In normal adult controls, plasma bicarbonate should range from 24 to

224

26 mmol/l. If values found are lower, down to 20 mmol/l or less, an adequate stimulus to the kidney to form an acid urine down to 5.3 or lower already exists.

Obviously, we must exclude bacterial contamination of the urine. Metabolic acidosis must furthermore be classified by the anion gap. In patients in an advanced state of chronic renal failure, the anion gap is increased, whereas in RTA the gap should be normal (hyperchloreamic acidosis). At the same time one should also investigate serum K levels.

As explained above, in proximal RTA urine pH can decrease to the required value if plasma bicarbonate is decreased to threshold levels.

In proximal RTA the renal bicarbonate threshold is decreased to a varying degree. Thus, for instance, Rodriguez-Soriano et al. (1980) reported threshold bicarbonate concentration in proximal RTA in the range 13.7 to 19.5 mmol/l. In other words, if an acid urine is formed with a marked decrease in plasma bicarbonate one cannot completely exclude proximal RTA.

In evaluating spontaneous acidification capacity, we also try to investigate the excretion of titratable acidity and ammonium.

Under normal circumstances, titratable acidity excretion in normal, healthy adults should be 10–30 mmol/24 hr (7–21 μmol/min) and ammonium excretion should be in the range 30–50 mmol/24 hr (21–35 μmol/min) (Pitts 1974, Krück 1958). At the same time bicarbonate excretion is very low, so that the sum of $(U_{TA}V + U_{NH_4}V)$ also represents the net acid excretion. The ratio NH_4/TA is on an average 1.28 ± 0.14 (Schwab, 1961, 1963).

The value of net acid excretion, therefore, under normal circumstances varies between 40–80 mmol/24 hr.

Tubular damage by various parenchymatous renal diseases is manifest by a decrease in the excretion of ammonium resulting from a decreased production of ammonia by tubular cells.

In proximal RTA, urinary excretion of ammonium and titratable acid are within normal limits or reduced. In distal RTA, the excretion of ammonium and titratable acid are subnormal.

In patients with metabolic acidosis and normal renal function a fairly high multiple occurs in the excretion of titratable acid and ammonium cation.

A RAPID AMMONIUM CHLORIDE TEST

According to Wrong and Davies (1959) this test is carried out as follows:

The investigation starts in the morning with a one-hour control urine collection period. This is followed by administration of NH_4Cl in a dose of 0,1 g/kg body weight. NH_4Cl is usually administered in coated tablets or capsules. The total dose is taken by mouth over one hour.

After the control urine collection period, further one-hour collection periods follow. For the rate of urine flow to be high enough, 500–600 ml water are taken orally, and this is repeated during the test according to need.

The number of one-hour collection periods ranges from 4 to 6, sometimes even longer. This latter factor depends upon when urine pH reaches 5.3 or less.

Urine is collected in a graduated cylinder under liquid paraffin. The characteristic time course of changes in urine pH, excretion of titratable acid and NH_4 in healthy controls is shown in Fig. 63.

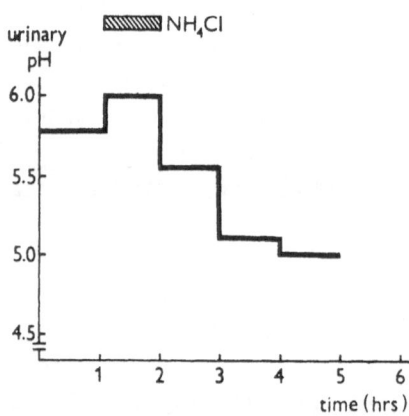

Fig. 63: Time-course of decrease of urinary pH in a healthy subject after the administration of NH_4Cl (0,1 g/kg).

In subjects with a normal acidification capacity, the required decrease in urine pH is achieved usually by 3–4 hours after the load.

As explained above, pH of the urine decreases under these conditions at least to 5.3. Excretion of titratable acid and NH_4 are increased after the load, but high values are not seen. To evaluate renal function from this aspect we would require several consecutive days of ammonium chloride loading.

Our own findings in this quick ammonium chloride test in healthy adult subjects, which agree with most of the published data, are shown in the following table:

urine pH 4.73 ± 0.23

$U_{TA}V$ (μmol/min) $= 31.2 \pm 7.6$

$U_{NH_4}V$ (μmol/min) $= 43.6 \pm 13.9$

$(U_{TA}V/C_{in})$ 100 (μmol/min/100 ml) $= 26.7 \pm 13.9$

$(U_{NH_4}V/C_{in})$ 100 (μmol/min/100 ml) $= 36.7 \pm 12.0$

ACIDIFICATION TEST WITH ARGININE HCl

In this test we give an i.v. infusion of arginine HCl in a dose of 200 mmol/m^2 over 4 hours (Lestraded et al. 1964, Caregaro et al. 1981). This means that the hourly dose is 50 mmol/m^2. In the control period before the infusion, urine is collected for 2 hours. The infusion is then set up for 4 hours and after this period urine is collected for a further 6 hours.

Under these conditions, pH of the urine decreases to 5.4 or lower. Excretion of titratable acid is increased to values about 50–150 μmol/min and the excretion of ammonium to values between 20 and 100 μmol/min.

SEVERAL DAYS TEST WITH NH$_4$Cl LOADING

The reaction of the kidney, in terms of ammonium excretion, after administration of ammonium chloride is relatively sluggish, and several days are required (usually 3–5) until this excretion value reaches a stable maximum for that subject (Sartorius et al. 1949). The main reason for this experimental approach is to evaluate the metabolic capacity of tubular cells to produce ammonia.

The test is carried out by giving the subject, for 3–5 days, NH$_4$Cl in a daily dose of 0.1 g/kg. This dose is subdivided over the 24-hr period. The diet is normal, but should be constant in composition. Water intake is ad libitum.

Urine is collected by spontaneous voiding in 12-hour periods. According to Gerok (1969), 3 days of intake of 100–200 mmol NH$_4$Cl/24 hour increases urine excretion of ammonium by 20–100 mmol/day/1.73 m^2, and increases excretion of TA by 10 to 30 mmol/day/1.73 m^2. Urine pH is decreased to 5.3 or less.

INVESTIGATION OF THE RENAL BICARBONATE THRESHOLD AND THE MAXIMAL TUBULAR REABSORPTION OF BICARBONATE

If plasma bicarbonate in healthy adult controls decreases below the lower level of the normal range, its excretion is nil. If the renal threshold for bicarbonate is decreased, urinary excretion is present even under the above conditions. Total bicarbonate excretion can, however, be low with a decreased threshold value because a decrease in plasma bicarbonate concentration may lead to the formation of a new balanced state in the ECF. Low urinary bicarbonate excretion therefore does not exclude the possibility of a marked decrease in the renal bicarbonate threshold.

Demonstration of a decrease in the renal threshold involves following the relation between urinary excretion and plasma levels during i.v. bicarbonate infusion.

According to Broyer et al. (1969) a bicarbonate test is carried out as follows:

After a 1-hour control period, an i.v. infusion is started with NaHCO₃ at a rate of 1-1.5 mmol/kg/hour. In adults of normal shape and size, the total hourly dosage is 70-100 mmol/hour. The infusion solution is usually 2.75% (w/v).

The duration of the infusion depends upon the renal reaction and the state of acid-base balance in the ECF. Usually we achieve a urinary pH of 7.5. Plasma bicarbonate should exceed the usual renal threshold value (24-26 mmol). However, it is undesirable for the patient if severe metabolic alkalosis is induced.

At the above infusion rate, plasma bicarbonate increases 1-2 mmol/hr. If the rate of rise is slower, Broyer et al. (1969) recommend an increase in infusion rate, with a bicarbonate dosage of 1.5-2.5 mmol/kg/hr.

In order to have an adeqaute rate of urine flow, 500 ml water is drunk at the start and then, during the test, according to the level of urine flow, more water is given.

Urine is collected in graduated cylinders under liquid paraffin. Samples of venous blood are collected anaerobically in the middle of each urine collection period.

HCO₃ levels are determined in the samples of urine and plasma. In all urine samples, and in one sample of plasma, we also measure the level of endogenous creatinine. On the basis of values of urinary excretion and the plasma levels, we construct a graph relating the two parameters (Fig. 64).

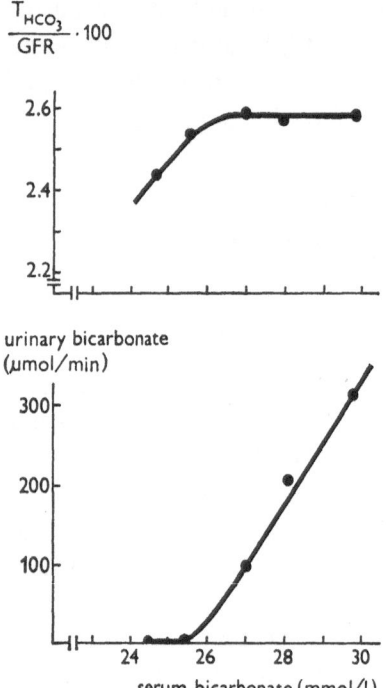

Fig. 64: Relationship between serum bicarbonate concentration and tubular reabsorption of bicarbonate (T_{HCO_3}/GFR 100) in a healthy subject (upper panel) and the relationship between serum concentration and urinary excretion of bicarbonate in the same subject (lower panel) during bicarbonate infusion.

There are occasionally difficulties in determining the minimal threshold level for bicarbonate excretion. In some patients this value cannot be determined because there is a continuous small excretion of bicarbonate (distal RTA). After reaching the desired level of P_{HCO_3}, there is a rise in $U_{HCO_3}V$ which is linearly related to P_{HCO_3}.

In an analogous manner to measurement of reabsorptive capacity for glucose (cf. pp. 234) one can determine the "mean" bicarbonate threshold. This latter value gives the plasma level of HCO_3 at which saturation reabsorption levels for the kidney occur. This value is shown by the intersection of the extrapolated line with the abscissa.

In patients with proximal RTA, with a rise in P_{HCO_3} there is a rapid rise in values of $U_{HCO_3}V/C_{cr}$. In patients with distal RTA, this latter rise is slower.

Sebastian and Morris (1979) recommend, for quantitative evaluation of changes in urinary bicarbonate excretion, calculation of changes in the fractional excretion of bicarbonate (FE_{HCO_3}). In an analogous manner with other solutes, we calculate FE_{HCO_3} according to the equation:

$$FE_{HCO_3} = \frac{U_{HCO_3}V}{GFR \times P_{HCO_3}}\ 100 \tag{1}$$

For interpretation of the findings, FE_{HCO_3} is important at the moment of attainment of a normal P_{HCO_3} value.

In patients with proximal RTA, FE_{HCO_3} exceeds 15%. In patients with distal RTA, FE_{HCO_3} does not exceed 5%. On the basis of values of $U_{HCO_3}V$, P_{HCO_3} and C_{cr}, we can further calculate tubular reabsorption of bicarbonate (T_{HCO_3}). As explained above, tubular transport of bicarbonate is characterized by a maximal value (T_{HCO_3}/GFR) after the threshold value is exceeded.

The calculation of T_{HCO_3}/GFR is as follows:

$$\frac{T_{HCO_3}}{GFR} = \frac{GFR \times P_{HCO_3} - U_{HCO_3}V}{GFR} \tag{2}$$

In healthy adult controls, T_{HCO_3}/C_{cr} ranges from 2.4 to 2.6 mmol/min/100 ml C_{cr}.

The relation between values of P_{HCO_3} and T_{HCO_3}/C_{cr} is shown in Fig. 64.

From the above calculations it is clear that T_{HCO_3}/GFR is identical with the mean threshold value of bicarbonate for the kidney.

Theoretically it is of interest that, as with other solutes, if the maximal reabsorption or secretory capacity of the tubules has been attained, one can determine GFR from the relation between urinary excretion and plasma concentration (for details see p. 235).

Indications for investigation

1. Metabolic acidosis of unknown origin

If the clinical picture does not give a clear reason for the presence of metabolic acidosis, one must exclude RTA. This comes into question if we are dealing with hyperchloremic acidosis with a normal anion gap.

Patients with RTA usually also have hypokalemia, but a normal K value does not exclude RTA. Urine pH should be measured. If in the presence of metabolic acidosis, urine pH is greater than 5.3 (with no signs of urinary infection), RTA is a probable cause.

GFR values are usually normal or slightly decreased. Further investigation is oriented towards which form of RTA may be involved. A normal state of acid-base balance in the ECF, however, does not exclude so-called incomplete forms of RTA. In such cases, metabolic acidosis can be sporadic and mild in degree. The diagnosis of RTA then requires an acidification test. Since RTA occurs in most cases as a result of renal disease, in particular with some generalized disease states, this possible diagnosis has to be considered in immunological diseases, adrenal damage (decreased production of aldosterone), hyperparathyroidism and hyperthyroidism, and in cases of liver cirrhosis. RTA in children comes into question with various congenital defects of tubular transport.

2. Urolithiasis

Since RTA (in particular distal RTA) is frequently complicated by urolithiasis and nephrocalcinosis, one must evaluate in patients with Ca urolithiasis whether renal acidification capacity is normal.

3. Tubulo-interstitial nephritis

In patients with various forms of tubulo-interstitial nephritis (phenacetine nephritis, pyelonephritis, interstitial form of transplantation nephropathy) RTA may result. In such cases there is the striking finding of metabolic acidosis despite the fact that GFR is only slightly decreased and there are no signs of renal failure.

4. Chronic renal failure

In these cases, metabolic acidosis is characterized by an increased anion gap. The defects in tubular function listed above play a role here.

In these patients, signs of proximal RTA may be striking (lowered bicarbonate threshold) or distal RTA may also be present.

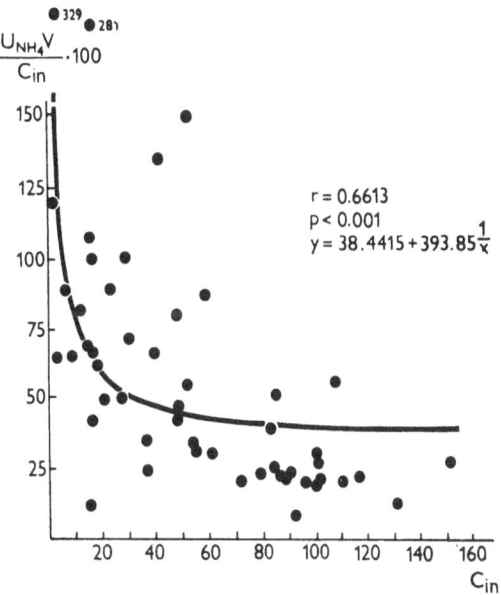

Fig. 65: Relationship between inulin clearance (C_{in}) and urinary amonium excretion related to glomerular filtration rate ($U_{NH_4}V/C_{in}$ 100) in patients with chronic renal diseases.

A decreased production of ammonia plays an important role in the metabolic acidosis of chronic renal failure. The total amount of ammonium cation excreted per day is decreased. The question is still open whether this decrease in ammonia production is related only to the decrease in functional renal parenchyma or whether there is a metabolic defect in the tubules of the residual nephrons.

In following the relation between the decrease in GFR (C_{in}) vs $U_{NH_4}V/C_{in}$, we find a hyperbolic curve, as shown in Fig. 65.

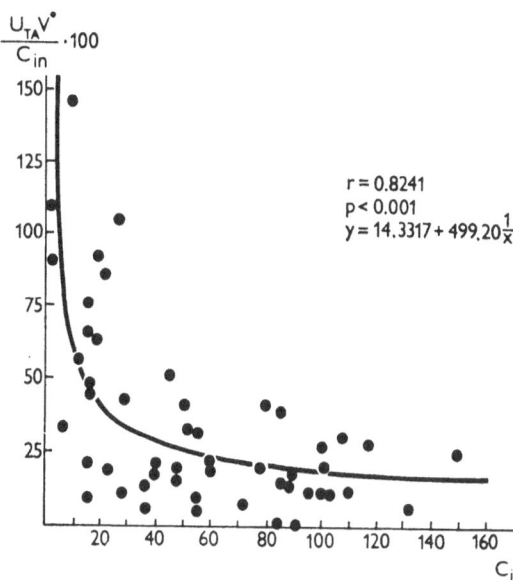

Fig. 66: Relationship between inulin clearance (C_{in}) and urinary excretion of titratable acidity related to glomerular filtration rate ($U_{TA}V/C_{in}100$) in patients with chronic renal disease.

231

The hyperbolic curve is also valid for C_{in} vs $U_{TA}V/C_{in}$ (Fig. 66).

For patients with chronic renal failure there is a characteristic decrease in $U_{NH_4}V/U_{TA}V$.

Contraindications to investigation

Rapid and extreme changes in acid-base balance represent a severe stress on the metabolism of the subject under investigation. As far as possible, we do not give loads (either acid or basic) until we have estimated the acidification capacity of the kidneys only on the basis of the "resting" acid-base balance and the renal reaction to it. Acute NH_4Cl or arginine HCl loads are not given to patients with severe metabolic acidosis at rest.

An NH_4Cl load is contraindicated in patients with liver damage. It is also undesirable in patients with gastrointestinal disease with severe "dyspeptic" complaints.

Infusion of $NaHCO_3$ is contraindicated in patients with cardiovascular disease and signs of Na and water retention.

Laboratory methods

Measurement of the acid-base balance in blood requires a good pH-meter and gas analyzer.

Urinary pH is measured with a glass electrode. At present, determination of total acid in the urine is carried out by the method of Jörgensen (1957), NH_4 and TA by the titration method of Chan (1972). These methods are sufficiently accurate and reproducible, but anaerobic sampling and rapid analysis are necessary.

REFERENCES

Gerok, W.: Primäre Tubulopathien. Stuttgart, Thieme 1969

Jörgensen, K.: Titrimetric determination of the net excretion of acid/base in urine. Scand. J. clin. lab. Invest. *9*: 287, 1957

Chan, J. C. M.: The rapid determination of urinary titratable acid ammonium and evaluation of freezing as a method of preservation. Clin. Biochem. *5*: 94, 1972

Adler, S., Lindeman, R. D., Yingst M. J. et al.: Effect of acute loading on urinary acid excretion by the aging human kidney. J. Lab. clin. Med. *72*: 278, 1968

Agarwal, B. N., Cabebe, F. G.: Renal acidification in elderly subjects. Nephron *26*: 291, 1980

Broyer, M., Proesmans, W., Royer, P.: La titration des bicarbonates chez l'enfant normal et au cours de diverses néphropathies. Rev. franc. Étud. clin. et biol. *14*: 556, 1969

Caregaro, L., Lauro, S., Ricci, G. et al.: Distal renal tubular acidosis in hepatic cirrhosis: clinical and pathogenetic study. Clin. Nephrol. *15*: 143, 1981

Dossetor, J. B., Gorman, H. M., Beck, J. C.: The diurnal rhythm of urinary electrolyte excretion I. Observations in normal subjects. Metabolism *12:* 1083, 1963

Edelmann, C. M. Jr., Boichis, H., Rodriguez-Soriano, J., Stark, H.: The renal response of children to acute ammonium chloride acidosis. Pediat. Res. *1:* 452, 1967

Glabman, S., Klose, R., Giebisch, G.: Micropuncture study of ammonia excretion in the rat. Am. J. Physiol. *205:* 127, 1963

Krück, F.: Titrierbare Urinazidität und Ammonium-Ausscheidung bei Störungen der Hydrogenbilanz. Klin. Wschr. *86:* 946, 1958

Lestradget, H., Correa, C. E., Broyer, M.: L'exploration de la fonction d'acidification du tubule rénal par une épreuve compte utilisant une surcharge intraveineuse de chlorhydrate de l'arginine. Rev. fr. Étud. clin. et bilo. *9:* 885, 1964

Lyons, H.: Acidosis in kidney disease. In: Acid-base and electrolyte balance. (Eds. Schwartz, A. B. Lyons, H.) New York, Grune and Stratton 1979

Mills, J. N., Stanbury, S. W.: A reciprocal relationship between K+ and H+ excretion in diurnal excretory rhythm in man. Clin. Sci. *13:* 177, 1954

Muldowney, F. P.: Renal acidosis. In: Renal disease (Ed. D. Black) Blackwell Scientific Publications 1979

Pitts, R. F.: The role of ammonia production and excretion in regulation of acid-base balance. New Engl. J. Med. *284,* 32, 1971

Pitts, R. F.: Control of renal production of ammonia. Kidney int. *1:* 297, 1972

Pitts, R. F.: Physiology of the kidney and body fluids. 3. ed. Chicago, Year book med. publ. inc. 1974

Pitts, R. F., Ayer, J. L., Schiess, W.: The renal regulation of acid-base balance in man III. The reabsorption and excretion of bicarbonate. J. clin. Invest. *28:* 35, 1949

Pitts, R. F., Lotspeich, W., Schiess, W., Ayer, J. L.: The renal regulation of acid-base balance in man. I. The nature of the mechanism for acidifying the urine. J. clin. Invest. *27:* 48, 1948

Rodriguez-Soriano, J., Edelmann, C. M. Jr.: Renal tubular acidosis. Am. Rev. Med. *20:* 363, 1969

Rodriguez-Soriano, J., Vallo, A., Garcia-Fuentes, M.: Distal renal tubular acidosis in infancy: a bicarbonate wasting state. J. Pediat. *86:* 524, 1975

Sartorius, O. W., Roemmelt, J. C., Pitts, R. F.: The renal regulation of acid base-balance in man IV. The nature of the renal compensation in ammonium chloride acidosis. J. clin. Invest. *28:* 423, 1949

Schwab, M.: Die renale Säureausscheidung bei chronischen Nephropathien. Verh. dtsch. Ges. inn Med. *67:* 595, 1961

Schwab, M.: Metodik und Indikation moderner Nierenfunktionsprüfungen. Verh. dtsch. Ges. inn. Med. *69:* 299, 1963

Schwartz, W. B., Hall, P. W., Hays, R. M., Relman, A. S.: On the mechanism of acidosis in chronic renal failure. J. clin. Invest. *38:* 39, 1959

Sebastian, A., McSherry, E., Morris, R. C. Jr.: Renal potassium wasting in renal tubular acidosis. J. clin. Invest. *50:* 667, 1971

Sebastian, A., Morris, R. C. Jr.: Renal tubular acidosis. In: Strauss and Welt's diseases of the kidney. 3. ed. (Eds. Earley, L. E., Gottschalk, C. W.) Boston, Little, Brown and Comp. 1979

Wrong, O., Davies, H. E. F.: The excretion of acid in renal disease. Quart. J. Med. *28:* 259, 1959

233

GLUCOSE EXCRETION

PHYSIOLOGY AND PATHOPHYSIOLOGY

Glucose freely penetrates the glomerular membrane, but under normal conditions does not appear in any appreciable amount in the final urine. With normal levels of blood sugar and GFR, about 170 g/day penetrate the glomerular membrane. Practically all the filtered load is reabsorbed in the tubules.

If blood sugar increases, either because there is a metabolic disease present or because glucose is being infused, urinary excretion starts and is dependent upon the blood level. Plasma glucose concentration at the threshold point of excretion gives the minimum value for tubular transport saturation. In healthy adults this value is 170–180 mg%.

Increasing plasma glucose above the minimum threshold level results in increasing amounts of excretion, but the relation between plasma glucose concentra-

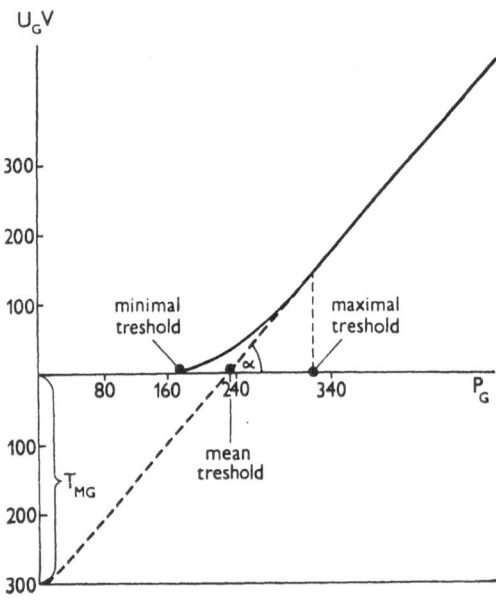

Fig. 67: Schematic presentation of the relationship between plasma glucose concentration and urinary glucose excretion in a helathy subject during glucose infusion designed to produce a linear rise of plasma glucose with time.

tion and urinary excretion (U_GV) is not a simple linear one. As can be seen in Fig. 67, the relation between U_GV and plasma glucose concentration (P_G) starts as a complex curve, and only with further increases in blood levels does a linear relation start to appear. The P_G value at which the U_GV vs P_G relation starts to be linear gives us the maximum glucose threshold value for the kidney. This latter value ranges from 330 to 400 mg%.

This curve suggests that the mechanism of reabsorption involves a maximal transport value. Attainment of this maximum transport level (Tm_G) results in the start of a linear relation between P_G and U_GV. Tm_G at P_G levels above the maximal threshold can be derived as follows:

$$Tm_G = GFR \times P_G - U_GV \tag{1}$$

For two levels of P_G: $(P_G)_1$ and $(P_G)_2$, which are both greater than the maximal threshold, we will have:

$Tm_G = GFR(P_G)_1 - (U_GV)_1$ and
$Tm_G = GFR(P_G)_2 - (U_GV)_2$

If we collect both equations, we have:

$$\Delta U_GV/\Delta P_G = GFR \tag{2}$$

It would appear from equation (2) that under these conditions, the relation between U_GV and P_G is linear, and further that the slope of the straight line = GFR.

The reasons for the "splay" in the initial portions of the curve in the region between minimal and maximal threshold values of P_G come into question. According to Smith (1951, 1956) the basis of this splay can be that each nephron does not have the same Tm value. Furthermore, it can be assumed that SNGFR is not the same in all nephrons. According to this view, with increasing P_G levels the Tm is first attained in nephrons which have a low tubular maximum transport, with a high filtered G load. Further rises in P_G result in saturation of tubular transport in other nephrons, until all nephrons are saturated and Tm for the entire kidney is attained.

"Splay" can also be explained on the basis of the kinetics of the reaction of glucose with a carrier molecule. According to the original view of Shannon (1939), the luminal membrane of the proximal tubule contains a "glucose carrier". The quantity of the carrier is finite and limited. The carrier complexes with glucose in the membrane, and then the complex breaks down in the cytoplasm. If we label the carrier B and glucose G, then:

At the luminal membrane there is the reaction:

$$G + B \rightleftarrows GB, \text{ and in the cytoplasm}$$
$$GB \rightarrow G + B .$$

This concept suggests that the amount of G which can be reabsorbed is limited by the amount of available B in the luminal membrane. In addition to the amount of B, the reabsorptive capacity will also depend upon the rate at which the complex GB breaks down to B + G.

The reaction in the luminal membrane can be characterized (according to mass action) by a dissociation constant K:

$$K = [G] \times [B]/[GB]$$

The lower the value of K, the greater the affinity of the carrier for glucose. The complexing reaction is therefore dependent upon the concentration of the substrate and can be expressed in a Michaelis-Menten formulation. This means that previous to the presence of a sufficiently high glucose concentration in the tubular lumen, part of the glucose will escape reabsorption.

Present knowledge suggests that splay will involve both of the above mentioned factors. Elucidation of this phenomenon is not just of theoretical importance — it allows us to characterize various types of abnormality of tubular transport of glucose.

The concept of a carrier is further of use in explaining competitive inhibition of tubular reabsorption. If two or more substances are transported by the same carrier, an increase in the transport of one will decrease the transport of a second substance. It has been shown that glucose, xylose, fructose and galactose are all transported by a common carrier mechanism.

Micropuncture data has shown that tubular transport of glucose occurs in the proximal tubule, and mainly in its proximal third. Thomas (1943) isolated from brush borders of rat kidneys a protein which binds glucose and phlorhizin. It would appear that there exist at least two hexose carriers, one in the luminal membrane and one antiluminal (peritubular). These carriers do not have the same specificity for hexoses. Tubular transport of glucose across the luminal membrane is Na--dependent (Brusse et al. 1972). Na ions probably change the conformation of the carrier and its affinity for D-glucose. Kinne et al. (1975) have also demonstrated a Na-dependent, phlorhizin-sensitive glucose transport in the luminal brushborder surface. On the other hand, Na-independent low affinity phlorhizin-insensitive transport is located in the basal and lateral membrane surfaces.

From the point of view of pathology, glucosuria can be subdivided into two basic groups:

1. Resulting from a high blood sugar so that the filtered G load is high. In this case, the source of the glucosuria is an extrarenal metabolic defect. In most cases this defect is diabetes mellitus.

Among nephrological aspects is the fact that this same type of glucosuria can occur in advanced stages of renal failure, at which time there is a decreased utilization of glucose (Dzúrik 1975). Patients treated with corticosteroids also have the same type of glucosuria.

2. Glucosuria can also result from a decreased ability of the tubules to reabsorb. In principle, this can be an isolated transport defect, or the defect can be part of a larger abnormality of transport processes in the kidney.

a) Renal glucosuria as a part of a generalized defect in tubular transport processes, as seen in the following pathologies:

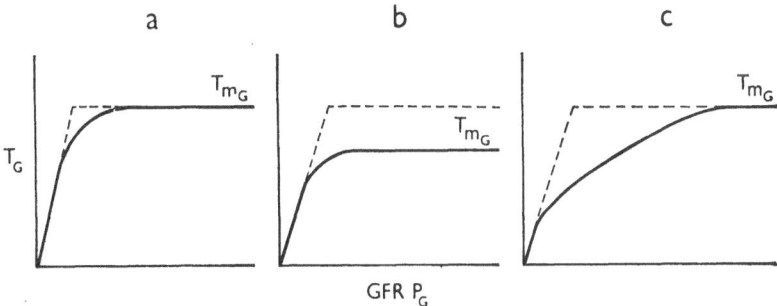

Fig. 68: Schematic presentation of the relationship between filtered amount of glucose (GFR P_G) and tubular reabsorption of glucose (T_G) in healthy subject (a), in a patient with renal glycosuria of type A (b), and in a patient with renal glycosuria of type B (c). (According to Reubi 1970).

Idiopathic Fanconi syndrome, Lowe syndrome, cystinosis, Wilson's disease, toxic renal damage (Pb, Ur, Cd, Hg, CN, lysol, maleic acid, oxalic acid) and shock kidney.

b) Familial renal glucosuria.

This pathology does not involve any other renal abnormality. Two types can be subdivided according to function: type A is characterized by a decrease in Tm_G; type B is characterized by a normal Tm_G but the splay is very much wider than normal. The relation between the filtered G load (GFR $\times P_G$) and reabsorption (T_G) in both types is schematically shown in Fig. 68.

Type A would appear to involve a deficiency in the quantity of available glucose carrier. Type B might well be related to a decreased G affinity of the carrier molecule (but the quantity of the latter is normal). Further observations on this will be necessary.

METHODS OF INVESTIGATION

1. QUALITATIVE DEMONSTRATION OF GLUCOSE IN THE URINE

Diagnostic test papers are used. The principle of the reaction involves oxidation of glucose by glucose-oxidase, in the presence of oxygen in the air, to gluconic acid and H_2O_2. The latter is catalyzed by peroxidase to oxidize colourless o-toluidine to a blue-coloured product. This reaction is specific and shows the presence of glucose in the range of 50–100 mg% (provided there is not an excess of inhibitors present in the urine).

In evaluation of glucosuria, one should take into account that the presence of glucose in the urine need not be a permanent feature. The morning urine can be negative, since blood glucose at this time of day is also lower, and glucose can appear in the urine at later times in the day. Any positive finding, however, requires a further workup — in particular a measurement of P_G.

2. GLUCOSE EXCRETION ($U_G V$)

Either we measure total glucose excreted per day, or urine is collected in three separate collection periods: usually 6–12 hr, 12–18 hr and 18–6 hr of the following morning. This approach allows us to judge the diurnal rhythm in the patient. Glucosuria must be related to the P_G level, measured in the morning on an empty stomach, at noon and in the afternoon.

On the basis of this test we know if the glucosuria is due to P_G levels or whether we have a case of renal glucosuria. In evaluating the former, we must take into account the general level of renal function and GFR in particular. With a marked decrease in the latter, sugar losses in the urine can be relatively small even with clear hyperglycaemia.

3. GLUCOSE "TITRATION" AND THE Tm_G

The test is carried out in the morning on an empty stomach. About 1 hr before the test onset one liter water is drunk and the bladder is catheterized. A blank sample of urine is taken. We then introduce, usually into the femoral artery, an indwelling needle to allow for repeated sampling. A blank sample of blood is drawn. C_{in} is measured at the same time (the analytical method must be specific enough so that glucose does not interfere in high concentrations). An indwelling needle is introduced into the antecubital vein and a priming inulin load, followed immediately by a maintenance infusion, is started (cf. p. 15). After one hr of maintenance infusion, the first urine collection period is started. After 2–3 control collections, each 10–15 min in duration, a further i.v. infusion is started in the contralateral antecubital vein with 20% glucose. An arterial blood sample is taken in the middle of each urine collection period.

Glucose "titration" is started by having the initial i.v. glucose infusion run in at 5 ml/min. Five 10-min collection periods are run at this infusion rate. The times of all blood samplings and termination of urine collection periods are carefully recorded. A total of 50 g glucose is given in this period.

Tm_G is approached, but not reached in this first loading period. This portion of the test should reveal the "splay" of the glucose concentration vs excretion curve.

Tm_G can be estimated only when we have attained a P_G value of 500 to 700 mg%. In order to achieve this, the next portion of the test involves an increase in the i.v. infusion rate of 20% glucose to 10 ml/min for 15–20 min. This delivers a further 30–40 g glucose to the patient and P_G is increased above the level of the maximal threshold. Reubi (1970) gives 200–300 ml of 40% glucose in this phase of the test in rapid i.v. infusion.

We then slow the infusion rate to 1–4 ml/min, and a further three urine collection periods are followed — the latter should be definitely at the level of Tm_G. Blood is sampled in all collection periods.

On the basis of the urine flow rate and values of P_G, U_G and C_{in} we calculate for each collection period U_GV and T_G. The latter is calculated according to the equation (1).

We then graph U_GV vs P_G. An example is shown in Fig. 67. From this we determine the minimal and maximal threshold values for glucose and the degree of "splay" can be observed. In patients with type B renal glucosuria, the splay is markedly widened and the maximal threshold is higher, usually greater than 400 mg%.

$\Delta U_GV/\Delta P_G$ at the point at which the curve becomes a straight line (the maximal threshold value) = GFR. Extrapolation of this straight line to the abscissa gives us the "mean threshold" for glucose. The latter gives us the glucose concentration at which maximal threshold exists for all nephrons. It is given by the ratio $Tm_G/$ /GFR. It is useful to reconstruct the curve using known GFR values (either C_{in} or C_{Cr}).

Tm_G can be calculated from the "mean glucose threshold" as determined on the abscissa intercept in the graph.

We can graph the filtered glucose load (GFR $\times$ P_G) and the amount reabsorbed (T_G). An example is shown in Fig. 68.

Our findings can be summarized as follows:
minimal threshold in healthy controls = 170–180 mg%
maximal threshold   = 330–400 mg%.
Normal values in healthy controls for Tm_G are (Smith 1956):
males   375 $\pm$ 79.7 mg/min/1.73 m^2
women 303 $\pm$ 55.3 mg/min/1.73 m^2
In the newly born Tm_G is lower, ranging from 30 to 80 mg/min/1.73 m^2. In the fourth month of life, the infant attains about 50% of the adult level (Tudvad 1949). In the elderly, Tm_G is decreased by as much as 7% over each decade. In males aged 80 years, it decreases to about 225 mg/min/1.73 m^2 (Miller et al. 1952).

Tm_G decreases in chronic renal disease. The cause is a decrease in the number of functional nephrons.

Indications for investigation

Measurement of Tm_G used to be carried out as a part of any complex series of renal tests to determine the quantity of functional parenchyma. Tm_G, however, decreases in chronic renal disease in proportion to GFR, and knowledge of this value alone is not of additional use to evaluate a given patient. In addition, this measurement stresses the subject and it cannot be considered as part of a routine workup.

In any diagnostic workup, glucosuria must be determined as a function of either hyperglycaemia or of a defect in tubular G transport.

If glucosuria is related to hyperglycaemia, further tests are oriented towards the blood glucose level and why it is raised.

If there is blood-sugar-related glucosuria, we must find out if there is any further relation to chronic renal failure or administration of glucocorticoids. If blood sugar is repeatedly normal, then glucosuria is related to tubular transport. The minimal threshold for glucose will be lowered. Further tests should try to define the tubular transport defect. Renal glucosuria can occur in relation to:

1. A generalized abnormality of the renal tubules (see p. 254). It is important for differential diagnosis to know whether renal glucosuria is associated with abnormal excretion into the urine of amino acids. In the first orientational test we can determine the excretion of amino nitrogen. Under normal conditions, urinary excretion of amino nitrogen does not exceed 200 mg/day (cf. p. 256). In patients with a general abnormality of proximal tubular function, urinary excretion of amino nitrogen is increased.

2. Toxic damage to the kidneys. This type of glucosuria is transitory and disappears with restitution of renal function.

3. Glucosuria after acute tubular anuria in relation to shock states. This disturbance of tubular function is also transitory.

4. Rare renal glucosuria in some chronic renal diseases (Reubi 1970).

If none of the above causes can be determined, we can consider a diagnosis of familiar renal glucosuria. This is an isolated transport defect. All other renal functions are normal.

Glucose "titration" can determine whether Type A or Type B familial disease is involved. This does not, however, have practical importance since the principles of management do not differ between the two types. The following findings are diagnostic (Elsas and Rosenberg 1979):

a) glucosuria exists without a raised blood sugar,
b) an oral glucose tolerance test gives normal result,
c) patients on a normal diet excrete more than 500 mg/day/1.73 m² of glucose (the diet should be 30 cal./kg body weight and 50% carbohydrate),
d) GFR, tubular function and all other renal tests (including i.v. urography) are normal.

Routine investigation of patients with moderate glucosuria may give rise to doubt as to whether this is associated with normal blood sugar levels. A small glucose load is recommended in such cases (Reubi 1970). 20 g are given per os in 300 ml water, and a possible glucosuric response is followed.

Differential diagnostic problems can arise when diabetes mellitus or another hyperglycaemic variant of glucosuria is combined with renal glucosuria in the same patient. This can be considered when the urinary glucose loss is far greater than the hyperglycaemia would suggest. In such cases we should test whether glucosuria remains if we get the blood sugar down to normal. If glucosuria persists with a normal blood sugar, a simultaneous tubular defect can be diagnosed. Such patients usually have an abnormal oral glucose tolerance test which suggests abnormal carbohydrate metabolism.

Glucosuria in pregnancy can result from hyperglycaemia or a tubular transport defect. The physiological rise in GFR in pregnancy with a relatively small decrease in the minimal glucose threshold value can result in glucosuria.

Contraindications to investigation

Measurement of Tm_G is contraindicated in patients with cardiovascular disease and fluid retention. A sudden and marked increase in blood sugar is very unphysiological, and this test does not belong to a routine workup at present.

Glucose "titration" gives us only a basis for differentiating between types A and B renal glucosuria, which has no practical significance.

Laboratory methods

For glucose determination the glucose-oxidase method is suitable (Trinder 1969), or the method of Richterich et al. (1974) can be recommended.

REFERENCES

Busse, D., Elas, L. J., Rosenberg, L. E.: Uptake of D-glucose by renal tubule membranes. I. Evidence for two transport systems. J. biol. Chem. *247*: 1188, 1972

Dzúrik, R.: Uraemia. The pathophysiology of carbonhydrate metabolism. Bratislava Publ. House of the Slovak Acad. Sci., 1973

Elsas, L. J., Rosenberg, L. E.: Renal glycosuria. In: Strauss and Welt's diseases of the kidneys. L. E. Earley, C. W. Gottschalk (Eds.) Little, Brown and Co. Boston 1979, pp. 1021–1028

Goaverts, P., Lambert, P. P., Lebrun, A., Heinzelin de Braucourt, C. M.: Mésure de la filtration glomérularie chez l'homme par l'injection intraveineuse de glucose. Bull. Acad. roy. Med. Belg. *13*: 253, 1948

Kinne, R., Murer, H., Kinne-Saffran, E., et al.: Sugar transport by renal plasma membrane vesicles. Characterization of the systems in the brush-border microvilli and basa-lateral plasma membranes. J. Membr. Biol. *21*: 375, 1975

Miller, J. H., McDonald, R. K., Shock, N. W.: Age changes in the maximal rate of renal tubular reabsorption of glucose. J. Geront. 7: 195, 1952

Reubi, F.: Nierenkrankheiten. Bern, Stuttgart, Wien, H. Huber 1970

Richterich, R., Küffer, H., Lorenz, E., Colombo, J. P.: Die Bestimmung der Glucose in Plasma und Serum (Hexokinase/glucose-6-Phosphatdehydrogenase-Methode) mit Greiner Electronic Selective Analyzer GSA II. Z. klin. Chem. klin. Biochem. *12*: 5, 1974

Shannon, J. A.: Renal tubular excretion. Physiol. Rev. *19*: 63, 1939

Smith, H. W.: The kidney: structure and function in health and disease. New York, Oxford Univ. Press 1951

Smith, H. W.: Principles of renal physiology. New York, Oxford Univ. Press 1956

Thomas, L.: Isolation on N-ethylmaleimide-labelled phlorizin-sensitive D-glucose binding protein of brush border membrane from rat kidney cortex. Biochim. Biophys. Acta *291*: 454, 1973

Trinder, P. A.: Determination of glucose in blood using glucose oxidase with an alternative oxygen acceptor. Ann. clin. Biochem. *6*: 24, 1969

Tudvad, F.: Sugar reabsorption in premature and full term babies. Scand. J. clin. Lab. Invest. *1*: 281, 1949

URIC ACID EXCRETION

PHYSIOLOGY AND PATHOPHYSIOLOGY

Uric acid (a metabolic end-product from endogenous and exogenous nucleo-proteins) is excreted by the kidneys by a special mechanism. On the basis of present knowledge (Lassiter 1975, Weiner 1979) it is believed that the mammalian kidney allows uric acid through the glomerular membrane and then intensively reabsorbs it in the proximal tubule. At the same time the proximal tubule also secrets uric acid, so that its transport in this segment, including the pars recta and perhaps also part of the loop of Henle, is bidirectional. Part of the secreted amount is reabsorbed at a site more distally placed — so-called post-secretory reabsorption (Diamond and Paolino 1973, Diamond and Meisel 1977, Steele and Boner 1973). Tubular transport of uric acid is carrier mediated. Under normal conditions this transport mechanism is not saturated.

Reabsorption and secretion of uric acid can be influenced separately by drugs. Pyrazinamide, and its active metabolite pyrazinoic acid (PZA), have a powerful inhibitory action on tubular secretion (Ÿu et al. 1961). With an adequate dose of PZA there is practically a complete stop of uric acid excretion. For this reason Ÿu and Gutman (1959) believed that the total filtered load of uric acid was reabsorbed in the proximal tubule and that secretion took place distal to the reabsorption site.

Tubular reabsorption of uric acid can be influenced by Probenecid. The details of transtubular transport of uric acid by the proximal tubule are still not completely, clear.

Several possible mechanisms can be considered to increase uric acid excretion. Increased uricosuria can result from increased secretion or decreased reabsorption, or both effects working together. The plasma concentration is of importance for this. With increasing concentrations the filtered load and the tubular load for secretion are both increased.

From the clinical and pathophysiological points of view it is important to distinguish hyperuricosuric states with and without a raised plasma level of uric acid.

Increased excretion into the urine can come about in patients with gout, but hyperuricosuria does not usually occur in this state. Seegmiller et al. (1961) showed a significant rise in uricosuria in 25% of patients with gout. In the remainder, urinary excretion of uric acid was either normal or depressed. Nephrolithiasis is a common complication of gout. It has been reported that 10–20 % of pateints with gout have a much higher frequency of stone formation (Ÿu and Gutman 1967). Whether hyperuricaemia plays a role in the lithiasis directly in the kidneys, in addition to the basic metabolic disease, remains an unknown factor. Gutman and Ÿu (1957) found that in such patients the fractional reabsorption of uric acid is increased. The net reabsorption in these patients was, on the average, 93.1% in comparison with healthy controls who had a mean of 91.9%.

Increased urinary excretion of uric acid from raised blood levels occurs with excessive production of purines and with proliferative diseases of the haematopoietic system.

According to Talbot (1959) 10% of gout patients have as the cause of hyperuricemia a blood disease.

Hyperuricaemia has been reported (Blahos 1969) in heamolytic anaemia, thalassemia, sickle cell disease, pernicious anemia, myelofibrosis, polycythemia secondary polyglobulinaemia, myeloid metaplasia, acute leukaemia, chronic leukaemia, myeloma, Hodgkin's disease and lymphosarcoma, among the blood diseases. The development of hyperuricaemia and uricosuria is also found when cytostatic drugs are used. Both the high blood and urine levels are more extreme with secondary than with primary gout.

Of the non-haematological diseases, hyperuricaemia has been described in psoriasis, in which there is extensive cell proliferation (Eisen and Seegmiller 1961). Both metabolic defects and renal excretory defects contribute to hyperuricemia during chronic lead poisoning (Serre and Simon 1963).

Hyperuricosuria due to hyperuricemia is dangerous to the kidney for a number of reasons. The high blood levels can result in precipitation of uric acid in the renal parenchyma. The tendency to precipitate in tissue is not a simple function of the uric acid blood level — a number of other factors probably play a role. Renal precipitation of uric acid is followed by interstitial inflammation and can progress to interstitial nephritis (urate nephropathy). Kidney biopsies from gout patients can sometimes show urate crystals. Gonick et al. (1965) believe that gout patients develop histological changes characterized by a uniform fibrillar thickening of the basal membrane of capillaries with proliferation of nuclei in the capillary loops.

Hyperuricosuria can result in renal stone formation, and obstruction of the urinary passages has even been observed. Hyperuricosuria without a raised plasma uric acid level can occur in so-called hyperuricosuric Ca-oxalate urolithiasis (Coe 1978). The disease affects mainly males and is probably a function of an increased purine intake — in some cases there may be an increased end-metabolic production of purines. This syndrome involves the formation of Ca-oxalate crystals. Renal excretion of Ca is in the normal range. The mechanism by which hyperuricosuria results in the formation of Ca-oxalate crystals is not known. Pak et al. (1977) and Coe et al. (1978) have shown a direct effect of uric acid in aqueous solution on the nucleation of Ca-oxalate.

Robertson (1976) believes that Na-acid-urate may promote Ca-oxalate disease by forming a gel phase in urine which adsorbs or interferes with naturally occurring inhibitors of Ca-oxalate crystal growth. These inhibitors may be acid mucopolysaccharides.

Increased renal excretion of uric acid may be the result of a number of renal pathologies Hyperuricosuria has been described in Fanconi syndrome in adults with light-chain disease (Lee et al. 1972). Diamond and Meisel (1977) assume that uricosuria in Fanconi syndrome is the result of a decrease in post-reabsorptive secretion of uric acid. Of the most commonly used drugs, aspirin causes an increase in uric acid excretion.

Hypouricaemia can be caused by the isolated defect in renal tubular uric acid transport (Benjamin et al. 1977).

A decrease in urinary excretion and increase of blood levels of uric acid occurs in advanced stages of chronic renal disease (Fig. 69). Plasma uric acid concentration remains normal in this state up to a decrease in GFR to values of about 20–30 ml/ /min. If GFR decreases, there is a compensatory increase in the uric acid excretion fraction (FE_{UA}) (Steele and Reisselbach 1967). If GFR decreases below 20–30 ml/

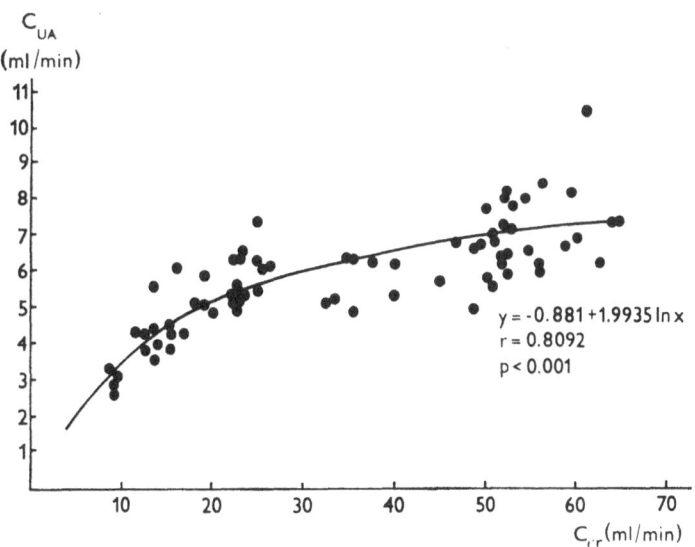

$$y = -0.881 + 1.9935 \ln x$$
$$r = 0.8092$$
$$p < 0.001$$

Fig. 69: Relationship between endogenous creatinine clearance (C_{cr}) and renal clearance of uric acid (C_{UA}) in patients with chronic renal diseases.

min, this compensation mechanism is not sufficient, and hyperuricaemia results. The mechanism of the increase in FE_{UA} with a gradual reduction in GFR is not yet known. It is of interest that FE_{UA} in these patients shows a direct relation to the increase in FE_{Na} (Malý and Schück 1973). The findings of Lang et al. (1980) suggest that in patients with chronic renal failure there is decrease in tubular reabsorption of uric acid in the residual nephrons.

Renal excretion of UA is influenced by the rate of tubular Na reabsorption, and thus is dependent upon changes in ECF volume (Steele 1969). Factors which increase tubular Na reabsorption also decrease the renal excretion of UA, and vice versa.

The frequent finding of hyperuricaemia developing after a diuretic course of tratment can be explained as a result of ECF volume depletion, with an associated decrease in urinary UA excretion because of the increased tubular Na reabsorption. On the other hand, a salt load and ECF volume expansion results in an increased UA excretion and a decrease in plasma levels.

Tubular transport of UA can be affected by the anions of many organic acids. The inhibitory action of lactate is of particular importance (Yu et al. 1957) along with a similar effect of keto-acids (Goldfinger et al. 1965). This mechanism obviously plays an important role in the development of hyperuricaemia during fasting (in addition to the factor of dehydration).

METHODS OF INVESTIGATION

1. URINARY CONCENTRATION OF URIC ACID (U_{UA})

U_{UA} depends upon the rate of urine flow and the amount of total UA excreted. U_{UA} decreases in hyperbolic relation to a rise in urine flow rate. This relation, under conditions of water diuresis, is shown in Fig. 70. It is clear that with a urine flow rate of about 1 ml/min, U_{UA} ranges about 50 mg%. At the height of water diuresis U_{UA} decreases to values about those of the plasma concentration or lower. There is a rapid decrease in U_{UA} with a rise in urine flow rate to values about 3 ml/min. A further increase in urine flow rate is associated with a slow decrease in U_{UA}.

A similar hyperbolic relation exists under conditions of induced osmotic diuresis (Fig. 71). With a mannitol diuresis, U_{UA} is higher than with water diuresis, which is a function of a simultaneous increase in uric acid excretion ($U_{UA}V$).

Measurement of U_{UA} is important in patients with urolithiasis and helps us to judge whether the recommended water intake regimen is associated with the desired decrease in U_{UA}. Measurements in a morning urine sample (before breakfast) allows us to discover to what degree U_{UA} increase during the night and whether

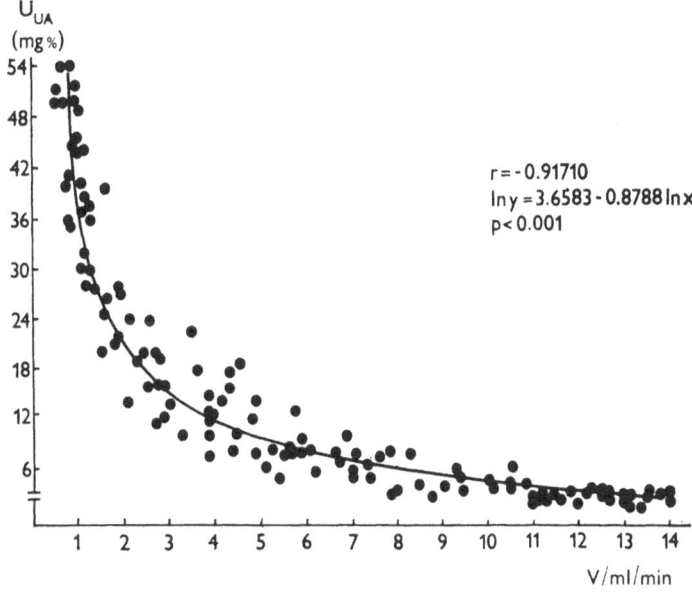

Fig. 70: Relationship between urine flow rate (V) and urinary concentration of uric acid (U_{UA}) in healthy subjects under conditions of water diuresis.

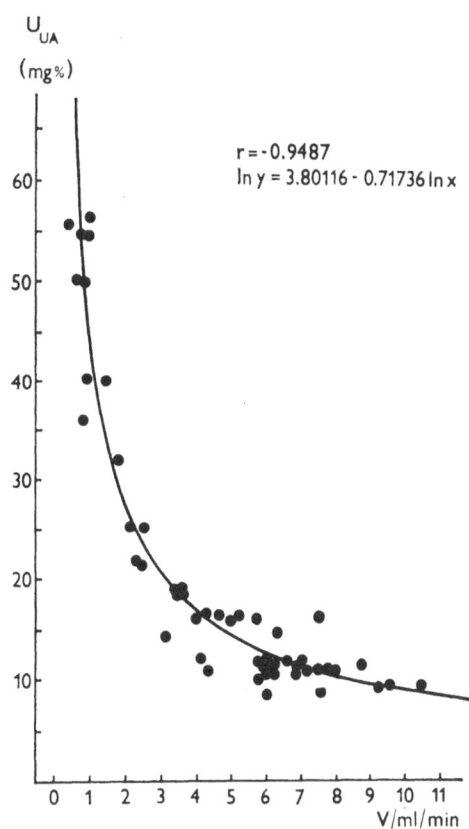

Fig. 71: Relationship between urine flow rate (V) and urinary concentration of uric acid (U_{uA}) in healthy subjects under conditions of mannitol osmotic diuresis.

the necessary degree of urine flow rate at night exists. Pak et al. (1977) have shown that urine is metastable with respect to Na-H-urate when total uric acid concentration exceeded 30 mg%. This could become a basis for the clinical diagnosis of an adequate uric acid level.

2. URINARY EXCRETION OF UA ($U_{UA}V$)

This is measured over 24 hr., with analysis of UA concentration in the mixed urine sample. The value of $U_{UA}V$ depends upon the dietary intake. Reliable results usually require measurement of daily UA excretion for 2–3 days consecutively, on a known and constant diet. The question of whether $U_{UA}V$ is normal or high depends upon precise knowledge of intake.

According to Seegmiller (1974), under conditions of a so-called non-purine diet $U_{UA}V$ on the third day of consecutive measurement should not exceed 600 mg/day.

A non-purine diet is one which contains no meat, fish, fowl, tea, coffee, beer or leguminous vegetables. Obviously, no drugs which influence renal UA excretion can be given. If possible, no drugs should be given at all during the test period.

Gutman (1968) considers the upper limit of normal of $U_{UA}V$ in males on a normal diet to be 800 mg/day, in females 750 mg/day. Coe (1978) reports, for the same conditions, the following subject distribution data for $U_{UA}V$:

$U_{UA}V$ (mg/day)	males	females
200	0	0
200–400	2	36
400–600	38	54
600–800	48	9
800–900	6	0

Pak et al. (1980) report normal values for $U_{UA}V$ to be 603 ± 166 mg/day. It would appear that on a normal diet the upper limit of normal uric acid excretion should be taken as 800 mg/day for males and 750 mg/day for females. If uricosuria is investigated on a non-purine diet, 600 mg/day would appear to be the upper limit of normal. The non-purine diet must be held to for at least 3 days.

3. CLEARANCE OF URIC ACID (C_{UA})

The test is carried out in the A.M. on an empty stomach. A water load of one liter is drunk one hr before the test starts. (Water diuresis has no significant effect on $U_{UA}V$).

Urine is collected for 1–2 hr. The bladder is emptied by spontaneous voiding. Venous blood is sampled in the middle of the collection period. For the calculation see p. 262. Normal values in healthy adult controls range from 6 to 12 ml/min (Pitts 1974).

In our own laboratory (Malý and Schück 1972) 66 healthy adults on a normal diet showed a mean C_{UA} of 8.68 $\pm$ 2.18 ml/min. In other words, most values in healthy controls should range between 4.3 and 13.0 ml/min. Plasma UA concentration was 5.13 $\pm$ 0.94 mg%. The mean ± 2 SD showed a range of 3.25 to 7.01 mg%. Precise measurements have shown that a small fraction of UA is bound to plasma protein (Klingberg and Kippen 1970).

FRACTIONAL EXCRETION OF UA (FE_{UA})

This gives us the relation between urinary excretion and the filtered load of UA. The result is the algebraic sum of a number of transport processes in the nephron.

Tubular reabsorption exceeds secretory processes so that the resulting C_{UA} is significantly less than GFR.

Measurement of FE_{UA} is carried out in the same manner as C_{UA} — one needs only to analyze for cr in the same urine and blood samples.

In healthy controls on a normal diet, FE_{UA} was 7.82 $\pm$ 1.72%. The mean ± 2 SD was 4.4 to 12.2%. These findings are in agreement with other data in the literature.

Indications for investigation

1. Urolithiasis

P_{UA} and $U_{UA}V$ should be determined. The possibility of urate urolithiasis must be ruled out (particularly if the patient has hyperuricaemia) with and without the presence of Ca-oxalate stones. The effect of therapy in such patients can be judged from U_{UA}.

2. Diuretic treatment

ECF volume depletion, and the resulting increased tubular Na reabsorption and decreased $U_{UA}V$, can produce hyperuricaemia. Plasma UA levels should therefore be followed during diuretic therapy.

3. Gout

P_{UA} and $U_{UA}V$ should be followed in these patients. The effectiveness of therapy can also be followed in the same manner.

4. Hyperuricaemia in blood diseases

Because of the danager of urolithiasis and obstruction of the renal passages, U_{UA}, urine pH and the rate of urine flow must be followed in blood diseases.

5. Chronic renal failure

With a sharp decline in GFR, the increase in FE_{UA} is not sufficient to maintain P_{UA} within normal limits. Measurement of P_{UA} and $U_{UA}V$ should be used to follow patients under treatment with allopurinol.

Laboratory methods

The specific uricase methods are used for urine and plasma samples. For clinical use the method of Kageyama (1971) and the method of Hoeckel and Heinz (1975) can be recommended.

REFERENCES

Benjamin, D., Sperling, O., Weinberger, A., Pinkhas, J., de Vries, A.: Familial hypouricaemia due to isolated renal tubular defect. Nephron 18: 220, 1977

Blahoš, J.: Kyselina močová. Praha, Státní zdrav. nakl. 1968

Coe, F. L.: Hyperuricosuric calcium oxalate nephrolithiasis. Kidney int. 13: 418, 1978

Diamond, H. S., Paolino, J. S.: Evidence for a post-secretory absorptive site for uric acid in man. J. clin. Invest. 52: 1491, 1973

Diamond, H. S., Meisel, A. D.: Classification of uricosuric states based upon response to pharmacologic inhibitors of urate transport. Adv. exp. Med. Biol. 76 B: 61, 1977

Eisen, A. Z., Seegmiller, J. E.: Uric acid metabolism in psoriasis. J. clin. Invest. 40: 1486, 1961

Goldfinger, S., Klinenberg, J. R., Seegmiller, J. E.: Renal retention of uric acid induced by infusion of beta-hydroxybutyrate and acetoacetate. New Engl. J. Med. 272: 351, 1965

Gonick, H. C., Rubini, M. E., Gleason, I. O., Sommers, S. C.: The renal lesion in gout. Ann. intern. Med 62: 667, 1065

Gutman, A. B., Yu, T. F.: Renal function in gout. Am. J. Med. 23: 600, 1957

Haeckel, R., Heinz, F.: Die Bestimmung der Harnsäurekonzentration mittels Uricase, Katalase und NADH-abhängiger Aldehyddehydrogenase. Z. klin. Chem. klin. Biochem. 13: 244, 1975

Kageyama, N.: A direct colorimetric determination of urine in serum and urine with unicase-catalase system. Clin. chim. Acta 31: 421, 1971

Klinberg, J. R., Kippen, I.: The binding of urate to plasma proteins determined by means of equilibrium dialysis. J. lab. clin. Med. 78: 503, 1970

Lang, F., Gregor, R., Oberleithner, H. et al.: Renal handling of urate in healthy man in hyperuricaemia and renal insufficiency: cirdcadian fluctuation, effect of water diuresis and uricosuric agents. Europ. J. clin. Invest. *10*: 285, 1980

Lee, D. B. N., Drinkard, J. P., Rosen, J. R. et al.: The adult Fanconi syndrome. Observations on etiology, morphology, renal function and mineral metabolism in three patients. Medicine *51*: 107, 1972

Lassiter, W. E.: Kidney. Ann. Rev. Physiol. *37*: 371, 1975

Malý, J., Schück, O.: Vliv vodní a osmotické diuresy na renální vylučování kyseliny močové u člověka. I. U lidí s normálními renálními funkcemi. Čas. Lék. čes. *111*: 2, 1972

Malý, J., Schück, O.: Renal uric acid excretion in patients with chronic pyelonephritis. Int. Urol. Nephrol. *5*: 209, 1973

Pak, C. Y. C., Walters, O., Arnold, L., et al.: Mechanism for calcium urolithiasis among patients with hyperuricosuria: supersaturation of urine with respect to monosodium urate. J. clin. Invest. *59*: 426, 1977

Pitts, R. F.: Physiology of the kidney and body fluids. Third edition. Year book, Medical publishers Chicago 1974

Robertson, W. G.: Urinary acid mucopolysaccharide inhibitors of calcium oxalate crystallization. In: Urolithiasis Research Fleisch H., Robertson, W. G., Smith, L. H., Vahlensieck, W. (Eds.) London, Plenum Press 1976, pp. 331–334

Seegmiller, J. E.: Diseases of purine and pyrimidine metabolism. In: P. K. Bondy, L. E., Rosenberg (Eds.), Duncan's Diseases of Metabolism (7th ed.) Philadelphia, Saunders, 1974, pp. 655–774

Seegmiller, J. E., Grayzel, A. I.; Laster, L., Liddle, L.: Uric acid production in gout. J. clin. Invest. *40*: 1304, 1961

Serre, H., Simon, L.: La goutte secondaire. In: La goutte. Paris. Masson Cie. Ed. 1963, pp. 240–286

Steele, T. H.: Evidence for altered renal urate reabsorption during changes in volume of the extracellular fluid. J. lab. clin. Med. *74*: 288, 1969

Steele, T. H., Boner, G.: Origins of the uricosuric response. J. clin. Invest. *52*: 1368, 1973

Steele, T. H., Reisselbach, R. E.: The renal mechanism for urate homeostasis in normal man. Am. J. Med. *43*: 876, 1967

Talbott, J. H.: Gout and dyscrasias. Medicine *38*: 173, 1959

Weiner, I. M.: Urate transport in the nephron. Am. J. Physiol. *237*: F 85 – F 92, 1979

Yu, T. F., Berger, L., Gutman, A. B.: Suppression of tubular secretion of urate by pyrazinamide in the dog. Proc. Soc. exp. Biol. Med. *107*: 905, 1961

Yu, T. F., Gutman, A. B.: Study of the paradoxical effects of salicylate in low, intermediate and high dosage on renal mechanism for excretion of urate in man. J. clin. Invest. *38*: 1298, 1959

Yu, T. F., Gutman, A. B.: Uric acid nephrolithiasis in gout (predisposing factors). Ann. intern. Med. *67*: 1133, 1967

Yu, T. F., Sirota, J. H., Berger, L., et al.: Effect of sodium lactate infusion on urate clearance in man. Proc. Soc. exp. Biol. Med. *96*: 809, 1957

AMINO ACIDS EXCRETION

PHYSIOLOGY AND PATHOPHYSIOLOGY

Amino acids freely penetrate the glomerular membrane and are intensively reabsorbed in the tubules. Under normal conditions tubular reabsorption of amino acids is 95–100% of the filtered load. Micropuncture studies show that tubular amino acid reabsorption takes place in the proximal tubule. Transtubular amino acid transport is active, the details of which still require investigation.

The fact that in tubular cells in the renal cortex higher amino acid concentrations occur than in plasma (Baerlocher et al. 1970) bears evidence for active transport. Concentrations of amino acids in tubular fluid and final urine are far lower than in plasma (Brown et al. 1961, Gayer and Gerok 1961, Young and Freedman 1971). The rate of tubular transport of individual amino acids depends upon their chemical structure. L-isomers of amino acids (the naturally occurring form in mammals) are transported more intensively than D-isomers (Crampton and Smyth 1953). The rate of transport is further dependent upon the length and charge of the side-chain. Reabsorption of amino acids increases with increased hydrophobicity. There is an inverse relation between the clearance and the length of the hydrophobic side-chain (Short and Rosenberg 1979).

The energetic basis of transtubular amino acid transport is not clear. The question of the interrelations between amino acids and Na has been intensively studied in recent years. On the basis of the socalled Na-gradient hypothesis (Crane 1962, 1965) it would appear that motion of Na ions in the direction of the electrochemical gradient into tubular cells is coupled to amino-acid influx and provides the driving force for concentrative uptake of the amino acids. The findings of Evers et al. (1976) support this view. On the basis of other reports (Silbernagel and Deetjen 1972, Young and Freedman 1971) it would appear that tubular transport of amino acids is associated with oxidative phosphorylation. Rosenberg and Scriver (1974) believe that Na ions form a tertiary complex with a carrier molecule and the amino acid molecules.

The concept of a carrier molecule for transtubular amino acid transport agrees with a number of experimental reports. The relation between filtered and reabsorbed amino acid loads can be analyzed on the basis of the Michaelis-Menten formula, which gives rate of uptake vs concentration of substrate.

Uptake rate increases with the concentration of substrate up to a given plateau value. It would appear that when the maximal plateau rate is attained (V_{max}), this represents the maximal reabsorption rate (Tm). This view can be used to analyze tubular transport of different amino acids. The assumption can be made that in the luminal membrane of tubular cells of the proximal tubule there is a finite number of recognition or transport sites.

Since there is competitive inhibition of different amino acids for transport (if the chemical structure is similar), it would appear that tubular transport of any group of amino acids involves a common carrier mechanism. Studies of genetic defects in amino acid transport have assisted in the analysis of transport mechanisms in general.

Present knowledge would appear to subdivide various transport mechanisms for amino acids. There are systems which are high capacity and low affinity, and vice versa. Each is specific for a given group of amino acids. The human kidney would appear to contain the following 5 high capacity-low affinity transport systems (Short and Rosenberg 1979):

1. alpha-amino-neutral amino acids
2. beta-amino-neutral amino acids
3. dibasic-cystine transport system
4. dicarboxylic transport system
5. iminoglycine transport system

These transport systems process the reabsorption of large amounts of amino acids of similar structure.

In addition, each system has sub-systems which are specialized for the transport of one or only a few amino acids. The latter are low-capacity, high-affinity.

This classification is due to studies of competitive inhibition of amino acids for transport, analysis of nephron "titration" with increasing concentrations of individual amino acids and analysis of various congenital defects of tubular transport of individual amino acids.

Using the Michaelis-Menten formulation for tubular transport of amino acids allows us to distinguish, just as with analysis of renal glucosuria (cf.p. 237), abnormalities which are based upon carrier capacity and affinity for substrate. If the quantity of carrier is decreased, there is a decrease in the maximal tubular transport (Tm). Abnormalities due to a decreased carrier affinity are manifest by a widened splay (when titrating the nephron with the amino acid in question) but Tm is normal.

In various pathological states, there is an increase in urinary excretion of amino acids. Two types of amino-aciduria can be distinguished:

1. Amino-aciduria based upon *increases in plasma levels* of one or more species. In this case the filtered load of the amino acid species in question is also increased. Since reabsorption in the tubules is not quantitative, increased urinary excretion can result. This type is referred to as "overflow".

An increased load of one amino acid and an increase in its tubular reabsorption can, because of competitive inhibition, produce a decrease in tubular reabsorption of other amino acids (with normal plasma concentrations).

2. *Renal-tubular amino aciduria* results from a tubular defect in reabsorption of amino acids.

The definition of amino-aciduria often leaves us without a clear answer to whether a change in the absolute excretion of some amino acids is involved (mg/day), or whether a change in renal clearance (expressed on the basis of 1.73 m² surface area) or a change in fractional excretion of the amino acids (% of the filtered load) is involved.

From metabolic and nutritional aspects it is important to measure the absolute amino acid losses. Knowledge of fractional excretion or fractional reabsorption of the amino acids is necessary to recognize tubular defects, since absolute excretion can, but need not, be raised. As an example we can cite the increased fractional excretion of practically all amino acids in patients with chronic renal failure, even though the absolute levels of excretion may be raised only for a few molecular species (citrulline and proline).

It is clear that as with other types of excretion, the absolute excretion of amino acids and the clearances depend upon both GFR and plasma levels. For these reasons, if tubular reabsorptive defects are to be recognized, attention must be given to GFR levels.

Amino-aciduria on the basis of increased plasma levels can have a number of causes. There are congenital defects in amino acid metabolism which are associated with increased plasma levels of one or more species. This is usually based upon a congenital enzyme defect. They are rare, and further characterization is outside the scope of this monograph.

Extrarenal amino-aciduria can occur with a number of diseases of the liver or the bones.

Renal amino-aciduria is subdivided into two large sub-groups:

a) Generalized amino-aciduria

This type involves increased excretion of practically all amino acids. There are also other signs of proximal tubular defects, such as renal glucosuria, phosphaturia, bicarbonate handling and even increased excretion of uric acid. This is also referred to as Fanconi syndrome (De Toni-Debré-Fanconi).

Generalized amino-aciduria can develop in relation to various congenital metabolic diseases, such as cystinosis, galactosaemia, glycogenosis, Wilson's disease, hereditary fructose intolerance, tyrosinaemia. It can also be related to Lowe's syndrome, osteogenesis imperfecta, congenital RTA, hereditary anaemia or to idiopathic Fanconi syndrome. It is more frequently related to various intoxications, such as with heavy metals (Cd, Pb, Hg, Ur) or organic substances (salicylates, lysol, nitrobenzine, maleic acid or outdated tetracyclines).

Generalized amino-aciduria has also been described after burns, in diabetes mellitus, multiple myeloma, Kwashiorkor, K depletion and the nephrotic syndrome.

b) Specific renal amino-aciduria

This variant involves an increased renal excretion of one amino acid or one chemical group of amino acids transported by a common carrier. These specific defects are all genetically related. In a number of these, the same amino acids are subjected to transport defects by the gut mucosa.

Short and Rosenberg (1979) distinguish the following congenital specific amino-aciduriae:
a) Cystinuria with raised excretion of cystine, lysine, arginine and ornithine. There would appear to be a defect in a common carrier mechanism for cystine and dibasic amino acids.
b) Hypercystinuria — in these cases only cystine is affected. It would thus appear that a specific carrier system exists only for cystine.
c) Dibasic amino-aciduria. This involves increased excretion of Lys, Arg, Orn.
d) Imino-glycinuria. The increased excretion is of proline, hydroxyproline and glycine.
e) Hartnup's disease. This involves increased excretion of neutral amino acids (with the exception of imino-acids and glycine).
f) Dicarboxylic amino-aciduria. This involves increased excretion of glutamic and aspartic acids.

Amino-aciduria in chronic renal failure is of clinical significance. Present knowledge has it that changes in amino acid excretion by residual nephrons involve some residues on the basis of a raised plasma level, other residues have tubular transport defects (Schück et al. 1979). It is possible that amino-aciduria in chronic renal failure represents both types (overflow and renal) combined. It is characteristic that defects in tubular transport of most amino acids in renal failure is not associated with an absolute increase in excretion — only the excretion fractions are raised (Gulyassy et al. 1970, Betts and Green 1977, Nádvorníková et al. 1978, Schück et al. 1979).

In renal failure there is a characteristic increase in urinary excretion of proline and citrulline. Excretion of other residues is unchanged or decreased. In our own series, we found a significant decrease in urinary excretion of lysine, histidine, aspartic acid, cystine, tyrosine and tryptophane.

There were significantly increased plasma levels of Cit, Pro, Gly. The plasma levels of Tyr, Thr, Leu, Lys and Trp were found to be decreased.

The renal clearances of citrulline and proline in patients with chronic renal failure were increased in hyperbolic relation to the decrease in C_{in}. The clearances of His, Glu and taurine were decreased in relation to C_{in}. The FE values of all amino acids increased in hyperbolic relation to the decrease in C_{in} (except for Arg where this could not be demonstrated).

There is a sudden increase in the FE of amino acids with a decrease in C_{in} below 30 ml/min. The mechanisms involved in residual nephrons are not yet clear.

METHODS OF INVESTIGATION

DEMONSTRATION OF INCREASED CYSTINE EXCRETION

The most common clinical task is demonstration of an increase in cystine excretion for the early diagnosis of cystine urolithiasis. The urine sediment is important, since it can contain characteristic hexagonal crystals. The maximal solubitily of cystine at urinary pH 4.5–7.5 ranges about 300 mg/l. As an orientational test of cystine concentration, the cyanide-nitroprussic test is used (Lewis 1932). This is carried out by adding to 3–5 ml urine (pH alkaline by addition of NH_4OH) 2 ml 5% NaCN. The mixture is left for 10 min, and then several drops of freshly prepared sodium nitroprusside solution are added. The positive reaction is a purple colour.

There are a number of screening tests for amino acids in the morning urine. Such tests will detect the more common specific hyperaminoaciduria.

URINARY EXCRETION OF ALPHA-AMINO-N

This is a useful orientational test which can reveal an increased urinary excretion of free amino acids. Under normal conditions, in healthy adults on a normal diet, urinary excretion of alpha-amino-N ranges about 100–150 mg/day.

Normal excretion of lapha-amino-N does not exclude isolated excretion of excessive amounts of one or more separate amino acids.

256

RENAL CLEARANCE OF SEPARATE AA (C_{AA})

Measurement of C_{AA} requires determination of urinary excretion and plasma levels of individual AA. The test is carried out on an empty stomach in the A. M. The C values are calculated in the usual manner and are expressed per 1.73 m^2 (important in children in particular).

The average C_{AA} values $\pm$ SD for separate AA in healthy adults are given in Table 1, which also gives the normal values for plasma levels. These data show that the renal clearance of most AA does not exceed 2 ml/min. The highest values were shown by taurine, His and Gly. In the newly born and in children normal C values were collected from a number of sources by Short and Rosenberg (1975).

Table I

	P μmol/l	C ml/min.	FE %
Asp	6.0 ($\pm$ 3.2)	3.9 ($\pm$2.4)	3.4 ($\pm$2.0)
Ser	129.1 ($\pm$26.0)	2.5 ($\pm$1.0)	2.1 ($\pm$0.8)
Pro	187.4 ($\pm$21.9)	0.05 ($\pm$0.05)	0.04 ($\pm$0.04)
Glu	80.5 ($\pm$19.6)	1.3 ($\pm$0.5)	1.2 ($\pm$0.4)
Gly	247.4 ($\pm$35.7)	5.2 ($\pm$3.2)	5.2 ($\pm$2.2)
Ala	455.0 ($\pm$112.4)	0.6 ($\pm$0.2)	0.6 ($\pm$0.2)
Cys	76.8 ($\pm$32.8)	2.0 ($\pm$1.1)	1.6 ($\pm$0.7)
Tyr	55.6 ($\pm$5.7)	1.9 ($\pm$0.8)	1.6 ($\pm$0.7)
His	91.4 ($\pm$21.3)	7.2 ($\pm$3.2)	6.5 ($\pm$3.6)
Arg	54.4 ($\pm$18.0)	0.3 ($\pm$0.1)	0.2 ($\pm$0.1)
Thr	122.9 ($\pm$17.9)	1.3 ($\pm$0.5)	1.1 ($\pm$0.4)
Val	216.0 ($\pm$32.1)	0.2 ($\pm$0.2)	0.2 ($\pm$0.2)
Ile	58.0 ($\pm$14.1)	0.3 ($\pm$0.2)	0.2 ($\pm$0.2)
Leu	123.9 ($\pm$25.6)	0.4 ($\pm$0.1)	0.4 ($\pm$0.1)
Phe	60.8 ($\pm$16.0)	1.2 ($\pm$0.4)	1.0 ($\pm$0.4)
Lys	173.3 ($\pm$22.9)	1.2 ($\pm$0.5)	1.1 ($\pm$0.4)
Trp	46.9 ($\pm$14.1)	1.3 ($\pm$0.1)	1.4 ($\pm$1.1)
Tau	62.8 ($\pm$20.7)	10.5 ($\pm$5.0)	13.6 ($\pm$9.3)
Cit	48.7 ($\pm$23.0)	0.3 ($\pm$0.4)	0.2 ($\pm$0.3)
Asn + Gln	760.8 ($\pm$124.5)	0.4 ($\pm$0.2)	0.3 ($\pm$0.2)
Orn	115.2 ($\pm$22.9)	0.7 ($\pm$0.4)	0.6 ($\pm$0.4)

FRACTIONAL EXCRETION OF AA (FE_{AA}).

FE_{AA} expresses the proportion of the filtered load which is excreted. The test is carried out in the A.M. after a night's fast. Urine is collected for 2–3 hr. Venous blood is sampled in the middle of the period. For calculations see p. 262.

Mean values in normal adults on a normal diet are given in Table 1. Significant differences can occur in patients with a decreased GFR. Expressing the renal excretion of AA is further of advantage in this way because one need not calculate C values per 1.73 m².

Indications for investigation

1. The metabolic base of urolithiasis

Cystinuria represents 1–2% of all cases of urolithiasis (Herring 1962). In typical cases there is formation of large stones which can be localized in the renal pelvis, ureter or the bladder. Pure cystine stones show a low level of contrast in X-rays. In a relatively high fraction (40%) the stones combine cystine and Ca salts, and these give a good contrast level in X-rays. Suspicion of cystinuria can arise from microscopic investigation of the urinary sediment. Hexagonal crystals are characteristic and they form mainly in concentrated urine. Sulfonamide crystals must be excluded (history taking). The cyanide-nitroprussic test is further used. A false positive reaction can occur if acetone is present. Homocystinuria also gives a positive test.

Demonstration of cystinuria requires a quantitative measure. With cystine we can also have increased amounts of Lys, Orn and Arg.

The upper limit of normal cystine excretion is 70 mg/gcr.

For differential diagnosis one must distinguish cystinuria from cystinosis with intracellular cystine deposition in the liver, kidneys, bone marrow and the cornea. The latter disease involves a generalized amino-aciduria and cystine stones do not form.

2. Detailed investigation of proximal tubular function

Many types of kidney disease can alter tubular AA transport. Amino-aciduria has been described in patients with the nephrotic syndrome (Hooft and Herpol 1959, Strickler et al. 1968). Amino-aciduria with toxic renal damage is usually not quantitatively important and disappears when renal function returns. In these cases amino-aciduria can be combined with renal glucosuria or other tubular defects. If normoglycaemic glucosuria is present along with amino-aciduria, tubular damage must be considered, particularly if RTA or hyperphosphaturia are present.

3. Measurement of renal AA excretion as part of a detailed metabolic workup

This sub-chapter is concerned with a number of varied metabolic defects (presented in the Introduction) with which we meet mainly in Paediatrics. In adults these tests are indicated in the diagnosis of Wilson's disease, uncertain neurological symptomatology and pellagroid skin changes (Hartnup's disease).

Proximal tubular damage should also be suspected with the use of some drugs such as expired tetracycline antibiotics or azauridine. We have also seen transitory amino-aciduria after administration of azosemide.

4. Chronic renal failure

Measurement of P_{AA} is important to evaluate the metabolic state of the patient. This measurement is indicated in patients under conservative treatment (to judge the adequacy of protein intake) and in patients on a regular dialysis program (who lose AA through the dialysis membrane).

The ratio of essential and non-essential AA is also of use. Values of this ratio lower than 0.46 are considered pathological.

Measured P_{AA} levels are interpreted with reference to transferrin, albumin and total plasma protein levels.

Laboratory methods

Thin layer two-dimensional partition chromatography is used to measure AA in urine and plasma (Efron 1960, Moore et al. 1958, Shih et al. 1967). Greater accuracy is obtained with column chromatography and gas-liquid chromatography.

REFERENCES

Baerlocher, K., Scriver, C., Mohyuddin, F.: Ontogeny of iminoglycine transport in mammalian kidney. Proc. Nat. Acad. Sci. USA *65*: 1009, 1970

Betts, P. R., Green, A.: Plasma and urine amino acids concentration in children with chronic renal insufficiency. Nephron *18*: 132, 1977

Brown, J. L., Samig, A. H., Pitts, R. F.: Localization of amino-nitrogen reabsorption in the nephron of the dog. Am. J. Physiol. *200*: 370, 1961

Crampton, R. F., Smyth, D. H.: The excretion of the enantiomorphs of amino acids. J. Physiol. (London) *122*: 1, 1953

Crane, R. K.: Na+-dependent transport in the intestine and other animal tissues. Fed. Proc. *24*: 1000, 1965

Crane, R. K.: The gradient hypothesis and other models of carrier mediated active transport. Rev. Physiol. Biochem. Pharm. *78*: 99, 1977

Efron, M. L.: High voltage paper electrophoresis. In: I. Smith (ed.) Chromatographic and electrophoretic techniques. Vol. 2. New York, Interscience 1960, pp. 158–189

Evers, T., Murer, H., Kinne, R.: Phenylalanine uptake in isolated renal brush border vesicles. Biochem. biophys. Acta *426*: 598, 1976

Gayer, J., Gerok, W.: Die Lokalisierung der L-Aminosäuren in der Niere durch step flow Analysen. Klin. Wschr. *39*: 1054, 1961

Gulyassy, P. F., Aviram, A., Peters, J. H.: Evaluation of amino acid and protein requirements in chronic uremia. Arch. intern. Med. *126*: 855, 1970

Hooft, C., Herpol, J.: Aminoaciduria in the course of lipoid nephrosis in children — in influence of ACTH. Acta Pediat. *48:* 135, 1959

Herring, C. C.: Observations on the analysis of ten thousand urinary calculi. J. Urol. *88:* 545, 1962

Hytter, F. E., Chyne, G. A.: The aminoaciduria in pregnancy. J. Obst. Gyn. Brit. Commonw. *79:* 424, 1972

Milne, M. D.: Renal tubular dysfunction. In: M. B. Strauss and L. G. Welt (eds.) Diseases of the kidney (2nd ed.) Boston, Little, Brown 1972, pp. 1071–1138

Moore, S., Spackman, D. H., Stein, S.: Chromatography of amino-acids on sulfonated polystyrene resins. Ann. Chem. *30:* 1185, 1958

Nádvorníková, H., Schück, O. Malý, J. et al.: Renal clearance of amino acids in patients with severe chronic renal failure. Nephron *20:* 83, 1978

O'Brien, S., Butterfield, L.: Further studies on renal tubular conservation of free amino acids in early infancy. Arch. Dis. Child. *38:* 437, 1963

Rosenberg, L. E., Scriver, C. R.: Disorders of amino acid metabolism. In: P. K. Bondy and L. E. Rosenberg (eds.) Diseases of Metabolism (7th ed.) Philadelphia, Saunders 1974, pp. 465—653

Schück, O. Nádvorníková, H., Tomková, D., Teplan, V.: Urinary excretion of amino acids in patients with chronic renal failure. Proc. 2nd Prague Symp. on chron. renal failure 1979

Shih, V., Efron, M. L., Mechanic, G. L.: Rapid short column chromatography of amino acids: A method for blood and urine specimens in the diagnosis and treatment of metabolic diseases. Ann. Biochem. *20:* 299, 1967

Short, E. M., Rosenberg, L. E.: Renal aminoacidurias. In: Strauss and Welt's diseases of the kidney. 3rd edition. (Eds. L. E. Earley and C. W. Gottschalk) Boston Little, Brown and Co. 1979, pp. 975–1020

Silbernagel, S., Deetjen, P.: The tubular reabsorption of L-cystine and L-cysteine. Pflüger's Arch. ges. Physiol. *337:* 277, 1972

Strickler, G. B., Hayles, A. B., Power, M. H., Ulrich, J. A.: Renal tubular dysfunction complicating nephrotic syndrome. Pediatrics *26:* 75, 1960

Young, J. A., Freedman, B. S.: Renal tubular transport of amino acids. Clin. Chem. *17:* 245, 1971

GLOSSARY

A_I	Angiotensin I
A_{II}	Angiotensin II
ADH	Antidiuretic hormone
AP	Arterial pressure
AUC	Area under the curve
C_X	Renal clearance of X
C_{tot}	Total plasma clearance
D	Administered dose
DV_X	Apparent volume of distribution of X
E_X	Extraction of X
ERBF	Effective renal blood flow
ERPF	Effective renal plasma flow
f_X	Diffusable fraction of X
FE_X	Fractional excretion of X
FF	Filtration fraction
FR_X	Fractional reabsorption of X
GFR	Glomerular filtration rate
k	Effective hydraulic permeability
K_{elim}	Elimination constant
K_f	Ultrafiltration coefficient
P_X	Plasma concentration of X
RBF	Renal blood flow
RPF	Renal plasma flow
RVR	Renal vascular resistance
T_X	Tubular transport of X
T_{mX}	Maximal tubular transport of X
t 1/2	Biological half-life
U_X	Urine concentration of X
V	Urine flow rate
VP	Vasopressin

FORMULAE

1. $C_x = \dfrac{U_x V}{P_x}$

2. $C_{H_2O} = V - C_{osm}$

3. $T^c_{H_2O} = C_{osm} - V$

4. $FE_x = \dfrac{U_x V}{GFR\, P_x} \, 100 = \dfrac{C_x}{GFR} \, 100 \doteq \dfrac{\dfrac{U_x}{P_x}}{\dfrac{U_{cr}}{P_{cr}}} \cdot 100$

5. $FR_x = 100 - FE_x$

6. Net tubular reabsorption of X
   $T_x = GFR\, P_x f_x - U_x V$

7. Net tubular secretion of X
   $T_x = U_x V - GFR\, P_x f_x$

8. $K_{elim} = \dfrac{\ln P_1 - \ln P_2}{t_2 - t_1} = 2.3 \dfrac{\log P_1 - \log P_2}{t_2 - t_1}$

9. $t\,1/2 = \dfrac{0.693}{K_{elim}}$ or $K_{elim} = \dfrac{0.693}{t\,1/2}$

10. $DV_x = \dfrac{D}{P_0}$

11. $C_{tot} = K_{elim} \dfrac{D}{P_0} = \dfrac{0.693}{t\,1/2} \dfrac{D}{P_0}$

    or $C_{tot} = \dfrac{D}{AUC}$

12. $RVR = 1328 \dfrac{\overline{AP}}{RBF}$

13. $FF = \dfrac{GFR}{RPF} \, 100$

INDEX

268